CLINICAL NEURO-OPHTHALMOLOGY

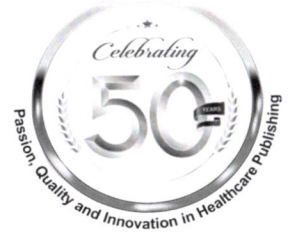

CLINICAL NEURO-OPHTHALMOLOGY

Editor

Ambar Chakravarty MD FRCP
Honorary Professor and Emeritus Consultant
Department of Neurology
Vivekananda Institute of Medical Science and Park Clinic
Kolkata, West Bengal, India

Foreword
SM Katrak

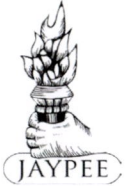

JAYPEE BROTHERS MEDICAL PUBLISHERS
The Health Sciences Publisher
New Delhi | London | Panama

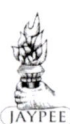

Jaypee Brothers Medical Publishers (P) Ltd

Headquarters

Jaypee Brothers Medical Publishers (P) Ltd
4838/24, Ansari Road, Daryaganj
New Delhi 110 002, India
Phone: +91-11-43574357
Fax: +91-11-43574314
Email: jaypee@jaypeebrothers.com

Overseas Offices

J.P. Medical Ltd
83 Victoria Street, London
SW1H 0HW (UK)
Phone: +44 20 3170 8910
Fax: +44 (0)20 3008 6180
Email: info@jpmedpub.com

Jaypee-Highlights Medical Publishers Inc
City of Knowledge, Bld. 235, 2nd Floor, Clayton
Panama City, Panama
Phone: +1 507-301-0496
Fax: +1 507-301-0499
Email: cservice@jphmedical.com

Jaypee Brothers Medical Publishers (P) Ltd
17/1-B Babar Road, Block-B, Shaymali
Mohammadpur, Dhaka-1207
Bangladesh
Mobile: +08801912003485
Email: jaypeedhaka@gmail.com

Jaypee Brothers Medical Publishers (P) Ltd
Bhotahity, Kathmandu, Nepal
Phone: +977-9741283608
Email: kathmandu@jaypeebrothers.com

Website: www.jaypeebrothers.com
Website: www.jaypeedigital.com

© 2019, Jaypee Brothers Medical Publishers

The views and opinions expressed in this book are solely those of the original contributor(s)/author(s) and do not necessarily represent those of editor(s) of the book.

All rights reserved. No part of this publication may be reproduced, stored or transmitted in any form or by any means, electronic, mechanical, photocopying, recording or otherwise, without the prior permission in writing of the publishers.

All brand names and product names used in this book are trade names, service marks, trademarks or registered trademarks of their respective owners. The publisher is not associated with any product or vendor mentioned in this book.

Medical knowledge and practice change constantly. This book is designed to provide accurate, authoritative information about the subject matter in question. However, readers are advised to check the most current information available on procedures included and check information from the manufacturer of each product to be administered, to verify the recommended dose, formula, method and duration of administration, adverse effects and contraindications. It is the responsibility of the practitioner to take all appropriate safety precautions. Neither the publisher nor the author(s)/editor(s) assume any liability for any injury and/or damage to persons or property arising from or related to use of material in this book.

This book is sold on the understanding that the publisher is not engaged in providing professional medical services. If such advice or services are required, the services of a competent medical professional should be sought.

Every effort has been made where necessary to contact holders of copyright to obtain permission to reproduce copyright material. If any have been inadvertently overlooked, the publisher will be pleased to make the necessary arrangements at the first opportunity. The **CD/DVD-ROM** (if any) provided in the sealed envelope with this book is complimentary and free of cost. **Not meant for sale.**

Inquiries for bulk sales may be solicited at: jaypee@jaypeebrothers.com

Clinical Neuro-Ophthalmology / Ambar Chakravarty

First Edition: **2019**

ISBN: 978-93-5270-557-3

Printed at Repro India Limited

Dedicated to

The memory of my teacher
Late Professor Shyamal Kumar Sen
(1922–2011)

CONTRIBUTORS

Editor

Ambar Chakravarty MD FRCP
Honorary Professor and Emeritus Consultant
Department of Neurology
Vivekananda Institute of Medical Science and Park Clinic
Kolkata, West Bengal, India

Contributing Authors

Arnab Biswas MS
Consultant Ophthalmologist
Kolkata, West Bengal, India

Sandip Chatterjee DNB FRCS FRCS
Professor and Head
Department of Neurosurgery
Vivekananda Institute of Medical Sciences and Park Clinic
Kolkata, West Bengal, India

Sudip Chatterjee MD DNB FRCP
Professor
Department of Endocrinology
Vivekananda Institute of Medical Science and Park Clinic
Kolkata, West Bengal, India

Ravindranath M Chowdhury MD DM
Associate Professor
Department of Neurology
National Institute of Mental Health and Neuroscience
Bengaluru, Karnataka, India

Ajitesh Das MD DM
Assistant Professor
Department of Endocrinilogy
Vivekananda Institute of Medical Sciences
Kolkata, West Bengal, India

Angshuman Mukherjee MD DM
Professor and Head
Department of Neurology
Vivekananda Institute of Medical Science
Kolkata, West Bengal, India

Arabinda Mukherjee MD DM
Honorary Professor and Consultant
Department of Neurology
Vivekananda Institute of Medical Science
Kolkata, West Bengal, India

Koushik Pan MD DM
Assistant Professor
Department of Neurology
Vivekananda Institute of Medical Science
Kolkata, West Bengal, India

Debasish Roy MD DM
Current Designation
Department of Neurology
Vivekananda Institute of Medical Science
Kolkata, West Bengal, India

Jayanta Roy MD DM, Director
Department of Neurology
AMRI Hospital, Mukundapur
Kolkata, West Bengal, India

Pushpita Sahu FRCS FCOpth
Honorary Consultant
Department of Ophthalmology
Vivekananda Institute of Medical Science
Kolkata, West Bengal, India

Barun K Sen MD DM
Assistant Professor
Department of Neurology
Vivekananda Institute of Medical Science
Kolkata, West Bengal, India

KK Sinha MD FRCP
Senior Consultant Neurologist
Advanced Diagnostic Centre
Ranchi, Jharkand, India

Sanjib Sinha MD DM
Professor
Department of Neurology
National Institute of Mental Health & Neurosciences
Bengaluru, Karnataka, India

FOREWORD

It is with a sense of honor and privilege that I write the foreword for the book "Clinical Neuro-ophthalmology," edited by Professor Ambar Chakravarty. This book is a vastly updated version of an earlier book on the same subject edited by Professor Ambar Chakravarty and published in 2004 on behalf of the *Journal of the Association of Neurologists of Eastern India*. The first half of this book begins with the basics of a neuro-ophthalmological examination and then takes the reader to the problems with each part of the visual pathways, starting with the optic nerves and going all the way to the higher function disorders of vision involving the retrochiasmal region of the vision pathways. The latter half of the book deals with the problems of ocular motility, covering the neural mechanisms of gaze and all the ophthalmoplegias—supranuclear, nuclear, and infranuclear. I must compliment the authors for including a chapter on optical coherence tomography in neurological practice and problem oriented neuro-ophthalmology, offering pearls to achieve the correct diagnosis and avoiding the pitfalls.

This book will prove to be useful not only to postgraduate students in neurology and ophthalmology, but also to neurologists and ophthalmologists of all ages. It will serve as a good "textbook" for the growing subspecialty of neuro-ophthalmology in India. Information is not knowledge and knowledge is not necessarily wisdom. But, the information and knowledge imparted by the authors in a lucid style will surely empower the reader with enough wisdom to understand the nuances of a complicated subject like neuro-ophthalmology. I am sure that this book will be highly appreciated and will find a place in the personal library of many neurologists, as it will be in mine.

Professor SM Katrak
Director, Department of Neurology
Jaslok Hospital and Research Centre
Professor Emeritus
GMC and Sir JJ Group of Hospitals
Mumbai, Maharashtra, India

PREFACE

In 2004, while I was the Founder Editor of the *Journal of the Association of Neuroscientists of Eastern India*, I first ventured into writing and editing a comprehensive clinically oriented book on neuro-ophthalmology, which perhaps had been the first of its kind written solely and published in India. A rather limited number of copies were published due to financial constraints, which were mostly sent to senior neurologists of the country and a lesser number of copies were sold at a nominal price to postgraduates in training in neurology. A few copies were handed over to the Ophthalmological Society for distribution among its members. The publication was an astounding success and I was flooded with requests from all corners of the country to provide trainees with the book which I could not comply with due to shortage of the number of copies published.

The result was that photocopies of the book came into circulation and I witnessed that when I attended a neuro-ophthalmology teaching course in a very reputed institute in the country. I felt bad and decided on the need for an updated volume published in larger numbers to cater to the needs of young neurologists and trainees in the country. Finance stood up as the major hurdle. I had no dearth of material and no dearth of very helping and dedicated colleagues willing to write.

Fortunately, more recently a significant educational grant was made available from Intas Pharmaceuticals through the good offices of Mr Jagrup Singh, Senior Vice President, who very kindly agreed to take up not only the responsibility of publishing the book but also promised arranging its distribution to all members of the Indian Academy of Neurology. My heartfelt thanks to the company and to Mr Singh for this kind gesture.

What is new in the present volume? This volume contains 23 chapters which probably covers almost all aspects of clinical neuro-ophthalmology. All the chapters which were covered in the previous volume have been much updated keeping in pace with recent developments. Couple of chapters from the previous book have been omitted; some new chapters have been incorporated and some new enthusiastic authors have been inducted. I would specially mention about a short chapter on optical coherence tomography in neurological practice, major modification in the chapter on diplopia to include phorias and squint, and at the end an interesting discourse on problem oriented neuro-ophthalmology. In all, I have tried to make the volume as compressive as possible. Unfortunately I had to sacrifice a chapter on visual electrodiagnosis to avoid making the book too voluminous.

I must thank all the contributors, mostly my colleagues at Vivekananda Institute of Medical Science, for contributing their best in updating the book and also to the publishing team for their efforts in bringing out the book in time.

I only wish and pray that that this book becomes as useful to all sections of readers as its previous version and even more.

Ambar Chakravarty
Kolkata
2nd July 2018

CONTENTS

1. **Assessment of Visual Acuity** — 1
   Arnab Biswas

2. **Optical Cohererence Tomography In Neurological Practice** — 4
   Pushpita Sahu

3. **Ophthalmoscopy in Clinical Practice** — 8
   Ambar Chakravarty

4. **Visual Field Examination for the Neurologist** — 19
   Ambar Chakravarty, Pushpita Sahu

5. **Examination of Pupil** — 30
   Ambar Chakravarty, Debasish Roy

6. **Unexplained Visual Loss** — 41
   Ambar Chakravarty

7. **Transient Visual Loss** — 48
   Jayanta Roy

8. **Optic Neuritis** — 58
   Debasish Roy, Ambar Chakravarty

9. **Neuromyelitis Optica Spectrum Disorders** — 68
   Debasish Roy, Ambar Chakravarty

10. **Non-inflammatory Optic Neuropathies** — 77
    Debasish Roy, Sandip Chatterjee, Ambar Chakravarty

11. **Chiasmal Disorders** — 93
    Sandip Chatterjee

12. **Retrochiasmal Visual Impairments** — 105
    KK Sinha

13. **Visual Illusions and Hallucinations** — 117
    Ambar Chakravarty

14. **Nuclear and Infranuclear Ophthalmoplegias** — 127
    Ambar Chakravarty

15. **Phoria. Squint and Diplopia** — 153
    Pushpita Sahu, Ambar Chakravarty

16. **Gaze and Supranuclear Oculomotor Disorders** — 163
    Angshuman Mukherjee, Ambar Chakravarty

17. **Ocular Oscillations** — 187
    Angshuman Mukherjee, Ambar Chakravarty

18.	Ptosis and Blepharospasm *Ravindranath M Chowdhury, Sanjib Sinha*	199
19.	Proptosis *Ajitesh Das, Sudip Chatterjee*	208
20.	Psychogenic Neuro-ophthalmological Disorders *Ambar Chakravarty*	218
21.	Idiopathic Intracranial Hypertension *Barun K Sen, Arabinda Mukherjee*	225
22.	The Eye and Headache *Koushik Pan, Ambar Chakravarty*	246
23.	Problem Oriented Neuro-Ophthalmology: Pearls and Pitfalls *Koushik Pan, Ambar Chakravarty*	254
	Appendix 1: Dynamic Visual Acuity: A Simple Test for Vestibular Function *Arnab Biswas*	267
	Appendix 2: Strabismus Terminology *Pushpita Sahu, Ambar Chakravarty*	268
	Appendix 3: A Note on Ocular Motor Disorders in Multiple Sclerosis *Pushpita Sahu, Ambar Chakravarty*	270
	Index	275

PLATE-1

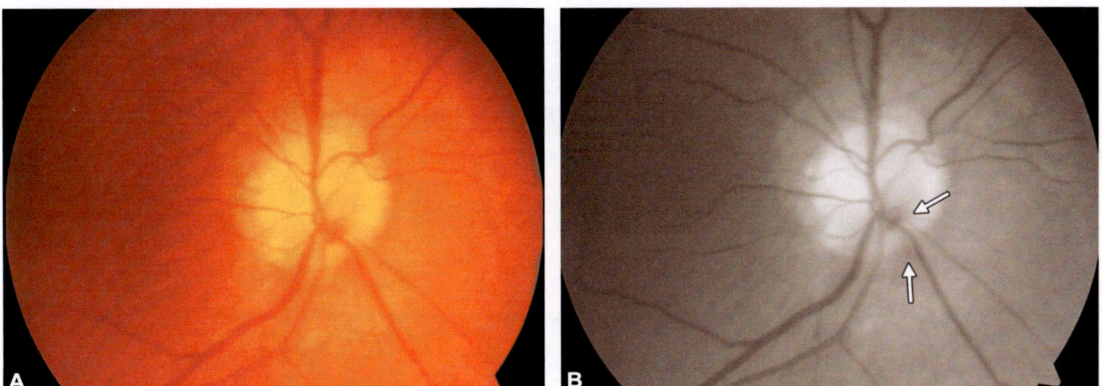

FIG. 4: Fundoscopy in a case of anterior ischemic optic neuropathy showing discal and peripapillary hemorrhages (Fundus anterior ischemic optic neuropathy). *(Chapter 10)*

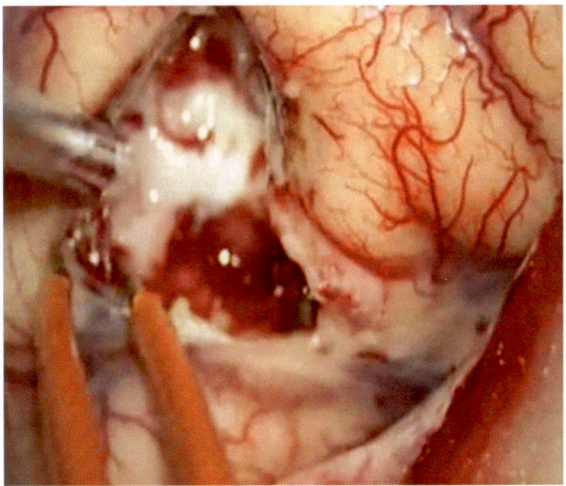

FIG. 10: Optic pathway glioma in a probable Neurofibromatosis 1 patient. *(Chapter 11)*

PLATE-2

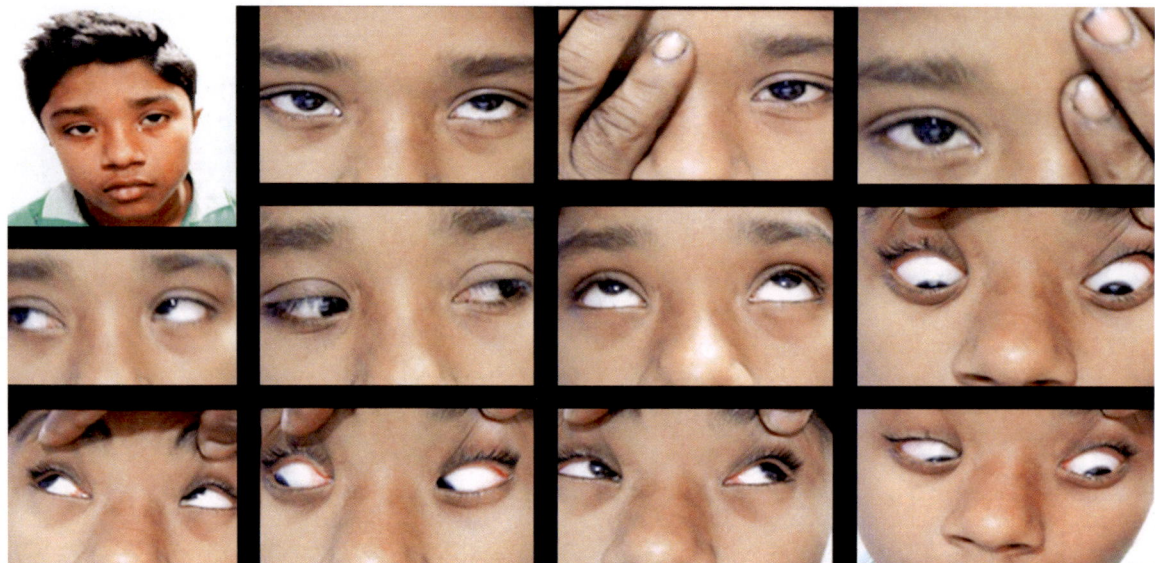

FIG. 6: A 12-year-old boy with head tilt to right for 2 months. He had no double vision. But complained of the surrounding environment to be tilted, to correct it, he adopted the right head tilt. A closer look at him revealed a skew deviation with the right eye at a lower position compared to the left (Ocular tilt). This eye position reversed when his eyes were covered alternately (Ocular counter-roll). Eye movements in all directions were full and there had been no abnormal torsional movement of the left eye on looking down in the adducted position; thus excluding a left trochlear palsy. This combination of head tilt, skew deviation, ocular tilt and ocular counter-roll on alternate cover test is called ocular tilt reaction (OTR). Interestingly, the tilt disappeared on making the boy lie flat on bed. There was no environmental tilt either, confirming the diagnosis of OTR. No cause for this occurrence could be found. *(Chapter 16)*

Miscellaneous

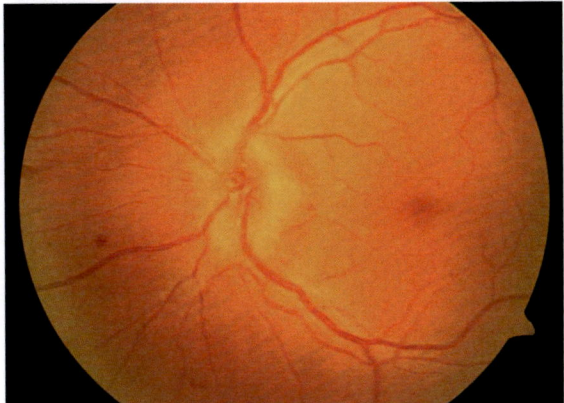

Anterior ischemic optic neuropathy (AION).

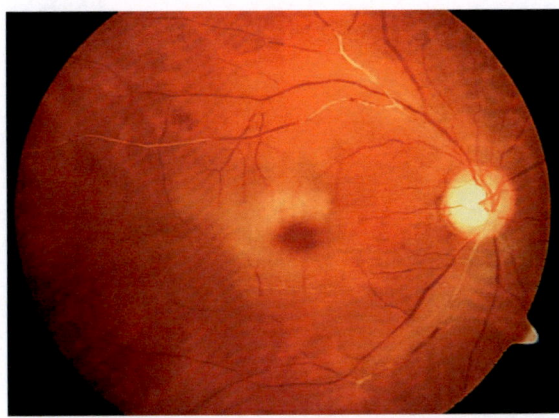

Central retinal artery occlusion (Macular cherry red spot).

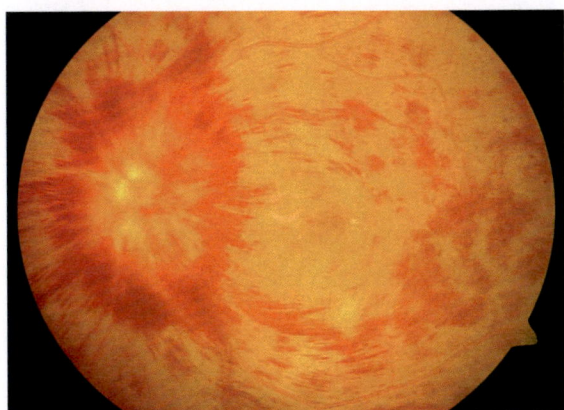

Central vein occlusion (CRVO).

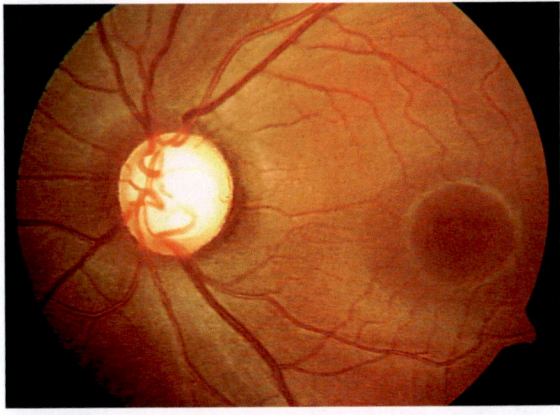

Glaucomatous cupping and optic atrophy.

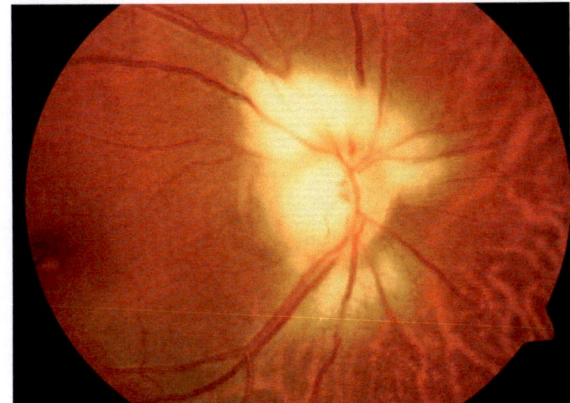

Myelinated nerve fibers.

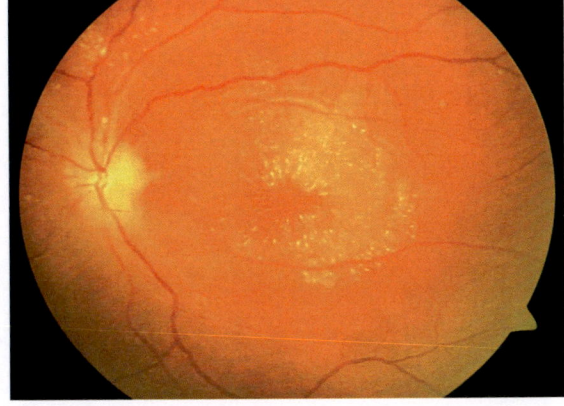

Neuroretinitis—macular star.

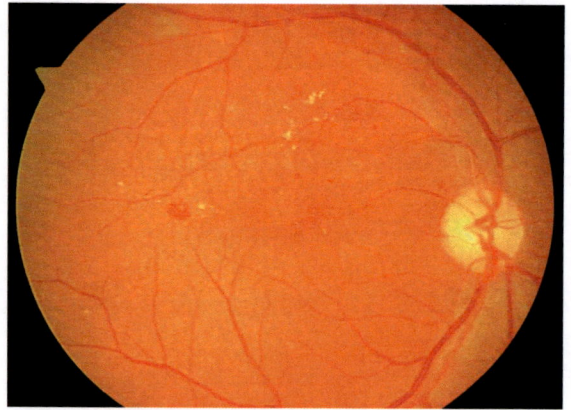

Nonproliferative diabetic retinopathy.

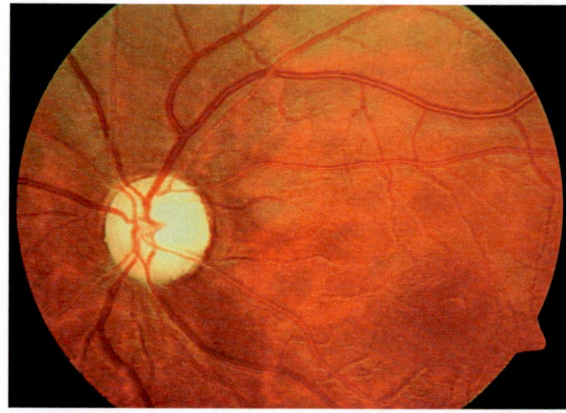

Optic atrophy.

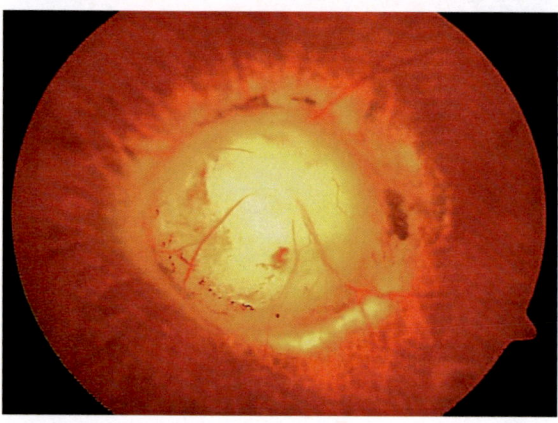

Optic disc Coloboma.

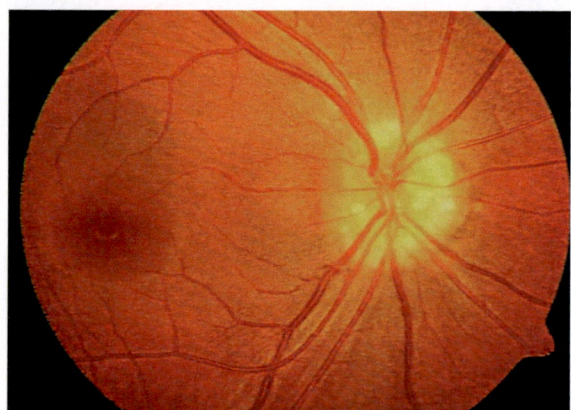

Optic disc Drussen.

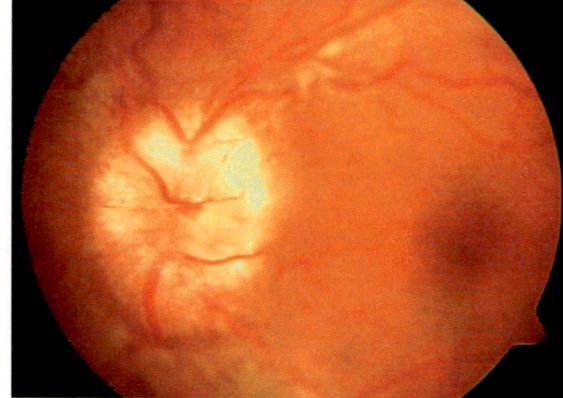

Papiledema.

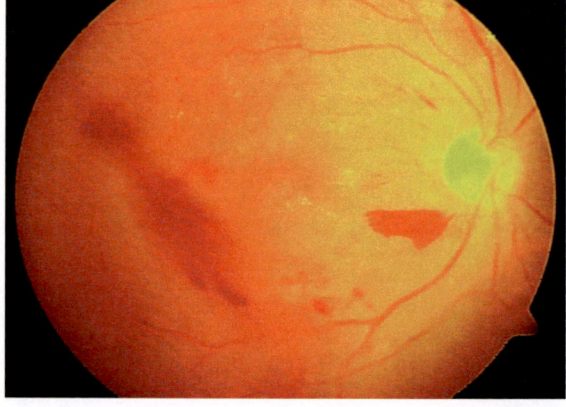

Proliferative diabetic retinopathy with vitreous hemorrhage.

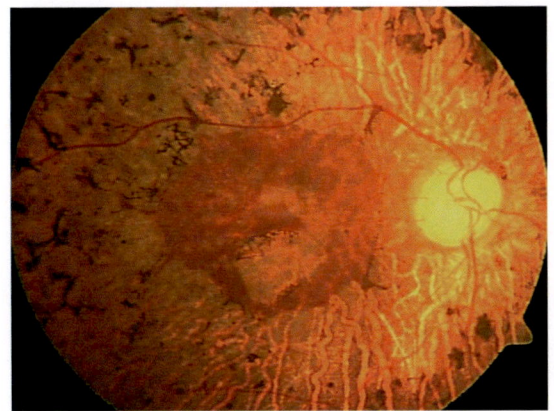
Retinaitis pigmentosa.

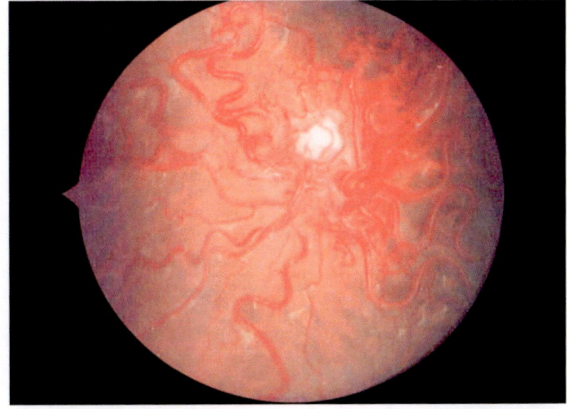
Retinal angiomatosis in Wyburn-Mason syndrome.

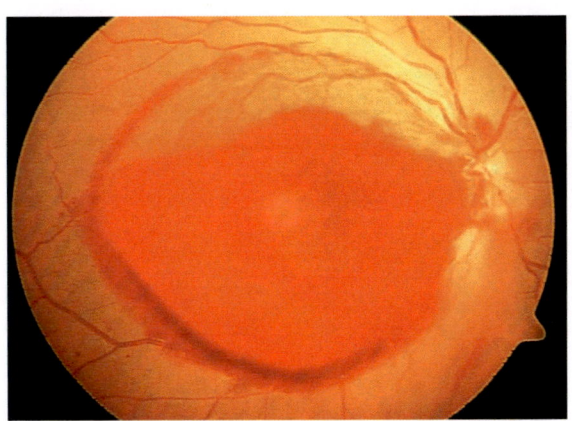
Sub Hyaloid hemorrhage.

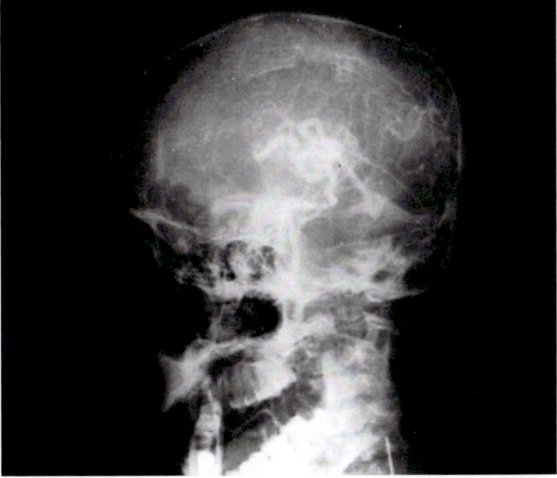
Cerebral vascular malformation in Wyburn-Mason syndrome.

CHAPTER 1

Assessment of Visual Acuity

Arnab Biswas

DEFINITION

Acuity of vision is defined as the power of the eye to see an object or letter clearly and distinguish it at a specified distance. It describes the sharpness of central vision. It is basically assessment of one of the properties of retina and optic nerve.

Vision should be tested with and without glasses on a standard chart. Each eye should be tested independently. A normal eye can easily distinguish two points separated by an angle of one minute to the eye. This is the standard of normal visual acuity (VA). Perfect acuity of vision requires two other basic factors—the light sense and color sense. The acuity of vision is tested by standard vision chart known as Snellen's chart.

SNELLEN'S CHART

Dutch ophthalmologist Herman Snellen developed the Snellen's eye chart in the 1860s. The Snellen's chart is used almost universally in testing the acuity of vision. The chart consists of Snellen's specially formed letters of the alphabet arranged in rows of decreasing letter size. The size of the letters is standardized so that letters in each row will be clearly legible at a designated distance to a person with normal vision.

Principles of Snellen's Chart

Each letter is of such a shape that it can be enclosed in a square. The size of the square is five times the thickness of lines composing the letter. The square subtends an angle of five minutes at a specified distance. The Snellen's chart should be placed at a distance of 6 m or 20 feet. The rays of light from that distance are parallel for practical purposes. Half this distance may also be used, but in that case the test types should be visualized reflected through a plain mirror, kept at a distance of 3 m or 10 feet from the patient. The chart consists of a series of letters of diminishing size.

The letters are so constructed that the angle of 1 minute is formed when:
- First letter or line is at 60 m distance
- Second line is at 36 m distance
- Third line is at 24 m distance
- Fourth line is at 18 m distance
- Fifth line is at 12 m distance
- Sixth line is at 9 m distance
- Seventh line is at 6 m distance
- Eighth line is at 5 m distance.

The right eye is tested conventionally first, except where the patient's complaint is particularly of defective vision in left eye. The patient is asked to read down the chart as far as he can and then this is repeated with the other eye. Finally both eyes are tested together. If the visual acuities of the two eyes are about equal, it is usually found that they reinforce each other so that the binocular vision is slightly better than the uniocular vision.

TYPES OF VISUAL ACUITY

- Distant
- Near
- Pinhole.

Distant Visual Acuity

It is the ability of a person to distinguish an object or letter whose rays are parallel and where no accommodation is required. Various distant VA charts are:
In adults:
- Snellen's chart
- Early treatment diabetic retinopathy study (ETDRS) chart (LogMAR chart).

In illiterates:
- E-chart/pictures chart
- Landolt's broken rings chart
- Multiple pictures chart.

In children:
- Cake decorations
- Teller acuity cards

Interpretation of Visual Acuity

Visual acuity is recorded as a fraction. The numerator indicating distance in meters at which the patient can read clearly the smallest possible letters/characters in the chart and the denominator indicating the distance in meters at which a normal person can read the same letters/characters in the chart. The normal VA is 6/6
- If the patient is unable to read two letters of the last line it should be indicated as 6/6–2
- If the patient is unable to read last line at 6 m but reads the previous lines then VA is 6/9
- If the patient is unable to read last two lines but able to read other letters, the VA is 6/12
- If unable to read last three lines then VA is 6/18
- If unable to read last four lines then VA is 6/24
- If they can read only the first two lines the VA is 6/36
- If the patient is unable to read even the first line, the VA is less than 6/60
- If the patient is not able to read even the top letter of the Snellen chart, he is asked to count fingers, and the VA is recorded as the distance at which he is able to count fingers (CF 3 m or 3/60)

Snellen's chart is useful and most accurate in literate people above the age of 6 years. For illiterates and children below 6 years of age, other test charts based on Snellen's principles are useful.

Testing Methods of Near Visual Acuity

It is the power of the eye to clearly see and distinguish smallest object or letters from a normal reading distance. It measures the accommodation of the eyes. The standard normal reading distance is considered to be 40 cm. When the distance vision has been tested, the VA at reading distance is checked. Special near vision charts are available with various side of print size. The smallest print the person can read at the near working distance is taken as the best corrected near acuity.

How to Perform the Near Acuity Test?

Patients who wear glasses or contact lenses should wear them for the test. The near vision should be checked with and without glasses.
- Instruct the patient to be seated
- After the patient is comfortably seated, printed test card is given to them
- Ask the patient to hold the test card at the distance specified on the card, usually 40 cm
- Have the patient cover the left eye with an occluder or the palm of the hand
- Ask the patient to read with the right eye the line of the smallest characters legible on the card
- Repeat the same procedure with the other eye occluded
- Record the near acuity value for each eye separately.

Pinhole Visual Acuity

The pinhole disc is a small circular disc with a small central opening that reduces the peripheral rays and allows the central rays to reach the retina. The standard trial pin hole is 1 mm in size. The pinhole permits the most central rays to enter and provide a good image, just as the pinhole camera gives a fine image without a lens system. The pin hole helps to differentiate visual loss caused by refractive errors from poor vision resulting from disease of the retina/optic nerve. In the latter condition vision will not improve when a pinhole disk is placed before the eye.

Bedside Visual Acuity Examination

In order to accurately assess VA, the patient should be conscious and cooperative. A Snellen's chart is routinely not available in the ICU or a nonophthalmological clinic. How many fingers can the patient see or looking at the bedside clock are rather crude methods, but certainly quite informative for a rapid bedside identification of major deficits. Other crude methods (e.g., the identification of routine objects) can also be employed, but ultimately, nothing beats the Snellen's chart in terms of repeatability, reproducibility, and accuracy.

Rather than focusing on subtle deficits of vision, the neurologist usually wants to know whether the patient is blind or not. Close one of the patient's eyes. The other eye, remaining open, gets an object moved in front of it. If the patient's eyes track that object, an idea that the optic nerve is intact (as well as most of the rest of the visual pathway) can be made.

Amsler Grid Test

The Amsler grid, used since 1945, is a grid of horizontal and vertical lines used to monitor a person's central visual field (Fig. 1). The grid was developed by Marc Amsler, a Swiss ophthalmologist. It is a diagnostic tool that aids in the detection of visual disturbances caused by changes in the retina, particularly the macula (e.g., macular degeneration), as well as the optic nerve and the visual pathway to the brain.

In the test, the person looks with each eye separately at the small dot in the center of the grid. Patients with macular disease may see wavy lines or some lines may be missing (Fig. 2).

Amsler grids are supplied by ophthalmologists, optometrists or from web sites, and may be used to test one's vision at home.

The original Amsler grid was black and white. A color version with a blue and yellow grid is more sensitive and can be used to test for a wide variety of visual pathway abnormalities, including those

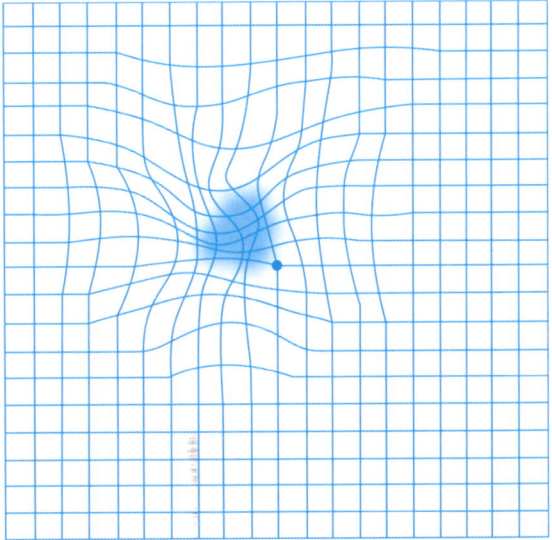

FIG 2: An Amsler grid, artist's conception, as it might be viewed by a person with age related macular degeneration.

associated with the retina, the optic nerve, and the pituitary gland.

Dynamic visual acuity: A simple test for vestibular function is summarized in appendix 1.

SUGGESTED READINGS

1. Agarwal LP. Agarwal's Principles of Optics and Refraction. CBS Publishers and Distributors 5th Edition 2007.
2. A Text Book on Optics and Refraction. Arvind Eye Care System Madurai 2007.
3. Brian T. Peters, Ajitkumar P. Mulavarab Helen S. Cohenc, Haleh Sangi-Haghpeykar, and Jacob J. Bloomberg. Dynamic visual acuity testing for screening patients with vestibular impairments. J Vestib Res. 2012 January 1; 22(2): 145–151.
4. Abrams D. Duke-Eldor's Practice of Refraction, Elsevier, 10th Edition 1993.
5. Goebel JA. The ten-minute examination of the dizzy patient. Seminars in Neurology. 2001; 21:391-8.
6. Peters BT, Bloomberg JJ. Dynamic visual acuity using "far" and "near" targets. Acta Otolaryngol. 2005; 125: 353-7.
7. Khurana AK. Theory and Practice of Optic and Refraction. Elsevier 2016.
8. Vital D, Hegemann SCA, Straumann D, Bergamin O, Bockisch CJ, Angehrn D, Schmitt KU, Probst R. A new dynamic visual acuity test to assess peripheral vestibular function. Arch Otolaryngol Head Neck Surg. 2010; 136:686-91.

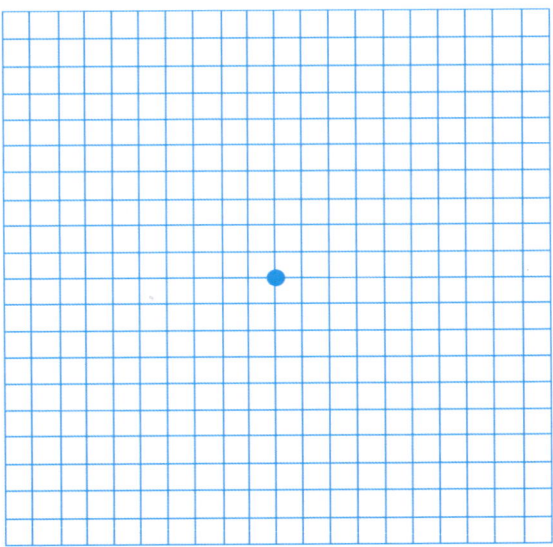

FIG. 1: An Amsler grid, as seen by a person with normal vision.

CHAPTER 2: Optical Coherence Tomography in Neurological Practice

Pushpita Sahu

INTRODUCTION

Optical coherence tomography (OCT) is a relatively new noninvasive imaging technique, which uses near infrared light to take images of cross section of the retina and optic nerve head. It is widely used by ophthalmologists for various conditions. Early detection of glaucoma before visual field defects become evident especially in glaucoma suspects is a common indication for OCT. The retinal nerve fiber layer (RNLF) plotting tells about any thinning of RNLF layer. The term preperimetric glaucoma is frequently used. Similarly diseases of macula-edema, atrophy, scarring, hole formation, or diseases/degenerations of layers of the retina is also identified by OCT.

Loss of neurons and nerve axons of the brain cannot be adequately quantitated with the available technology like magnetic resonance imaging. So, examination of the retina and optic nerve provides a window to the visualization of central nervous system. Optical coherence tomography is now being increasingly used by neurologists. Measurement of thickness of peripapillary RNLF in optic neuropathies, e.g., multiple sclerosis, documentation and follow up of disc edema of various etiology, differentiating between papilledema and pseudopapilledema, and optic neuropathy from maculopathy are some of the indications for neurologists to ask for OCT imaging.

There are two types of OCT—time domain and spectral domain. Let it suffice to say that spectral domain OCT provides a much faster rate scan and higher scan resolution. Using OCT, it is possible to clearly identify the different layers of retina and structural detail of optic nerve head and any pathology affecting them which is not detected clinically.

Optical coherence tomography operate on the principle of indirect interferometry, in which a beam of light is directed into the retina, and the resulting back-scattered light travels an unknown distance to a detector, which is compared to a reference beam of known length to calculate the echo time delay of light. In time domain OCT, the reference arm mechanically moves and the echo time delays are measured one at a time. Time domain-OCT involves a scanning technique using a low-coherent light source. A pulsed laser light source, passes through an optical splitter to divide it into two paths. Using a moving mirror, the light from one path is back reflected to travel a known path length and the time delay is measured which is variable. The second path light is directed over the eye and is scattered back by the internal structures producing interference patterns with the reference light. This provides in depth information and the locations of various structures from within the eye. The principle of spectral domain OCT is somewhat different. The reference arm in a spectral/frequency domain-OCT system has a static mirror instead of a moving one as in time domain-OCT. This results in higher speed of data acquisition than time domain optical coherence tomography.

CERTAIN FACTS ABOUT OPTICAL COHERENCE TOMOGRAPHY (FIG. 1)

- Optical coherence tomography can be performed for anyone above 5 years of age as certain positioning and cooperation is needed. It is done in a sitting position with the chin on the chin rest and head against the bar—similar to the one adopted for slit lamp examination
- Usually dilating drops are not needed unless the patient has very small pupil or there is

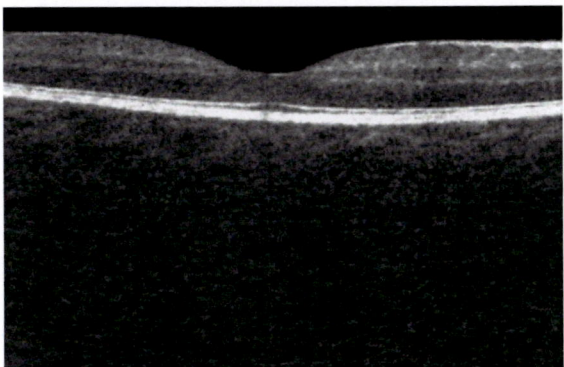

FIG. 1: Normal optical coherence tomography.

- medial opacity or cataract or poor vision interfering with fixation
- The test duration is usually 10 minutes for each eye
- Imaging of RNLF, optic nerve head, and macula is done. Imaging the peripapillary nerve fiber layer within 3.4 mm ring around the optic nerve measures the mean value of RNLF thickness, and average value of each quadrant inferior, superior, nasal, and temporal is given which is also color coded depending on the thickness
- Signal strength must be good for a good image. Signal strength of at least 7/10 by Cirrus imaging (Cirrus SD-OCT) and 15 for spectral domain OCT is considered acceptable. Corneal scar, cataract and dry eye can affect signal strength. It may be difficult to obtain good signal strength in patients of myopia more than 8 diopters because the peripapillary nerve fiber may be thinner and the anteroposterior length longer
- Thinning of peripapillary RNLF is consistent with optic neuropathy and elevation of peripapillary RNLF value occurs when there is disc edema. Retinal nerve fiber layer measurement can be compared with normal values, but one must be aware of the normal value of each specific model and instrument. The average RNLF measurement is the most extensively used measure and it can be normal, increased or decreased and may correspond ophthalmoscopically with a normal, swollen or pale disc.

USES OF OPTICAL COHERENCE TOMOGRAPHY IN NEUROLOGY

Optic Neuritis (Especially in Multiple Sclerosis)

Reduction of RNLF thickness is observed in patients of multiple sclerosis (MS). A large group of visually asymptomatic patients, may show thinning of RNLF. Thinning of RNLF is also seen in the fellow eye. Eyes with optic neuritis (ON) also have reduction of macular volume. Early detection of RNLF thinning thus give evidence of axon loss as well as retinal ganglion cell loss. Thinning of peripapillary RNLF has not only been observed in patients of MS with ON but also in the asymptomatic fellow eye of MS patients. Also thinning of RNLF has been seen in patients of MS without evidence of ON. There is a potential role of OCT in trials that examine efficacy of various neuroprotective and disease modifying therapies.

Neuromyelitis Optica Spectrum Disorders

In neuromyelitis optica spectrum disorders, thinning of peripapillary RNLF is noticed. Superior and inferior quadrants are more affected by RNLF thinning. And prominent microcystic macular edema may be seen with thickening of inner nuclear layer.

Alzheimer's Disease

In Alzheimer's disease, there is reduction of peripapillary nerve fiber thickness. This may help in early diagnosis thus identifying patients who would benefit most from clinical trials of new therapies.

Parkinson's Disease and Atypical Parkinsonian Syndromes

Peripapillary RNFL thinning has been demonstrated in some patients with Parkinson's disease, the temporal quadrant being identified as thinner compared with controls. Macular thinning and volume loss from the inner retina has also been observed. It seems in future there may be a scope to differentiate Parkinson's disease from atypical parkinsonism by OCT examination. Abnormalities have also been observed in progressive supranuclear palsy and system atrophy patients in way of thickening of outer nuclear and plexiform layer.

Different Types of Optic Neuropathies

Although thinning of RNLF can be seen in different types of optic neuropathies, it does not define the cause but has prognostic significance. In patients with compressive neuropathy due to chiasmal and parachiasmal lesions, it is found that those with RNLF thinning prior to surgery were less likely to recover visual acuity postsurgery compared to those who did not have RNLF thinning prior to surgery.

Papilledema

In combination with other clinical measures (vision, color vision, and visual field), OCT can play a part in monitoring disease progression.

In Idiopathic intracranial hypertension trial (IIHIT), eyes with macular ganglion cell layer/inner plexiform layer thinning had worse visual prognosis. Increased peripapillary RNLF thickness was associated with higher elevation of intracranial pressure.

Optical coherence tomography can be used to differentiate between papilledema and pseudopapilledema. A single OCT cannot distinguish true from apparent disc edema, but in a serial study changes are expected in true edema and stability is to be expected in pseudopapilledema. With autofluorescence optic nerve drusen may be seen.

Non-arteritic Anterior Ischemic Optic Neuropathy (Fig. 2)

Associated with disc at risk typified by a small or absent physiological cup, the cup area and the cup/disc ratio is significantly smaller than normal.

At onset of the disease, the RNLF thickness almost doubles compared with the fellow eye. At 2 months, more than 80% of eyes show RNLF thinning. This progresses over 2–4 months and stabilizes by 6 months.

However, ganglion cell layer (GCL) thinning occurred before RNLF thinning. So GCL thinning is a better marker for early structural loss in non-arteritic anterior ischemic optic neuropathy and optic neuritis.

Maculopathy

Maculopathy can cause central visual loss like optic neuropathy. Optical coherence tomography helps to differentiate between the two.

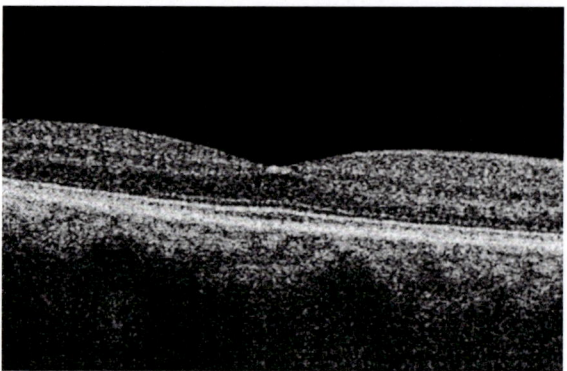

FIG. 2: Optical coherence tomography in patient with non arteritic anterior ischemic optic neuropathy.

Screening Guidelines for Hydroxychloroquine Toxicity

Following tests should be performed:
- Dilated fundus examination, 10-2 visual field test, spectral domain OCT, fundus autofluorescence, and multifocal electro-retinography. Visual field may show a cluster of paracentral points of decreased sensitivity
- Spectral domain OCT may show distinctive changes before clinical evidence of hydroxychloroquine toxicity like disruption or complete loss of outer nuclear layer, external limiting membrane, outer/inner junction, and retinal pigment epithelium in the parafoveal region.

CONCLUSION

As a clinical tool, OCT is particularly useful for the structural measurement of peripapillary nerve fiber thickness, optic nerve head volumetric analysis, and macular anatomy. OCT can be used to identify optic neuropathies of varied etiology especially MS, documentation, and follow up of disc edema of varied etiology (Papilledema and idiopathics intracranial hypertention), differentiating pseudo-papilledema from true disc swelling and differentiating optic neuropathy from maculopathy.

SUGGESTED READINGS

1. Bodis-Wollner I, Miri S, Glazman S. Venturing into the no-man's land of the retina in Parkinson's disease. Mov Disord. 2014;29(1):15-22.

2. Gelfand JM1, Goodin DS, Boscardin WJ, et al. Retinal axonal loss begins early in the course of multiple sclerosis and is similar between progressive phenotypes. PLoS One. 2012;7(5):e36847.
3. Kanamori A, Nakamura M, Escano MF, et al. Evaluation of the glaucomatous damage on retinal nerve fiber layer thickness measured by optical coherence tomography. Am J Ophthalmol. 2003;135(4):513-20.
4. Medeiros FA, Moura FC, Vessani RM, et al. Axonal loss after traumatic optic neuropathy documented by optical coherence tomography. Am J Ophthalmol. 2003;135(3):406-408.
5. Monteiro ML, Leal BC, Rosa AA, et al. Optical coherence tomography analysis of axonal loss in band atrophy of the optic nerve. Br J Ophthalmol. 2004;88(7):896-9.
6. Nolan RC, Narayana K, Galetta SL, et al. Optical coherence tomography for the neurologist. Semin Neurol. 2015;35:564-77.
7. Parisi V, Manni G, Spadaro M, et al. Correlation between morphological and functional retinal impairment in multiple sclerosis patients. Invest Ophthalmol Vis Sci. 1999;40(11):2520-27.
8. Trip SA, Schlottmann PG, Jones SJ, et al. Retinal nerve fiber layer axonal loss and visual dysfunction in optic neuritis. Ann Neurol. 2005;58(3):383-91.

CHAPTER 3

Ophthalmoscopy in Neurological Practice

Ambar Chakravarty

INTRODUCTION

The present chapter written mostly in an instructive manner would help practicing clinicians and trainees to recapitulate common and important opthalmoscopic findings encountered in neurological practice.

Direct ophthalmoscope was first used by Jan Purkinje of Prague in 1823 and by Hermann von Helmholtz of Germany in 1851 of whom Helmholtz got the credit for the discovery. There are two types of ophthalmoscopy—direct and indirect. The direct method gives a direct, erect image of a small area of the fundus. The indirect method is a little more complicated and requires more dexterity. The 20–30 diopter lens used in conjunction with the slit lamp provides a narrower angle of view, but one which is greatly magnified. Indirect method, primarily used by ophthalmologists, is used to look at the periphery of the retina and gives a wide angle, stereoscopic view, which is inverted and laterally reversed. Most neurologists use the direct ophthalmoscope as it is portable, battery operated, and gives a better-magnified view.

Direct ophthalmoscope helps to focus light to the back of the eye in order to view the disc and the vessels with a white light. Usually a smaller and a larger light source are available of which the smaller light is good for small, undilated pupils, but the larger light provides better illumination.

It is important that the size of the light source is smaller than the pupil at a focusing distance. If it is too big, you will induce too much glare from the light striking the outside of the pupil.

Instruments with a green light provides 450 nm monochromatic light which is particularly useful to view optic nerve drusen and for detecting nerve fiber defects. A vertical narrow beam light source is often provided to assess lesions which are in front of retina in contrast to lesions which arte on the retina. The wheel has red and black marked numbers. The red ones used for myopic eyes and the black ones foe hypermetropic eyes.

Patients should be examined in a dimly lit room to achieve maximal papillary dilation. In general, neurologists prefer not to dilate the pupil so as not to miss testing the papillary reflexes. This may be very relevant in an intensive care setting, but in the clinic a dilated ophthalmoscopy provides more information. Phenylephrine or tropicamide may be used.

Contraindications to dilation consist of known narrow angle glaucoma and impending surgery, or an unstable neurologic condition where watching pupillary change may be necessary, the latter situation would very rarely arise in an outpatient clinic. The patient should fixate on a distant object again to achieve maximal papillary dilatation. It is a good practice to train oneself to view the patient's right eye with the examiner's right eye and vice versa. With patient looking straight ahead, the optic disc would come into view. If the patient is now asked to look at the light source, the macula would be seen as it lies two disc diameters away on the temporal side. Next one should identify the central retinal and identify and trace its branches.

If you are having trouble finding the disc, find a major blood vessel and follow it. If you are going in the right direction, it will appear larger and lead you to the disc. To find the macula, just turn the ophthalmoscope a bit temporally about 2–3 disc diameters, and you will find the macula. Otherwise, ask the patient to stare directly at the light; if they can do it, you should be looking at or near the fovea.

COMMON ERRORS THAT PREVENT YOU FROM OBTAINING A CLEAR VIEW OF THE DISC AND RETINA

- The patient is not fixating at an object in the distance
- The light source is too large
- The pupil is too small, and should be dilated
- You are not close enough to the patient's eye
- You have not dialed in the correct power
- Your head is blocking the patient's view and the patient is moving around too much
- You lack the confidence to view clearly.

Optic nerve is formed by axons from ganglion cells in the retina. What we see when we peer into the eye with the ophthalmoscope is the optic disc and retina (Fig.1). The diameter of the optic nerve is 1.62 mm. There are about 1 million nerve fibers that form the optic disc.

The normal optic disc is a bit oval and has a slight pink hue. In about a third of subjects, the lamina cribrosa, a sieve-like structure is visible at the depth of the disc through which the fibers of the nerve fiber layer leave the eye to form the retrobulbar portion of the optic nerve. The optic cup needs to be identified and the cup/disc ratio assessed. Normally, it is around 0.3.

The cup to disc ratio is usually the same in each eye. The larger the cup, the larger the scleral opening at the back of the globe. The space between the cup and the edge of the disc is the neuroretinal rim. All around the disc you can see the scleral ring. The papillary area is the disc itself. The area around the disc is called the peripapillary disc area.

Can You Appreciate the Nerve Fiber Layer?

The surface layer is the nerve fiber layer from all over the retina. We try to examine the nerve fiber layer to determine whether there is any loss. Its appearance is like fine horsehair. The red-free filter will enhance your ability to see the nerve fiber layer.

Twenty-five percent of normal eyes have an optic crescent usually located temporally. Most pronounced crescents are seen in association with myopia. There are a variety of crescents. The crescent is just a regional area of retinal pigment epithelial thinning.

Vascular Supply of the Optic Nerve and Disc (Fig.2)

The optic disc is supplied by blood both from the choroidal artery as well as from the central retinal artery (CRA) and also the short ciliary arteries.

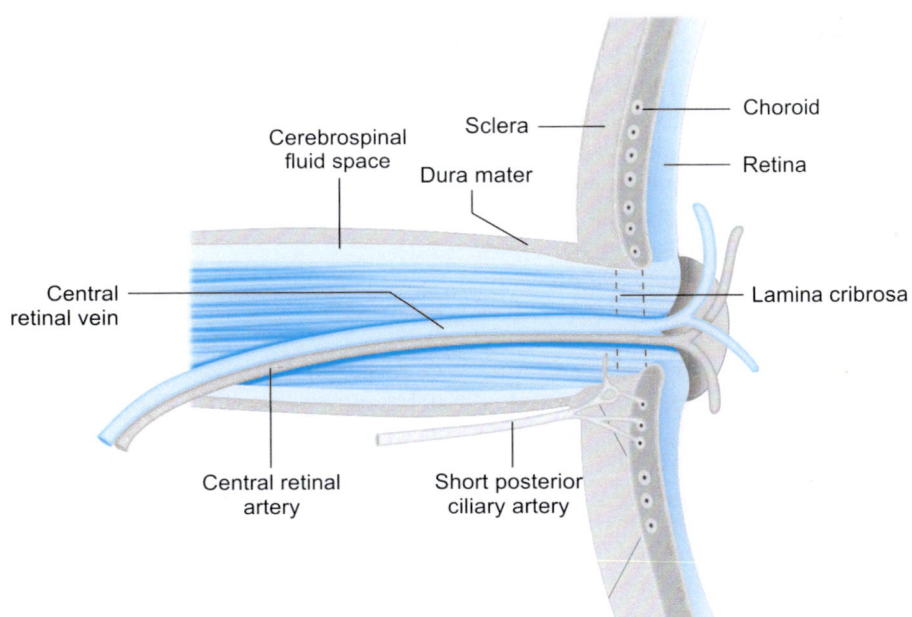

FIG. 1: Schematic sectional view of the optic nerve and the normal optic disc.

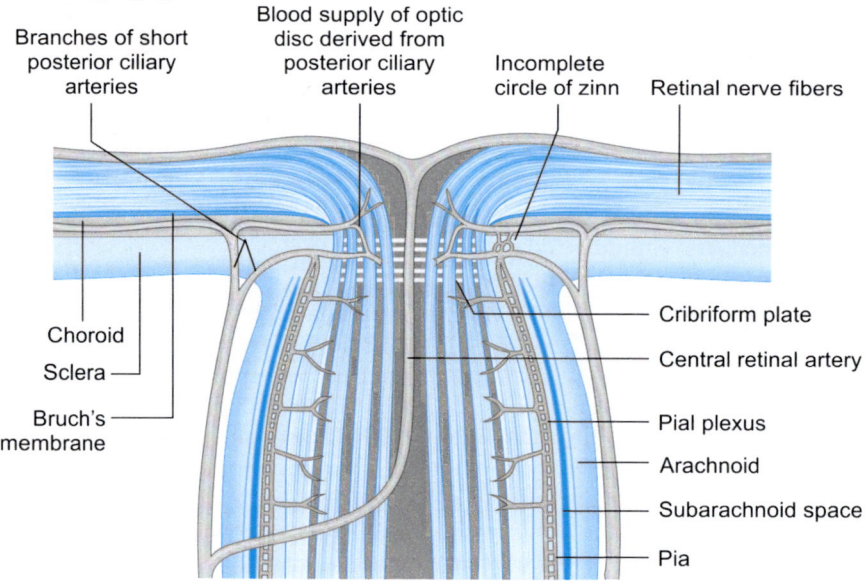

FIG. 2: Illustration of the vascular supply to the optic disc and retrolaminar optic nerve.

Lamina cribrosa supply is the short ciliary arteries. Posteriorly, there are recurrent branches from the ophthalmic artery and pial vessels. Venous drainage is through the central retinal vein (CRV) and the vortex vein through the choroid.

The CRA pierces the optic nerve about 1 cm behind the globe and enters the eye at the optic nerve head—usually nasal to the exit site of the CRV. It divides into superior and inferior branches. It further branches to supply four quadrants of the retina. Since the CRA has only minimal supply to the nerve fiber layer in the anterior-most segment of the optic disc, a CRA occlusion generally does not cause swelling of the optic disc. In contrast, ischemia of the optic disc from insufficiency of a posterior ciliary artery [i.e., anterior ischemic optic neuropathy (AION)] characteristically presents with optic disc edema.

In about a third of eyes, the hook shaped cilioretinal artery is visible, which usually supplies a small part of retina. It exits the disc separately from the CRA. The importance of the cilioretinal artery is that it can occlude and cause usually a central visual loss or during a CRA occlusion, its presence will spare central vision and the macula. Occlusion of a cilioretinal artery is a characteristic evidence of giant cell arteritis.

Spontaneous venous pulsations generally suggest that intracranial pressure is not increased. However, the reverse is not always true. Venous drainage from the eye is through the CRV and the posterior vortex vein. The latter is usually visible in hypopigmented discs. Ultimate drainage is in the cavernous sinus.

Normal Variations of the Disc and Fundus

Normal disc color is pink. It may look paler in blonde individuals. Color depends upon the amount of pigment in the choroid. With age, the pigment increases.

Effect of Refraction and Shape of the Globe

In myopia, due to elongation of the globe, the disc and the cup both look larger and paler which may be mistaken for optic atrophy. The reverse occurs in hypermetropia where the disc may look full due to shortening of the globe and may be confused with a swollen disc. Such variations are of much clinical importance.

Normally, myelination of the optic nerve starts once the nerve fibers pass through the lamina cribrosa. In many subjects, myelination starts early inside the globe where it appears as a feather edged bright white bundle which again may be confused with papilledema. This may also mimic soft exudates near the disc.

These two points are very practical ones. Myelinated nerve fibers are a developmental anomaly where myelination appears past the lamina cribrosa on nerve fibers of the disc and retina. It typically has "feathered" edges which follow the nerve fiber layer. It may be unilateral or bilateral and usually not associated with visual impairment. Myelinated nerve fibers can simulate papilledema or be mistaken for nerve fiber layer infarct (soft exudates). This point is equally important to remember.

Bergmeister Papilla

This is the remnant of tissues around the fetal hyaloid artery during development. Preretinal vascular loops may be seen and may cause transient mono-ocular blindness and retinal artery obstructions.

These form as proliferation of vascular system into Bergmeister's papilla. Remnants of fetal hyaloids artery tissues may be found on the discs and again confused with a swollen disc.

Is the Disc Swollen?

Several anomalies of the disc may give false impression of a swollen disc. These include tilted disc, optic disc drusen, hypermetropic discs, and so called "little red discs." Collectively, they are designated as pseudopapilledema.

Optic Disc Drusen

This is distinguished from true papilledema by absence of hyperemia, no obstruction of surface arteries on the disc margin, no physiologic cup, no spread of elevation to surrounding nerve fiber layer and irregular disc border. They are congenital, refractile bodies that may be buried; (i.e., below the surface of the superficial nerve fiber layer and, therefore, not visible using ophthalmoscopy) but tend to mineralize as the individual ages. Drusen is the German word for a geode, since drusen look like the crystals in a geode. A single drusen is a druse. Disc drusen can be associated with visual field defects—especially nerve fiber bundle defects and constriction. Drusen only rarely affects central visual function, so that acuity is usually normal and central scotomas usually do not arise. Drusen may occur with associated splinter or subretinal hemorrhages around the disc. It is thought that these discs may be more prone to serious visual loss with other conditions such as ischemic optic neuropathy, optic neuritis, or hemorrhagic retinopathy. Drusen are occasionally seen with other conditions such as retinitis pigmentosa and angioid streaks.

If you are suspicious of "buried drusen" based on the appearance of the optic disc, image the optic nerve with thin section computed tomography (CT) through the optic nerve, perform orbital ultrasound, or view the disc in the preinjection images of fluorescein angiography.

Tilted discs (nasal fundus ectasia) results from an oblique insertion of the optic nerve to the globe with vessels emerging in an oblique manner. Such individuals are often myopic, may have choroidal epithelium defects, situs inversus, and astigmatism. The defect results from faulty closure of the embryonic fissure. Such a disc may be confused with a swollen disc and field defects may be associated which does not respect the vertical meridian. Often the field defects resemble bitemporal hemianopia when smaller size targets are used.

OTHER VARIETIES OF ANOMALOUS DISCS

Hyperopic Discs and Little Red Discs

"Little red discs" are small and hyperemic and may be mistaken for papilledema. Hyperopic discs are usually small and have no cup. Recognize anomalous discs by looking for an absent cup, tortuosity of the blood vessels and too many blood vessels on the disc.

Papilledema (Fig. 3)

True papilledema is the disc swelling caused by increased intracranial pressure. The findings of papilledema include hyperemia, i.e., caused by dilation of the disc capillaries, and swelling of axons in the peripapillary nerve fiber layer and the nerve fiber layer of the surface of the disc which cause blurred disc margin and elevation and swelling of the disc. "Blurred disc margin" alone can be seen with anomalous elevation, but vessels are not obscured. Elevation of the disc usually occurs peripherally before centrally and there

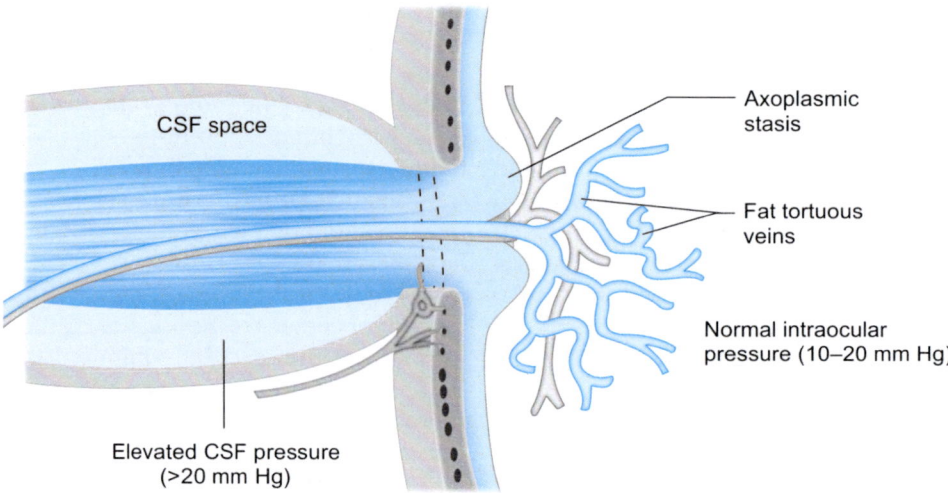

CSF, cerebrospinal fluid.
FIG. 3: Diagram to illustrate elevated cerebrospinal fluid pressure causing stasis of axoplasmic flow and disc swelling (papilledema).

may be an early appearance of a "red cell" shape or volcano. Peripapillary retinal nerve fiber layer hemorrhage may be present. Retinal veins appear dilated, elongated, and tortuous. Absence of spontaneous venous pulsations of retinal veins is often encountered but is not a consistent finding in early papilledema. Presence of venous pulsations, however, indicate that cerebrospinal fluid (CSF) pressure at the time of examination is less than 200 mm of water.

Lars Frisen classified papilledema grading as:
- Stage 0: Normal disc with blurring of nasal and temporal disc; no obscuration of the vessel and the cup is maintained
- Stage 1: A C-shaped blurring of the nasal, superior and inferior borders. Usually the temporal margin is normal
- Stage 2: Involves elevation of the temporal margin
- Stage 3: There is elevation of the entire disc with obscuration of the retinal vessels at the disc margin
- Stage 4: There is complete obliteration of the cup and partial obscuration of the vessels on the surface of the disc
- Stage 5: There is a dome-shaped appearance and all vessels are obscured.

Chronic Papilledema

As papilledema persists to the chronic phase, peripapilary hemorrhages and exudates resolve. The optic disc takes on a rounded, "champagne cork-like" appearance. Refractile bodies, resembling optic disc drusen, may appear in the disc substance. Disappearance of the physiologic cup is also a late sign in the evolution of papilledema.

Atrophic Papilledema

If the underlying cause of papilledema remains untreated, the disc swelling ultimately resolves. However, the optic disc itself becomes atrophic, or pale, and retinal blood vessels take on a narrow, sheathed appearance. The time course for the development of optic atrophy in the setting of papilledema is variable, and may require 5–6 weeks or longer depending on the underlying process and degree/duration of CSF pressure elevation. Optociliary shunt vessels, collateral vessels that develop in response to chronic pressure behind the optic disc, may appear during the transition from chronic to atrophic papilledema, but typically disappear when optic atrophy is complete. Prior to the onset of atrophic papilledema, and following treatment of increased intracranial pressure, optic disc swelling often requires up to 4–8 weeks to resolve to a baseline funduscopic appearance.

Papilledema is typically bilateral. On rare occasions, papilledema may be markedly asymmetric. Asymmetric disc swelling in papilledema results when the optic disc communicates poorly with the intracranial subarachnoid space. Disc swelling may also be asymmetric following the onset of unilateral optic atrophy, in which there are not enough viable axons in the atrophic nerve to produce disc swelling. In patients with the Foster–Kennedy syndrome, one optic nerve becomes atrophic from direct compression by a tumor (often a frontal or olfactory groove meningioma) while the fellow optic nerve becomes swollen secondary to increased intracranial pressure.

Differential Diagnosis of Papilledema (Box 1 and Table 1)

In the setting of bilateral optic disc swelling, the full spectrum of entities that cause increased intracranial pressure, as well as those that may mimic papilledema must be considered. Both common and less common etiologies for papilledema are listed in box 1.

Space-occupying intracranial lesions and venous sinus thrombosis must be excluded first and foremost; idiopathic intracranial hypertension (IIH, pseudotumor cerebri) may be diagnosed in patients of appropriate age and characteristics only when other entities have been reasonably excluded by neuroimaging and lumbar puncture.

> **Box 1: Differential diagnosis of papilledema**
> - Intracranial mass lesion
> - Venous sinus thrombosis/obstruction
> - Intracranial hemorrhage (subarachnoid, intraparenchymal, and subdural)
> - Hydrocephalus
> - Meningitis
> - Spinal cord tumor
> - Guillain–Barré syndrome and chronic inflammatory demyelinating polyneuropathy
> - Dural arteriovenous malformation
> - Idiopathic intracranial hypertension (pseudotumor cerebri)

In fact, the diagnosis of IIH may be formally established only when the following criteria (modified Dandy criteria) have been met:
- Signs and symptoms of increased intracranial pressure (headache, nausea, vomiting, transient visual obscurations, and papilledema)
- Normal neurologic examination with exception of unilateral/bilateral sixth nerve palsy
- Elevated CSF pressure (>250 mm water in adults) with normal constituents
- Modern neuroimaging (CT with and without contrast, or magnetic resonance imaging) excluding a mass lesion, hydrocephalus, venous sinus thrombosis, or other causes for increased intracranial pressure.

The differential diagnosis and underlying etiology for bilateral optic disc swelling in general may be further defined by the clinical history. Important features include the mode of onset, the effects on visual acuity and fields, and any associated signs or symptoms. When the disc swelling is bilateral and acuity is spared, papilledema, or pseudopapilledema is of prime consideration.

Malignant Hypertension

The ophthalmoscopic features of malignant hypertension may be difficult to distinguish from those of papilledema. In addition to elevated blood pressure and other systemic signs of end organ involvement (such as hematuria), retinal findings that are suggestive of malignant hypertension include cotton wool spots, lipid star formation, and macular serous detachment. Disc swelling in the setting of malignant hypertension has been previously related to elevated CSF pressures; however, more recent observations have indicated that an ischemic process may also be responsible.

Diabetic Papillopathy

Diabetic papillopathy is another entity that presents with bilateral optic disc swelling; this most often occurs in insulin-dependent type 1 diabetics. The occurrence of diabetic papillopathy apparently has no relation to the degree of diabetic retinopathy. Central visual acuity loss is generally modest, and the visual prognosis is good, with visual improvement preceding the resolution of

Table 1: Features which distinguish papilledema from pseudopapilledema

Papiledema	Pseudopapilledema
Physiologic cup is usually present	Physiologic cup is absent
Vessels arise nasally in the disc	Vessels arise from the center of the disc at the apex of disc swelling
Veins bifurcate normally	Anomalous branching and venous trifurcations occur
Peripapillary blurring of the NFL	Disc margin irregular, pigment changes
Hyperemia with capillary dilation	Absent capillary telangiectasia; disc color varies from pale to hyperemic
Diffuse elevation of the disc	Elevation irregular, refractile bodies (drusen)
Peripapillary NFL radial hemorrhage	Occasionally seen peripapillary subretinal hemorrhage or rare superficial hemorrhages
Retinal veins dilated	No retinal vein dilation
Exudates if the papilledema is chronic	No exudates
Not familial	Frequently familial
Absent SVP	SVP present
Appearance changes with time	Appearance stable over time

NFL, nerve fiber layer; SVP, spontaneous venous pulsation.

disc swelling. Some consider diabetic papillopathy to be a form of ischemic optic neuropathy; marked capillary telangiectasias on the optic disc surface may be a distinguishing feature for this entity.

Pseudopapilledema (or pseudodisc edema) has already been mentioned and important causes highlighted. The features which distinguish papilledema from pseudopapilledema are listed in table 1.

Causes of Unilateral Optic Disc Swelling

When encountering a patient with unilateral optic disc swelling, the most common and important entities to consider are optic neuritis (in younger patients) and AION (in older patients). Compressive and infiltrative optic neuropathies as well as central retinal vein occlusion (CRVO) should also be considered. Although such disorders usually present with unilateral disc swelling, bilateral or sequential optic nerve involvement may also occur.

Optic Neuritis

Optic neuritis refers to primary inflammation of the optic nerve. While the optic disc appears normal in most patients with acute demyelinating optic neuritis (retrobulbar optic neuritis), disc swelling may be present in 20–40% of cases. Optic disc swelling in the setting of optic neuritis indicates extension of inflammation to the optic nerve head (termed papillitis), and broadens the differential diagnosis to include other forms of inflammatory optic neuropathy. Although disc swelling was present in 35% of participants in the Optic Neuritis Treatment Trial (ONTT), peripapillary or disc hemorrhages were uncommon in these patients (6% of ONTT participants), and their presence should suggest an alternative diagnosis, such as AION. Macular lipid exudate (macular star), and/or vitreous cells (more than trace) in the setting of unilateral optic disc swelling are more consistent with neuroretinitis, sarcoidosis, syphilis, or other infectious/ inflammatory etiologies.

Anterior Ischemic Optic Neuropathy

Anterior ischemic optic neuropathy is the most common cause of unilateral optic disc swelling in patients over 50 years of age.

Optic disc swelling and neurologic complications may result from giant cell arteritis. Visual loss is characterized by a pallid appearance (occasionally hyperemic, particularly in arteritic

AION), flame or splinter hemorrhages, and peripapillary retinal arteriolar narrowing. The disc is most often diffusely swollen, with a segment of more prominent involvement. Although sectoral disc involvement may display an altitudinal distribution, it may not correspond consistently with the location of visual field loss. Diffuse or focal telangiectasia may be present on the edematous optic disc; this finding may represent microvascular shunting from ischemic to nonischemic regions of the nerve head. The fellow eye optic disc is often crowded and cupless, an anatomic feature that has been demonstrated to be a risk factor for non-arteritic AION. In contrast, the presence of bilateral or sequential disc swelling in any patient with suspected AION should greatly increase suspicion for giant cell arteritis.

Optic neuritis and AION have been discussed in detail elsewhere (Chapters 6 and 7).

Compressive/Infiltrative Optic Neuropathies

Patients with compressive optic neuropathy usually present with progressive visual loss. Optic disc swelling may resolve into optic atrophy. Optociliary shunt vessels support the chronic nature of the disc swelling. These shunt vessels are classically observed in the patient harboring an optic nerve sheath meningioma. In this setting, compression of the intraorbital optic nerve sheath by tumor results in impairment of axonal transport. Optic disc swelling (unilateral or bilateral) may also occur as a manifestation of infiltrative processes, such as lymphoma, leukemia, and plasma cell dyscrasias.

Central Retinal Vein Occlusion

Patients with CRVO demonstrate marked optic disc swelling in combination with dilated, tortuous retinal veins and retinal hemorrhages. While retinal hemorrhages in patients with other forms of optic disc swelling are often limited to the peripapillary region, peripheral intraretinal hemorrhages are characteristic of CRVO. Vascular risk factors such as hypertension and diabetes mellitus are frequently associated with unilateral CRVO in older patients. The presence of bilateral CRVO, or its occurrence in younger patients, should prompt evaluation for a hypercoagulable state.

Optic Atrophy

Optic atrophy may result from several conditions like inflammatory, vascular, toxic, or compressive in etiology. In such conditions, the disc has a full moon appearance with marked pallor and often the lamina cribrosa is prominent. Postpapilloedemic optic atrophy may also occur where the disc margin may appear a little fuzzy. There is visual loss, a deafferented pupil and relative afferent pupil defect if the condition is asymmetrical. Segmental atrophy may also occur. Visual field may show a central or centrocecal scotoma in demyelinating cases.

Ascending versus Descending Atrophy

Primary retinal disorders that destroy the retinal ganglion cells cause Wallerian degeneration of their axonal projections to result in "ascending" pallor of the optic discs. Some of the more common examples include retinitis pigmentosa, CRA occlusion, and metabolic neurodegenerative disorders (e.g., Tay Sachs disease). The optic disc may have more of a yellowing "waxy" pallor. Primary injury of the optic nerve, on the other hand, results in "descending" retrograde degeneration of the axons, producing the more commonly observed whitish pallor of the disc. In clinical practice, distinguishing the nature of the pallor and cause of it based on color alone is often not productive.

There are mimics of optic atrophy including large physiologic cups with exposure of the lamina cribrosa, and sloping ectatic discs. Myopic discs are paler than hyperopic discs.

Causes of Optic Atrophy

Acquired optic atrophy represents the nonspecific sign of injury to the optic nerve from a variety of insults. For example, the result of underlying optic nerve tumor, optic neuritis, and ischemic optic neuropathy. It may be generalized or altitudinal. Postpapilledemic optic atrophy leaves behind rippling lines in the peripapillary retina that signify the presence of previous papilledema. Also the disc margin often looks rather fuzzy in contrast to optic atrophy resulting from intrinsic diseases of optic nerve (primary optic atrophy).

Congenital optic atrophy can be caused by genetic conditions including a dominant form (presents age 4–8; mild loss), or recessive form (age 1–9; moderate-to-severe), recessive form with diabetes (severe). When associated with diabetes and deafness, consider Friedreich's ataxia, diabetes insipidus, Usher's syndrome, Refsum's syndrome, and Laurence–Moon–Biedl syndromes. Occasionally, it can also be the result of a perinatal (vascular) injury that may not be recognized clinically; this may be a retrospective diagnosis. Susac's syndrome is a very rare form of microangiopathy characterized by encephalopathy, branch RAOs and hearing loss. This is likely to be an autoimmune disease.

Leber hereditary optic neuropathy is a maternally inherited mitochondrial disorder producing initially unilateral and later bilateral primary looking optic atrophy. Some disc swelling may be evident in the early stage (see chapter 7).

Glaucomatous optic atrophy is characterized by progressive cupping of the disc with varied types of field defects caused by persistently raised intra ocular pressure.

The enlarged cup may give the appearance of disc pallor, but careful inspection of the neuroretinal rim will reveal that this portion of the disc is pink and healthy appearing. As neurologists we can think of it as papilledema in reverse.

Toxic optic neuropathy is usually a bilateral optic neuropathy which can be due to nutritional, methyl alcohol or drugs. Loss of the macular papillary bundle characterizes this neuropathy.

Recognize Vascular Disease

Retinal artery occlusions frequently cause symptoms of transient monocular blindness and can be related to conditions that can cause stroke. These occlusions can affect the central or branch retinal artery. If the CRA is occluded, the retina will appear pale, and a "cherry red spot" (over the macula) will be present due to visualization of the underlying vascular choroid. In acute central RAO, the optic disc is usually not swollen because the CRA contributes little blood to the blood supply to the optic disc. Weeks to months later, the disc becomes pale due to the process of ascending optic atrophy.

Retinal vein occlusions (branch or central) can be seen with hypercoaguable states, hypertension, and other vascular disease. Central RVO has already been mentioned in the section on unilateral papilledema. RVOs often give a dramatic appearance. Some describe the retina as looking like a "tomato splat". Also known as a "blood and thunder fundus," vision may or may not be affected. Central RVO/branch RVO is associated with hypertension, diabetes, arteriosclerosis, and hypercoaguable states. Patients with CRVO and arterial occlusion have permanent severe visual loss. Branch RVOs are characteristically found in hypertensive patients with venous crossing changes and stasis distally.

Hemorrhages on the Disc and in the Retina (Fig. 4)

Whenever you see "red," four questions should come to your mind:
1. Is it a hemorrhage?
2. Where is the hemorrhage—in which layer is it located?
3. What disease process may have produced the hemorrhage?
4. What do I need to do about it?

Locating the depth of the hemorrhage in the eye can be difficult unless you know the layers and characteristics of hemorrhage in the various layers of the retina or vitreous. The architecture of the retina usually dictates the shape of the hemorrhage. The most common form of hemorrhage is the "splinter hemorrhage." These are lines of beading radiating from the disc between the nerve fiber layer. The second most common hemorrhage is deeper in the retina and will appear to be circular dots and blots. Every layer will have a characteristic appearance.

Some hemorrhages are worth knowing about because they can be diagnostic.

Terson's Hemorrhage

It is usually a hemorrhage in the vitreous or subhyaloid region associated with subarachnoid hemorrhage. This syndrome got its name from A Terson (a French ophthalmologist) who first described the finding of vitreous hemorrhage associated with subarachnoid hemorrhage. If these hemorrhages are large, the retina and disc may not be visible. If the retina is visible, multiple hemorrhages may be seen at various levels (vitreal, subhyaloid, and intraretinal). Subhyaloid

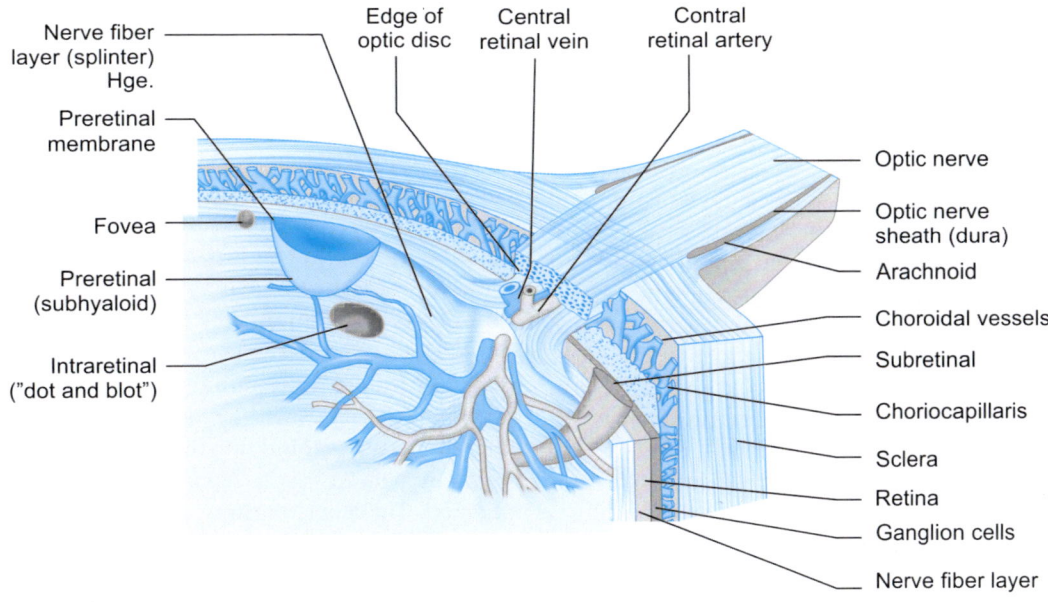

FIG. 4: Schematic representation of location of retinal hemorrhages.

hemorrhages often have a characteristic horizontal upper level.

Roth Spot

Roth spot is named for Dr M von Roth who described the hemorrhage in 1872; however, he did not make a connection with endocarditis. Dr M Litten made this observation in 1902 when he designated these white centered hemorrhages for Roth, his mentor. Roth spots are "white-centered" hemorrhages that occur either as round hemorrhages or flame-shaped hemorrhage, i.e., either bleeding in the nerve fiber layer or in the outer plexiform layer. Historically, a central core of inflammatory cells or fibrous tissue characterizes these hemorrhages. For a while, "Roth spots" were supposed to be pathognomonic for bacterial endocarditis; however, it is now known that white centered hemorrhages can be caused by diabetes, hypertension, anemia, pernicious anemia, myeloma, sickle cell anemia, leukemia, as well as trauma and emboli other than from infectious sources.

Congenital/Inherited Retinal Abnormalities

Retinitis pigmentosa may be inherited through several genes and characteristically exhibits pigmentary changes with bone spicule like formation and loss of peripheral vision. Atypical retinitis pigmentosa without bone spicule formation may be associated with several neurologic diseases like progressive external ophthalmoplegia, olivopontocerebellar atrophy, mitochondrial encephalopathy with lactic acidosis and stroke-like episodes (MELAS), myoclonus epilepsy with ragged red fibers, and Usher's syndrome. Here also peripheral vision is lost first.

RETINAL PHAKOMATOSES AND RELATED CONDITIONS

The phakomatoses are a group of disorders characterized by cutaneous lesions and hamartomatous growths elsewhere in the body. Ophthalmoscopically detectable retinal lesions can be seen in some of these.

In tuberous sclerosis, the main retinal abnormality is astrocytic hamartomas, which are typically smooth, dome-shaped, semitransluscent, grayish, and white lesions located anywhere in the retina, but found preferentially in the pericapillary region. Calcific lesions at this location may be mistaken for optic nerve drusen.

Neurofibromatosis type 2 often reveals retinal hamartomas, optic disc gliomas, retinal hemangiomas, medullated nerve fibers, choroidal naevi, uveal melanomas, and choroidal hamartomas.

Retinal lesions are uncommon in Sturge–Weber syndrome but choroidal hemangiomas occur in some resulting in unilateral glaucoma.

Von Hippel–Lindau disease is characterized by a predisposition to develop hemangioblastomas of the central nervous system and retina along with renal cell carcinoma, pheochromocytomas and cysts in other organs. The characteristic retinal lesion is retinal angiomatosis which are usually of the size of diabetic microaneurysms and consist of a tight network of small vascular channels, with an arterial feeding and venous draining vessel. Over time, these vessels become dilated and tortuous and ultimately exudative retinopathy and detachment may result fluorescein angiography is essential for early diagnosis.

Retinocephalic vascular malformation (Wyburn-Mason syndrome; Bonnet–Dechaume-Blanc syndrome) is not a phakomatoses. This is characterized by unilateral vascular malformation of the retina, brain, and parts of the face. This indeed is a very rare condition and a single case has been reported from India (Chakravarty et al.). The vascular malformation affects one or all retinal vessels which are markedly dilated and tortuous with mild proptosis and conjunctival congestion. Cranial bruit may be heard and the cerebral vascular malformation demonstrable by angiography.

Optic Disc Anomalies

Optic nerve hypoplasia exhibits the "double ring sign" with tiny discs with a paler peripheral ring. Several types of field defects may ensue. Hypoplastic discs may be associated with several conditions like in children of diabetic mothers, maternal drug ingestion, maternal infections during pregnancy, albinism, Klippel–Trénaunay–Weber syndrome, hemifacial atrophy, osteogenesis imperfecta, Aicardi syndrome, Apert syndrome, trisomy 18, fetal alcohol syndrome, and Dandy–Walker syndrome. It may also occur in hypopituitarism, agenesis of the septum pellucidum, cerebral palsy, epilepsy, head/face anomalies, deafness, chondrodysplasia, heart disease, trisomy 18, and septo-optic dysplasia (de Morsier syndrome).

Several endocrinological abnormalities may be associated.

Excavated Optic Disc Anomalies

Colobomas (from the Greek-Kolobos, a gap or hole where tissue is lacking) are usually congenital (occasionally acquired) defect, the lack of tissue causes a notch, gap, hole, or fissure. Colobomas are caused by failure of the closure of the embryonic fissure. Optic nerve colobomas and retinochoroidal colobomas result from incomplete closure of the embryonic fissure and may be associated with other congenital anomalies like congenital heart defects, choanal atresia, dysplastic ears, and less commonly sphenoidal encephalocele and thalidomide exposure *in utero*. Retinochoroidal colobomas occur inferior to the optic disc and have pigment around them. Vision may or may not be affected. However, at times retinal detachments may occur.

In morning glory disc anomaly, the disc looks like a funnel shaped flower with early branching of the CRA deep in the disc tissue with the branches coming out from the margin of the disc. Visual problems may or may not be prominent and the condition is unilateral.

SUGGESTED READINGS

1. Brodsky MC, Baker RS, Hamed LM. Pediatric neuro-ophthalmology. New York: Springer; 1995.
2. Brodsky MC. Congenital anomalies of the optic disc. In: Miller NR, Newman NJ, editors. Walsh and Hoyt's neuroophthalmology. Baltimore: Williams and Wilkins; 1998. pp. 775-823.
3. Brown G, Tasman W. Congenital anomalies of the optic disc. New York: Grune & Stratton, 1983.
4. Chakravarty A, Chatterjee S. Retino-cephalic vascular malformation. J Assoc Physicians India. 1990;38(12): 941-3.
5. Digre K, Corbett JJ. Practical viewing of the optic disc. Boston: Butterworth; 2003.
6. Liu GT, Vorpe NJ, Galetta SL. Optic disc swelling: Papilledema and causes. In: Neuro-ophthalmology - diagnosis and management. Philadelphia: WB Saunders; 2000.
7. Miller NR, Newman NJ. Papilledema: A sign of increased intracranial pressure. In: Walsh and Hoyt's clinical neuro-ophthalmology. Baltimore: Williams & Wilkins: 1998.
8. Rosen ES, Eustace P, Thompson HS, et al. Neuro-ophthalmology. London: Mosby; 1998.
9. Spalton D. Hitchings R, Hunter P. Atlas of clinical ophthalmology. 2nd ed. London: Mosby Year Book; 1994.

CHAPTER 4

Visual Field Examination For the Neurologist

Ambar Chakravarty, Pushpita Sahu

INTRODUCTION

Visual field is that portion of the space which is visible to an individual. Although this is perceived binocularly, the field of vision is plotted for each eye separately. Neurologists often make a major clinical distinction between "confrontation" and "formal" visual field testing. Confrontation testing usually involves fingers wiggling or various colored pins moving, and is invariably done well by a neurologist. The fundamental principle is comparing the field of the patient with that of the examinee's assuming that the examiner possesses a normal acuity and a normal visual field. Formal visual field testing involves large pieces of other people's expensive equipment and is usually done (eventually) by someone else. Although the underlying principles and anatomic correlations are essentially the same for all forms of visual field testing, the increased volume and sensitivity of the clinical information provided by formal "perimetry" makes the understanding and utilization of these techniques essential for all neuro-ophthalmic and most neurologic practitioners.

In 1947, Lloyd classified the visual fields obtained in his outpatient clinic under three broad headings:
1. Those interpretable on their own merits
2. Those that mean something to the person who took them
3. Those unintelligible to anyone.

He further stated that most of the difficulties in perimetry may be listed as follows:
- Inefficient explanation of what is required, either by the physician to the perimetrist, by the perimetrist to the patient, or both
- Uncomfortable, hungry, or frankly bored patient
- Large nose or dropping lid as causes of contraction
- Failure to watch the patient's eye to ensure proper fixation
- Moving test-object too fast or too slow
- Going on too long for the patient or the perimetrist
- Failure to give a separate explanation of what is required for the central field, particularly a demonstration of the blind spot and an assurance that this is normal where the patient shows signs of anxiety
- Failure on the part of the perimetrist to remember what he is looking for.

Despite subsequent passage of more than 50 years, and the advent first of Goldmann perimetry and then of automated perimetry, surprisingly little appears to have changed.

Critical to any attempt to produce a meaningful examination of the visual fields is the fundamental question: "Why are we doing this?" A clear goal must be defined before instituting the visual field testing. "We" is emphasized as a reminder that perimetry is always a collaborative team activity, which usually includes a patient, a nurse/technician, and an interpreting physician.

The two main indications for visual field testing in neurology are:
1. *Diagnostic:* What is the anatomical location and pathology of the lesion present?
2. *Prognostic:* Is there quantitative or qualitative change in a visual field defect that has previously been detected?

Currently, the two principal methods for formal neuro-ophthalmic visual field testing are Goldmann perimetry and automated (computerized) perimetry (e.g., Humphrey, Octopus systems). A simpler but now much less

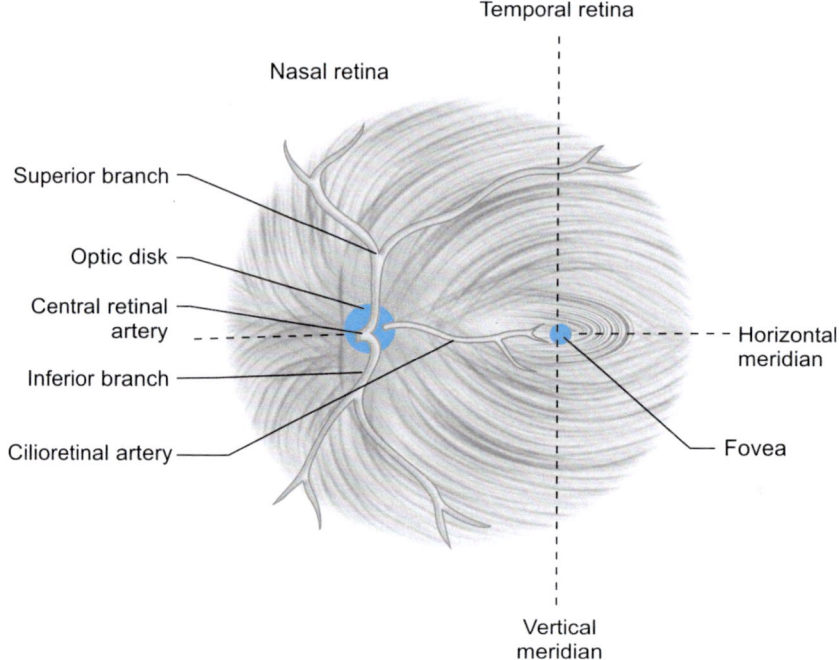

FIG. 1: Retinal nerve fiber layer and arteries. Note the arcuate distribution of temporal and nasal fibers as they coverage to the disc and the imagery horizontal and vertical meridians.

commonly used technique is the manual tangent screen (Bjerrum's). Goldmann perimetry is usually performed as a kinetic (moving target) test, while automated perimetry uses static testing. Each system has inherent advantages and disadvantages (Table 1).

However, no matter what technique is used, four sad but honest truths are likely to remain:
1. Any perimetry is a boring test for most patients
2. Intra- and intertest variation is an almost inevitable concomitant of perimetry
3. Automated perimetry is still a subjective test—just because the perimeter uses a computer, it does not alter the intelligence or capacity of the patient undergoing the test, the technician supervising the test or the physician ordering and interpreting it
4. There are still patients in whom visual field examination, by any testing method, may not be successful.

Frisén commented *"Perimetry is a demanding test for both the patient and the examiner. Both have the right to work under optimal conditions, with a minimum of distractions, and both work best if they know precisely what is expected from them. Perimetry is never performed in a vacuum, but represents one quantitative aspect of visual function testing, based on sound indications reached by careful history and detailed physician's examination. For maximum yield within a minimum time, the examination must be geared to the exact needs of the individual. However, repeated measurements with sufficiently finely graduated stimuli will nearly always give different results."*

TOPICAL DIAGNOSIS

Three golden rules to improve the interpretation of diagnostic field testing are:
1. Reject artefact
2. Respect the horizontal meridian (monocular field = retina or optic nerve)
3. Worship the vertical meridian (chiasmal/retrochiasmal)

Artefact

Artefact masquerading as meaningful neuro-ophthalmic visual field loss, comes from a number of sources including:
- Intra- or intertest fluctuation in responses

Table 1: Perimetry systems

Goldmann Perimetry	Automated Perimetry
Advantages	
• Shorter examination time	• Increased sensitivity (especially central field)

• Easier for "difficult" or "neurological" patients
  ○ Fixation monitoring
  ○ Hands-on patient/examiner interaction
  ○ Rapid re-examination of artefacts
	• Random presentation; avoidance of examiner bias

• Full-field examination	• Statistical data analysis possible (individual field and longitudinal comparisons)
• Rapid screening (e.g., normal; hemianopia)	• Easily operated
Disadvantages	
• Lower sensitivity (especially central field)	• Duration of testing ○ Often limits examination to central 24–30 degrees

• Interexaminer variability (e.g., target presentation, response detection)	• Poor with "difficult patients"
	  ○ Reduced compliance
	  ○ Increased fatigue

• Subjective examiner bias ("artistry")	• Hidden "neurological" peripheral field defects
• Difficulties with statistical analysis or longitudinal comparisons	• Poor intratest artefact detection
• Requires experienced operator	
Lesions of Choice	
• Retrochiasmal "neurological" fields	• Optic neuropathies
• Hysteria/malingering	• Chiasmal lesions
	• Assessment of change in (1) and (2)
	• Change in known retrochiasmal lesions (e.g., tumor therapy)

- Small pupil size causing peripheral field constriction
- Amblyopia, cataract or media opacity causing generalized or central field depression
- Omitting refractive correction for central 30 degree testing, causing central pseudoscotomata or depression
- Non-rimless refractive correction or lens holder poorly located, causing ring or hemi-ring scotomata
- Aphakia: Corrective lens causing ring scotomata or no correction causing erratic central responses
- Ptosis or heavy brow causing altitudinal field loss
- Inattentive, uncooperative, unreliable, or unsuitable patient producing strange or meaningless fields, especially with automated perimetry
- Hysteria or malingering causing particularly wide fluctuations in response

Horizontal Meridian

Optic Nerve or Retina

The horizontal meridian of the visual field reflects the horizontal raphe of the distribution of the optic nerve fiber layer across the retina. Visual field defects that respect the horizontal meridian are classically one of the hallmarks that help to distinguish anterior optic nerve (optic nerve head) lesions (e.g., glaucoma, anterior ischemic optic neuropathy) from retinal lesions (geographic scotoma) or macular lesions (central scotoma).

In cases of idiopathic or demyelinating optic neuritis, the classic (diagnostic) description of the visual field loss as a "central or cecocentral scotoma with intact peripheral field" has therefore been somewhat awkward to explain theoretically. However, this description was enshrined prior to the development of automated perimetry. More recently, an interesting and repeated observation in optic neuritis and other optic neuropathies has been that static, automated perimetry may sometimes define a patchy "Swiss-cheese type" of central vision field defect, while kinetic Goldmann perimetry is relatively normal despite reduced visual acuity (statokinetic dissociation). Now automated perimetry results from the recent optic neuritis treatment trial have shown that actually a wide variety of visual field defects can occur in optic neuritis, with altitudinal defects being the most common on visual inspection of the field testing results, and statistical analysis of the visual field defects suggesting evidence for some involvement of all components of the central 30 degrees of the visual field (Table 2).

An additional note of caution regarding a central scotoma as "diagnostic" of demyelinating optic neuritis in a recent report showing that some

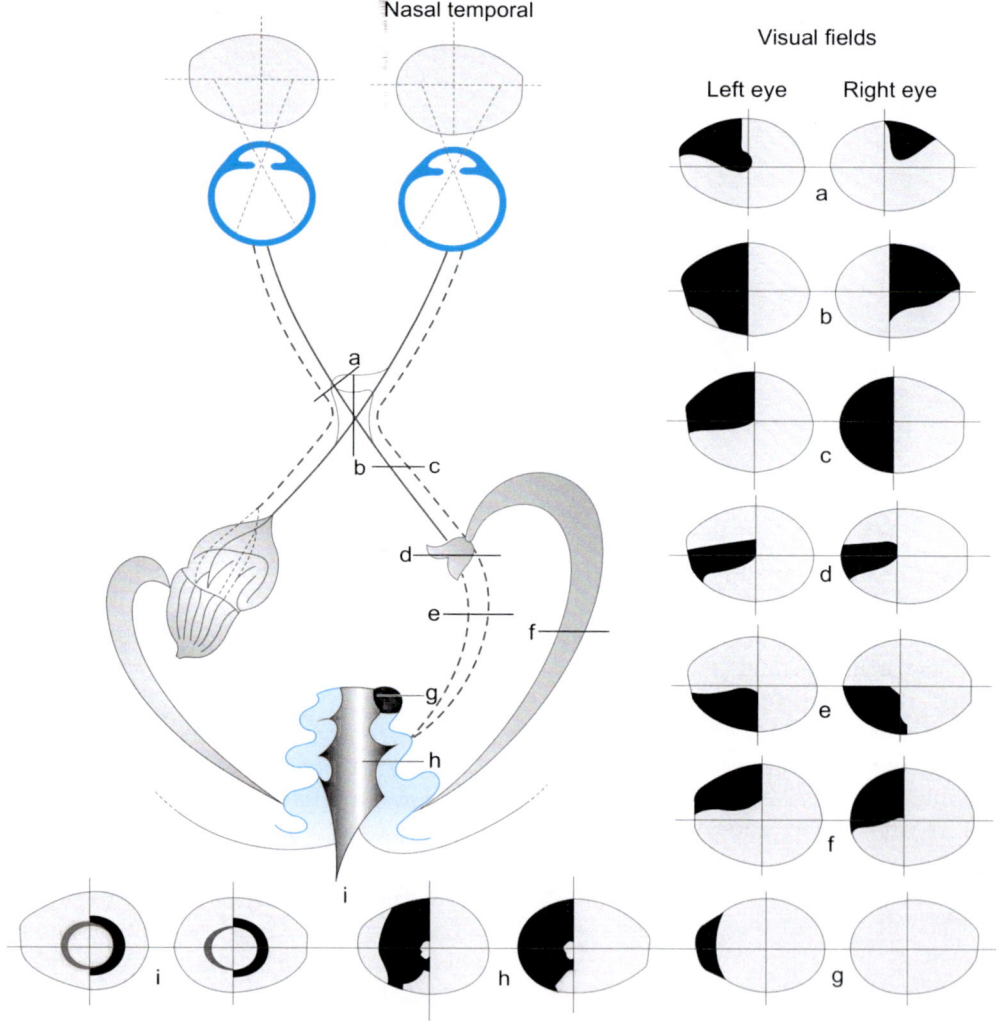

FIG. 2: Localization of lesions in the optic pathway (Chiasmal and retrochiasmal) causing various field defects. Visual fields from both eyes are usually abnormal but there is greater congruity with more posteriorly located lesions.

Table 2: Characteristics of pupils encountered in neuro-ophthalmology

Condition	General characteristics	Response to light	Room condition
Essential anisocoria	Round, regular	Both brisk	No change
Horner's syndrome	Small, round, unilateral	Both brisk	Darkness
Tonic pupil syndrome	Usually lager in bright light; sector pupil palsy, vermiform movement unilateral or less often bilateral	Absent to light, tonic to near; tonic redilation	Light
Argyll Robertson pupils	Small, irregular, bilateral	Poor to light, better to near	No change
Midbrain pupils	Mid dilated; May be oval; bilateral	Poor to light, better to near	No change
Oculomotor palsy	Mid-dilated, unilateral (rarely bilateral)	Fixed	Light
Pharmacologically dilated pupils	Very large round, unilateral	Fixed	Light

Source: Dorsolateral medullary infarct (Wallenberg's syndrome).

cases of anterior ischemic optic neuropathy may also present with a central scotoma rather than an altitudinal hemianopia.

Uncommon but important differential diagnoses that can masquerade as "optic nerve type" visual field defects which respect the horizontal meridian include retinal lesions such as retinal detachment, autosomal dominant retinitis pigmentosa, chorioretinal degeneration or branch retinal artery occlusions. In addition, neurologists need to be aware of retinal disorders such as the cone dystrophies, which cause progressive visual loss with central scotomas, impaired color vision and optic atrophy, and are therefore often misdiagnosed as an optic neuropathy, with subsequent extensive (and expensive) but unnecessary laboratory and radiological investigations.

One other retinal disorder of importance to neurologists is the peripheral visual field constriction associated with the use of the anticonvulsant vigabatrin, a GABA transaminase inhibitor. Although initially considered a rare complication, it has now been recognized that this visual field loss is extremely common, and that once it has developed it is usually irreversible, despite cessation of the drug. The visual field loss is almost never detected by confrontation visual field testing, and it is therefore essential that all patients receiving vigabatrin, or probably any of the GABAergic anticonvulsants, should have regular visual field testing performed using computerized or Goldman perimetry.

Vertical Meridian

The vertical meridian is the great visual field watershed that separates retinal and optic nerve lesions from chiasmal and retrochiasmal damage. It is essential to recognize even the most subtle visual field deficit that respects the vertical meridian.

Optic Chiasma

The classic description of the complete bitemporal field defect caused by a lesion of the optic chiasm needs little elaboration. However, in early chiasmal compression, asymmetric visual field involvement is the rule rather than the exception, with a wide variety of field defects possible, and examination of the central 15 degrees of visual field for bitemporal foreshortening or field loss respecting the vertical meridian is critical. The tilted optic disk syndrome is an important congenital anomaly that can masquerade as a bitemporal chiasmal field defect with "pseudorespect" for the vertical meridian, and its recognition is important to prevent unnecessary neurological investigations.

Unilateral temporal visual field defects that respect the vertical meridian are, until incontrovertibly proven otherwise, an invaluable warning of a chiasmal lesion. If overlooked, they can represent a major neuro-ophthalmic disaster.

Binasal Field Loss

This, in contrast, usually arises as a subset of field defects involving the horizontal meridian.

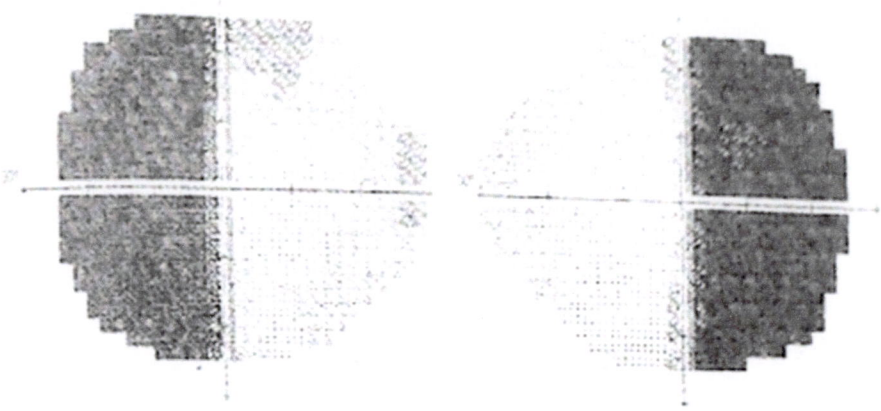

FIG. 3: Bitemporal visual field loss.

Common causes are:
- Glaucoma
- Optic nerve head drusen
- Chronic disk edema (e.g., papilledema)
- Optic nerve hypoplasia
  Also include:
- Retinoschisis or detachment
- Chorioretinal degeneration
  Historically cited but dubious:
- Dolichoectasia of the carotid or anterior cerebral arteries, with compression of the lateral sides of the optic chiasm or both optic nerves
- Chiasmal trauma
- Neurosyphilis
  Finally:
- Hysteria/malingering—the absence of an area of "pre-fixation blindness" helps to distinguish this from organic binasal loss.

Retrochiasmal Lesions

The hallmark of the visual field defects caused by retrochiasmal lesions is that they are homonymous, and as a general principle the pattern of the defect in each eye becomes increasingly congruous as the lesion approaches the occipital lobe. Visual acuity is unaffected by the hemianopia, but frequently patients are not aware that the field defect is in both eyes and they report that the vision is reduced in the eye on the side of the hemianopia.

Complete Homonymous Hemianopia

This in an individual patient essentially does not have anatomically localizing value, since it may arise from a lesion at any point in the retrochiasmal pathway. However, associated clinical deficits may suggest a localization (e.g., optic tract lesion with hemiparesis and hypothalamic dysfunction; optic radiation lesion with hemiparesis, hemisensory loss and aphasia). In 100 patients with homonymous hemianopia, Smith reported that 40% had occipital lobe lesions, 33% parietal lobe, and 24% temporal lobe lesions, but optic tract and lateral geniculate lesions were rare. Approximately 42% of cases had a vascular origin and 38% were caused by tumor. However, in patients presenting with an isolated homonymous hemianopia, 89% were of vascular origin, with 86% due to occipital lobe infarction caused by posterior cerebral artery occlusion. In contrast, all of the cases under 30 years of age had nonvascular causes.

Optic Tract Lesions

These usually cause grossly incongruous homonymous hemianopia, often associated with unilateral or bilateral impairment of central visual acuity and sometimes a classical ipsilateral temporal optic disk pallor and contralateral wedge or butterfly band pallor.

Lateral Geniculate Nucleus Lesions

These usually have a distinctive, rule-breaking congruous wedge-shaped homonymous defect that straddles the horizontal meridian in a pattern that reflects either lateral or anterior choroidal artery occlusion.

Occipital Lobe Lesions

These usually produce either a complete homonymous hemianopia, with or without macular sparing, or exquisitely congruous homonymous scotomata that can be anatomically localized within the architecture of the calcarine cortex. Midline tilting (deviation from the absolute meridian) of the field defect in patients with complete homonymous hemianopia is very common when careful perimetry is performed, but is rarely more than 15 degrees.

The classic map of the visual cortex created by Gordon Holmes is well known and depicts an orderly topographic representation of the contralateral hemifield of vision in the human striate cortex, with the central 15 degrees of visual field being allocated to approximately 25% of the surface area of the striate cortex. With the advent of high-resolution magnetic resonance scanning, this long-held clinical–anatomical correlation has undergone revision, with considerable expansion of the area of the striate cortex that subserves central vision and a concomitant reduction of the area devoted to peripheral vision. These changes help to explain why visual defects confined to the monocular temporal crescent are rare, since the anterior striate cortex subserving this monocular region of visual field constitutes less than 10% of the total striate cortex surface area. Similarly, the commonly used central 24–30 degree paradigms for computerized visual field testing actually assess 80–83% of the striate cortex, mitigating against failure to detect cortical occipital lesions with these programs.

The phenomenon of macular sparing with homonymous hemianopia is also more readily understood with this expanded central field representation, and is ascribed to the conjoint vascular supply of the occipital pole by the posterior and middle cerebral arteries that occurs in a minority of patients. Because the representation of the central vision field is so magnified in the posterior half of the striate cortex, perfusion by the middle cerebral artery with preservation of any portion of this region after posterior cerebral artery occlusion will variably spare cortex devoted exclusively to macular vision. Thus, the presence of a macular sparing homonymous hemianopia does suggest an occipital lobe origin for the deficit.

Several important clinical syndromes that involve lobe lesions warrant mention:
- Ipsilateral eye pain with contralateral homonymous hemianopia is an important indicator of occipital lobe infarction due to posterior cerebral artery occlusion (usually

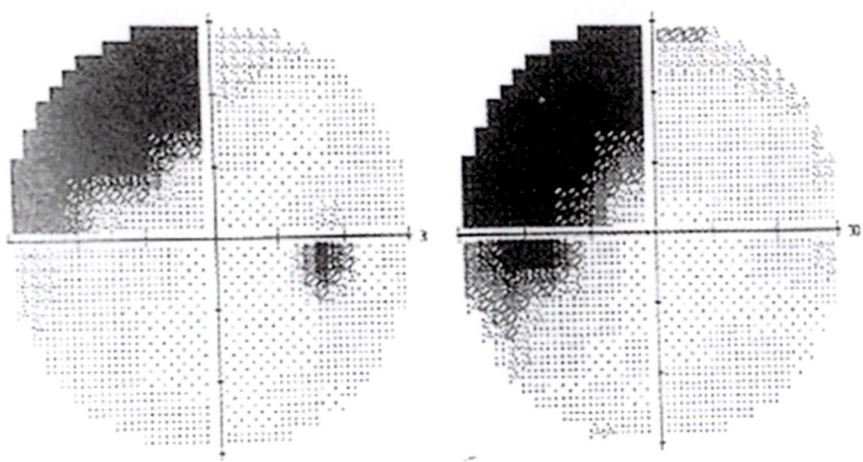

FIG. 4: Left superior homonymous quadranopia.

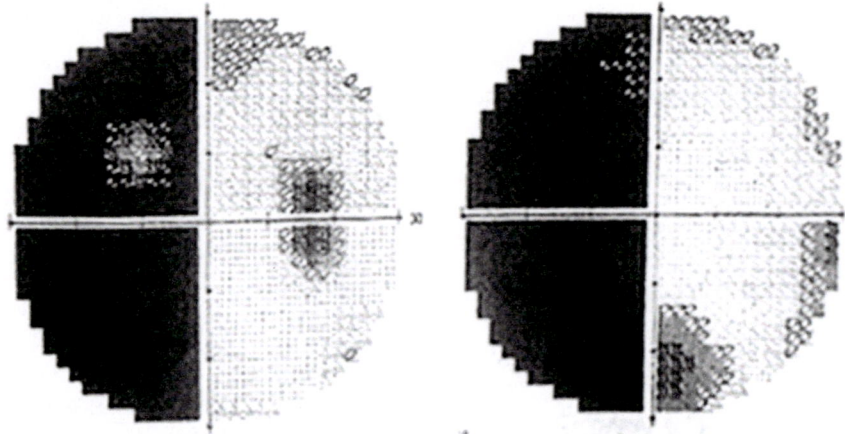

FIG. 5: Left homonymous hemianopia.

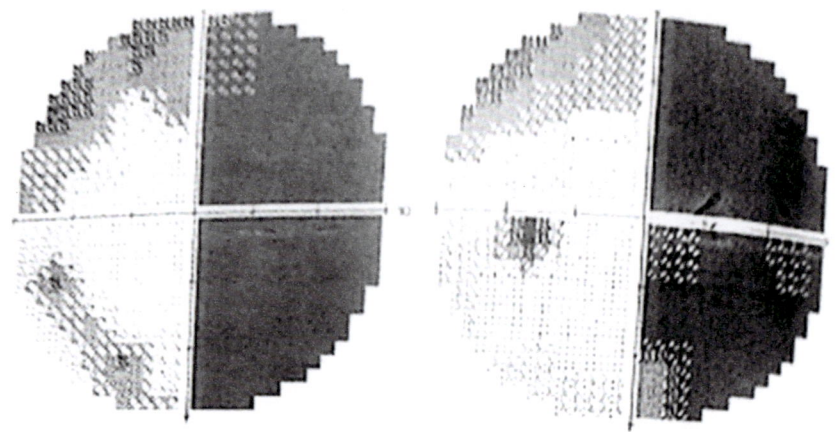

FIG. 6: Right homonymous hemianopia.

embolic). While cardiac investigation may be warranted, carotid studies are not directly indicated
- Alexia without agraphia and a right homonymous hemianopia indicates infarction of the left occipital lobe with extension to the splenium of the corpus callosum. All patients with a right homonymous hemianopia should have reading tested as part of their neurological examination
- Monocular peripheral field loss (temporal crescent) occurs with posterior optic radiation or anterior occipital lobe lesions that damage the projection of the unpaired peripheral nasal retinal fibers. Conversely, in a homonymous hemianopia, the monocular temporal crescent may be spared with posterior occipital lobe lesions that do not involve the anterior visual cortex. However, as discussed above, occipital lobe lesions causing visual field defects confined entirely to the monocular temporal crescent are rare. Monocular peripheral temporal visual field defects far more commonly arise from retinal lesions

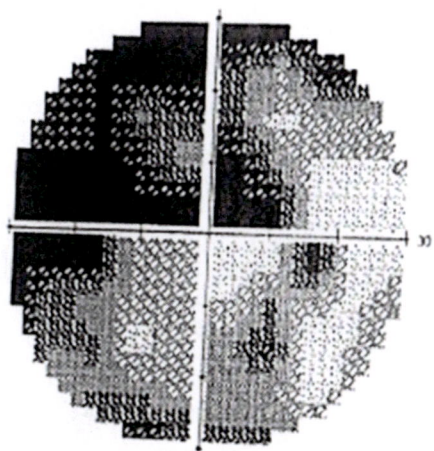

FIG. 7: Superior altitudinal defect in glaucoma. Similar defect may be seen rarely in AION.

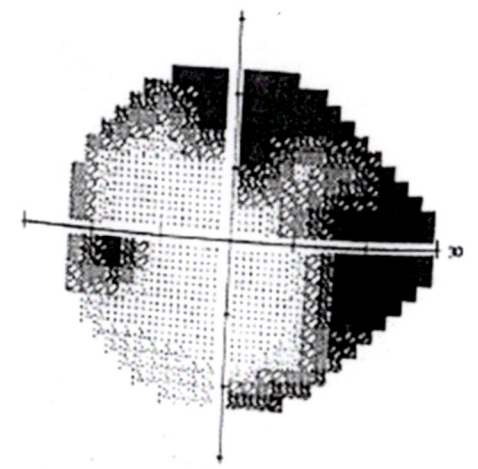

FIG. 8: Nasal step in glaucoma.

not occipital lesions, and the peripheral nasal retina should be carefully examined before a diagnosis of occipital pathology is made.

- Isolated homonymous congruous quadrantic visual field deficits with sharp horizontal borders have a high degree of specificity for lesions of the occipital lobe, rather than parietal or temporal lobes. When the field defect respects the horizontal meridian, it suggests specific involvement of the extrastriate (V2/V3) cortex as well as the upper or lower calcarine striate (V1) cortex. These lesions are often small, arise from vertebrobasilar disease and may escape detection by CT scan if presenting acutely. In contrast, the visual field defects caused by lesions of the optic radiations in either the parietal or temporal lobe are often incongruous and tend to have sloping borders that fail to respect precisely the horizontal meridian. Similarly, patients with optic tract lesions, such as those that occur occasionally following posterior GPi pallidotomy for Parkinson's disease, have incomplete homonymous quadrantic defects that do not respect the horizontal meridian and are often accompanied by homonymous paracentral scotomas.
- Rarely, occipital lobe lesions may cause bilateral homonymous paracentral scotomata that are mistaken for bilateral optic nerve lesions with cecocentral scotomas. With occipital lobe lesions, the pupil reflexes are normal.

Visual Field Defects in Glaucoma

Neurologists should acquaint themselves with at least the common forms of visual field defects produced by raised intraocular pressure. The common and important defects are only highlighted here.

Before discussing the field loss in glaucoma one must familiarize self with a few basic points. The retinal nerve fiber layer is constructed in such a way that no axon crosses the horizontal midline, and defects tend to localize to one side of the horizontal or the other. Fibers from macula run to the temporal side of the disk in the papillomacular bundle. The rest of the peripheral temporal retinal fibers arch above and below the macula to reach the upper and lower pole of the disk. The nasal fibers pass to the disk radically. It is the loss of the axon that results in visual field defect. The size and shape depend on the fibers affected. Loss of the arcuate temporal fibers will result in arcuate field defect and loss of radial nasal fibers will result in wedge defect. However due to the optics of the eye, the field defect will be reversed, i.e., the upper arcuate temporal fiber loss will produce a lower nasal arcuate defect and vice versa.

Damage to the optic nerve and hence the field defect in glaucoma may occur in one of two ways or a combination of both. Progressive nerve damage may occur diffusely with concentric enlargement of cup, progressive increase in cup: disc ratio and thinning of neuroretinal rim. The whole field may be diffusely affected showing an increase of threshold and lowering of sensitivity. This type of diffuse loss in early glaucoma is usually associated with high intraocular pressure. Damage may also occur focally with enlargement of the cup superiorly or inferiorly, or affection of part of neuroretinal rim producing nerve fiber bundle defect and corresponding field loss. This is mostly of vascular origin and seen in so-called "low tension glaucoma". With progress, both the features overlap.

Early glaucomatous damage therefore can show a diffuse lowering of sensitivity, or isolated paracentral scotoma in the same isopter as the blind spot, or a temporal wedge, even an early nasal step. With progress, there is enlargement of blind spot, Seidel scotoma, superior or inferior arcuate, double arcuate meeting in nasal step with or without peripheral breakthrough. With further progress an entire hemifield may be involved resulting in altitudinal defect. Finally, the patient may be left with a small central island and a small temporal crescentic field left.

Malingering and Factitious Visual Field Defects

Nonorganic (functional) visual loss is often accompanied by well-recognized indicators on manual (Goldmann/tangent screen) perimetry testing of the visual fields, including tubular or spiraling visual fields and crossed isopters. However, automated computerized visual field analyzers are becoming increasingly the instrument of choice for routine visual field screening and their output ostensibly has impressive controls for subject reliability and statistical analysis of deviation from the normal. Several reports are therefore important in demonstrating that malingerers without previous experience of visual field testing can easily produce automated visual fields that appear to reliably reflect organic patterns of visual field loss, including enlarged blind spots, quadrantic, hemianopic, altitudinal, and pseudo, chiasmal field defects. Neurologists suspecting factitious impairment must be guided by the summation of their whole examination, and not influenced by statistical output of a computerized field tester.

SUGGESTED READINGS

1. Anderson DR, Patella VM. Automated Static Perimetry. Mosby, St Louis, 2nd Edition, 1999.
2. Arndt CF, Derambure P, Defoort-Dhellemmes S, et al. Outer retinal dysfunction in patients treated with vigabatrin. Neurology. 1999;52:1201-5.
3. Biousse V, Newman NJ, Carroll C, et al. Visual fields in patients with posterior GPi pallidotomy. Neurology. 1998;50:258-65.
4. Fang JP, Donahue SP, Lin RH. Global visual field involvement in acute unilateral optic neuritis. Am J Ophthalmol. 1999;128:554-65.
5. Frisén L. Kinetic perimetry: Techniques and Strategies. Topics in Neuro-ophthalmology. Thompson HS. et al (eds). William & Wilkins Baltimore 1979, pp20-29.
6. Grochowicki M, Vighetto A, Berquet S, et al. Pituitary adenomas: Automatic static perimetry and Goldmann perimetry. A comparative study of 345 visual field charts. Br J Ophthalmol. 1991;75:219-21.
7. Horton JC, Hoyt WF. Quadrantic visual field defects. A hallmark of lesions in extrastriate (V2/V3) cortex. Brain. 1991;114:1703-18.
8. Horton JC, Hoyt WF. The representation of the visual field in human striate cortex. A revision of the classic Holmes map. Arch Ophthalmol. 1991;109:816-24.
9. Jacobson DM. The localizing value of a quadrantanopia. Arch Neurol. 1997;54:401-4.
10. Johnson MA, Krauss GL, Miller NR, et al. Visual function loss from vigabatrin. Effect of stopping the drug. Neurology. 2000;55:40-5.
11. Keltner JL, Johnson CA. Automated and manual perimetry–A six-year overview. Special emphasis on neuro-ophthalmic problems. Ophthalmology. 1984;91(1):68-85.
12. Lloyd JPF. Making perimetry pay. Tr Ophth Soc UK. 1948;67:409-22.
13. Luco C, Hoppe A, Schweitzer M, et al. Visual field defects in vascular lesions of the lateral geniculate body. J Neurol Neurosurgery and Psychiatry. 1992;55:12-5.
14. McFadzean R, Brosnahan D, Hadley D et al. Representation of the visual field in the occipital striate cortex. Br J Ophthalmol. 1994;78:185-90.
15. McFadzean RM, Hadley DM. Homonymous quadrantanopia respecting the horizontal meridian. A feature of striate and extrastriate cortical disease. Neurology. 1997;49:1741-6.
16. Rizzo JF, Lessell S. Optic neuritis and ischemic optic neuropathy. Overlapping clinical profiles. Arch Ophthalmol. 1991;109:1668-72.
17. Smith JL. Homonymous hemianopsia: A review of one hundred cases. Am J Ophthalmol 1962;54:616-22.

18. Stewart JFG. Automated perimetry and malingerers. Can Humphrey be outwitted? Ophthalmology. 1995;102:27-32.
19. The clinical profile of optic neuritis. Experience of the Optic Neuritis Treatment Trial. Optic Neuritis Study Group. Arch Ophthalmol. 1991;109:1673-6.
20. Thompson JC, Kosmorsky GS, Ellis BD. Fields of dreamers and dreamed-up fields. Functional and fake perimetry. Ophthalmology. 1996;103:117-25.
21. Trobe JD, Lorber ML, Schelzinger NS. Isolated homonymous hemianopsia. Arch Ophthalmol. 1973;89:377-81.

CHAPTER 5

Examination of the Pupil

Ambar Chakravarty, Debasish Roy

INTRODUCTION

Pupillary examination is a powerful tool in the neurological evaluation. The key in understanding the significance of pupillary findings is to know the anatomy of the system and to recognize the various reactions of the pupil. It is further important to correlate historical information with clinical findings in the context of known anatomy to arrive at a cogent diagnosis. The eye is a part of the central nervous system and it gives a clue about the nature of many central nervous system disorders. The pupil is the window to the eye and thus a thorough examination of the pupil forms the backbone of a comprehensive neurological examination. Pupillary examination gives information about the integrity of the anterior and posterior visual pathways. It also gives us an idea about the functioning of the second and third nerves and the integrity of the brain stem. Detailed pupillary examination can also yield useful information about the autonomic nervous system and even hemispheric function.

ANATOMY AND PHYSIOLOGY (FIGS 1 AND 2)

The normal pupil is situated inferomedial to center of cornea. When viewed in the natural state, the iris and pupil appear slightly larger (12.5% larger) because of the corneal magnification. The sphincter muscle is located at the pupillary border and is more powerful than the dilator muscle. Blood supply of iris is through the radially arranged vessels arising from the major arterial circle at the iris base. Pupillary control is essentially a balance between parasympathetic and sympathetic control. Although pupillary size and reactivity, as well as ciliary muscle tone, are basically controlled by the autonomic nervous systems, the major role is played by the parasympathetic system due to the mechanical superiority of the sphincter muscle.

Parasympathetic impulses arise in the Edinger–Westphal complex (EWc), a central paired subnucleus of the oculomotor nerve in the midbrain. Light directed into either eye usually produces bilateral pupillary constriction. The pupillary light reflex begins with hyperpolarization of the retinal photoreceptors.

Ultimately the retinal ganglion cells are activated. The retinal ganglion cells send their axons through the optic nerve, chiasm, and optic tract to synapse in the pretectal nuclei. Interneurons then connect the pretectal nuclei to the EWc. Efferent pupillary fibers arise from the EWc and traverse the mesencephalon in the rostral fascicles of the third cranial nerve. It enters the orbit as part of the inferior division of the nerve, and arrives at the ciliary ganglion by means of the motor nerve to the inferior oblique muscle. Most of the pupillomotor fibers synapse in the main or accessory ciliary ganglion and reach the iris sphincter muscle via the short ciliary nerves. Interruption in this pathway to the sphincter muscle will cause pupillary dilatation and decreased reactivity. Afferent visual system pathology does produce difference in pupillary size. Pupillary constriction is also a component of a number of synkinetic reactions involving parasympathetic activity—near reflex (miosis, accommodation, and convergence), Bell's phenomenon (levator inhibition, superior rectus muscle stimulation, and miosis) and Westphal-Piltz reaction (orbicularis spasm and miosis). The cortical region responsible for supranuclear generation of the near response remains uncertain. It probably rises from diffuse cortical projections. Ultimately supranuclear inputs for the near reflex converge upon the rostral

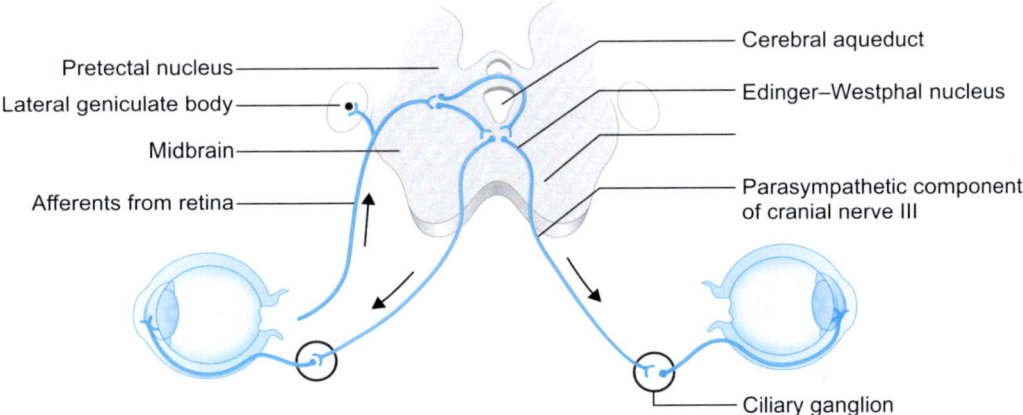

FIG. 1: Pupillary light reflex pathway from retina through optic pathway to lateral geniculate body and then on to Edinger–Westphal nucleus complex and then along third cranial nerve trunk to the iris sphincter.

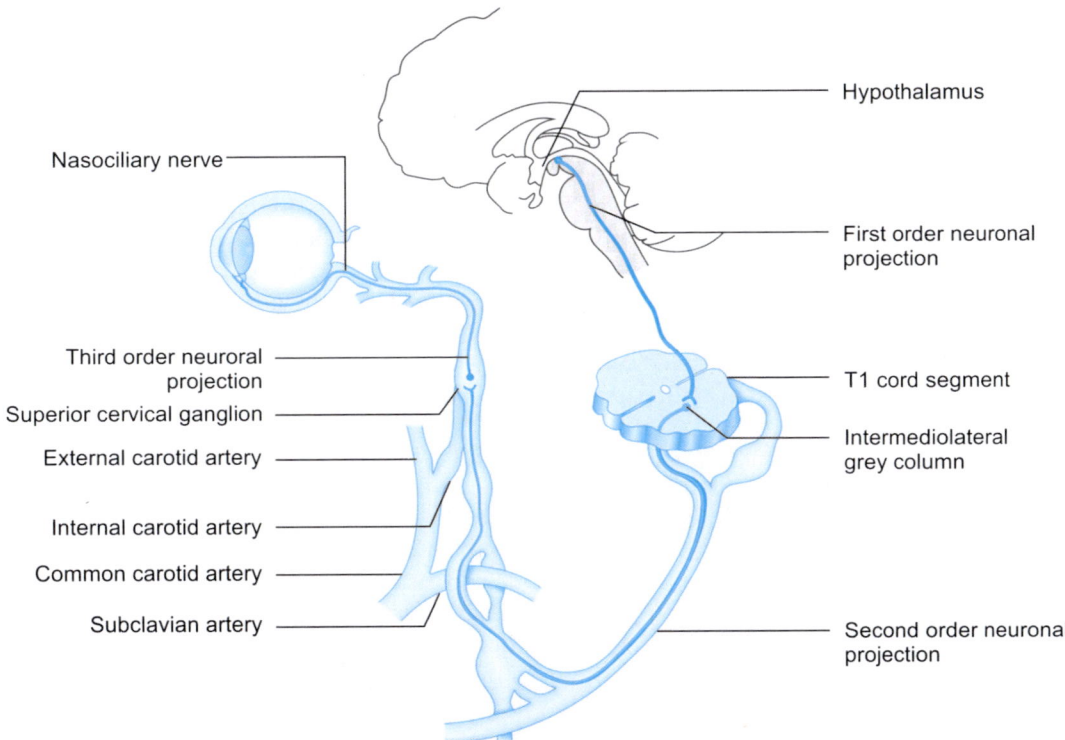

FIG. 2: Sympathetic pathway to the iris dilator muscle.

superior colliculus. From here, connections are made to the mesencephalic reticular formation, pretectum and EWc to generate the near triad- pupillary constriction, lens accommodation and convergence.

First order neuron of sympathetic pathway arises in the hypothalamus and descends through the reticular substance to synapse in the intermediolateral grey substance of the lower cervical and upper thoracic spinal cord (ciliospinal center of Budge–Waller, C8–T1). Second order neuron arises in the intermediolateral grey column and then ascends without synapse through the sympathetic paraspinal chain to the superior cervical ganglion. From the superior cervical ganglion the postganglionic or third order neuron travels on the surface of the common carotid artery. At the bifurcation of the internal and external carotid arteries, fibers controlling facial sweating follow the external carotid artery, while those destined for the eye and lid follow the internal carotid artery. In the cavernous sinus these eye and lid fibers join the fifth and sixth cranial nerves and enter the orbit via the superior orbital fissure. Fibers destined for the dilator muscle enter the eye via the long posterior ciliary nerves or short posterior ciliary nerves.

EXAMINATION OF PUPIL

There are some prerequisites to a good pupillary examination. The room light should be adequate, neither too bright nor dark. It should preferably be adjustable. The visual acuity in both eyes must be checked properly. The range of external ocular movements must be examined. The lid position must be noted to see if there is any evidence of ptosis. A proper history of any previous eye surgery or injury must be taken. A proper systemic and ocular medication history is essential as some medications can modify pupillary size and reactivity. The level of consciousness must be ascertained.

There are certain things which should not be overlooked in a thorough pupillary examination. The shape and size must be recorded and notes made about any abnormal shape or inequality in size. The margin should be smooth and the color of the iris should be noted. The light and accommodation reflex must be tested in both eyes separately. The swinging flashlight test must be done to look out for a relative afferent pupillary defect (RAPD). The ciliospinal reflex needs to be tested if there is suspicion of Horner's syndrome. Note should also be made about any abnormal movements like hippus.

The most important evaluation technique for pupil is the history. A careful history of known pupillary disorders is vital to establish whether a pupillary sign has any meaning in the context of the disorder under consideration. Rarely a patient will present with complaint of abnormality of pupil as a presenting symptom, hence the presenting complaints should be stressed upon to get a proper clue into the diagnosis of pupillary abnormality such as associated history of trauma, features of raised ICP, irritative lesions, visual acuity, lid lag, double vision, and use of drugs. Old photographs provide significant information and should be evaluated in all cases of long standing asymmetry documented on examination. Bedside evaluation of pupil and its reactions require a good visibility with comfort of patient and examiner. Examination of pupil requires a good illuminator which provides bright, even beam without hot spots or dim areas. Evaluation should begin in darkness or in very dim light as this allows the pupils to start their construction from a bigger size and increases the amplitude of the pupillary movement making it easier to see.

A brief comment must be made about a peculiar condition called hippus. It is a state of alternating dilatation and contraction of the pupil probably due to modulating signals from the Edinger–Westphal nucleus. Exaggerated hippus is found in aconite poisoning and also in liver and kidney diseases and is considered a poor prognostic sign in the intensive care unit.

There are three stages in the examination of the pupils:

Evaluation of Anisocoria

Pupillary inequality is usually due to an iris innervation problem. The best way to decide whether it is the sphincter muscle or the dilator muscle that is weak is to compare the amount of anisocoria in darkness and in light. No anisocoria in darkness or in light indicates an intact efferent arm of the light reflex arc. Virtually everyone has a measurable pupillary size difference if sensitive enough techniques are used; however, only 20% of normal individuals have enough asymmetry to be recognized clinically (i.e., 0.4 mm or more). Age plays a major role in pupillary size. Newborns have small hyporeactive pupils, young children have larger, briskly reactive pupils and as the age progresses the normal pupillary size and reactivity diminishes such that older individuals have miotic, relatively slowly reactive pupils.

Evaluation of the Afferent Arm of the Reflex Arc

Swinging light pupil test: The swinging light pupil test is a rapid, low cost, accurate, and objective method of identifying asymmetric optic nerve disease, but it is useless unless proper technique is used. The idea is to look for RAPD in one eye compared to the other by alternate projection of light over each eye.

The afferent pupillary defect is clinically manifested by the "swinging flashlight sign". In a normal pupil with intact sensory pathways there is constriction of both pupils when light is shown on one eye. In a deafferenated pupil the ipsilateral and contralateral constriction is absent when light is shown on the affected eye and pupillary constriction occurs in both eyes when light is shown on the healthy eye. When light is flashed from one eye to the other at regular intervals there may be apparent dilatation of the pupils when light is flashed on the affected eye (Fig. 3). This is called the Marcus Gunn pupil or the swinging flashlight phenomenon. It is found in optic neuritis, but may be found in any other clinical condition which causes deafferentation of the pupil.

Evaluation of the Near Response

The pupillary response to near effort must be checked. If the light reaction seems a little weak, the examiner should look to see if the pupils constrict better to a near stimulus than do to light. If they do, this is called "light-near dissociation" and may indicate underlying pathology like neurosyphilis, lesions of the dorsal midbrain (obstructive hydrocephalus, pineal region tumors), and aberrant regeneration (oculomotor nerve palsy, Adie's tonic pupil).

Features of common causes of pupillary asymmetry in neuro-ophthalmology have been given in table 1 and the sites of lesions causing pupillary abnormalities are shown in figure 4.

PUPILLARY ABNORMALITIES

Anisocoria

Local Ophthalmologic Conditions

Typically, patients with anisocoria due to local causes have a painful red eye with a small pupil and visual disturbance. Any conditions resulting in inflammatory response within the anterior chamber may cause spasm of the sphincter muscle, resulting in anisocoria.

Acute closed-angle glaucoma causes a red painful eye and visual disturbance. In this condition, the pupil is generally fixed in mid-position, with an impaired light reflex that may be misinterpreted as interruption of the parasympathetic nervous system. Prosthetic eyes do not show a brisk light reflex. Other important causes of irregular pupils and poor light reflex are congenital malformation of the iris, postoperative changes, and post-traumatic mydriasis due to traumatic tears in the iris and its sphincter muscle.

Episodic Anisocoria

Either parasympathetic or sympathetic paresis or overactivity may produce intermittent anisocoria. The common causes of episodic anisocoria due to parasympathetic paresis include uncal herniation, seizure disorder, and migraine. Parasympathetic hyperactivity conditions like cyclic oculomotor paresis, parasympathetic spasm are known to add to the episodic anisocoria. Other conditions producing the episodic anisocoria include sympathetic hyperactivity conditions, sympathetic dysfunction producing alternating anisocoria and pupillary dilatation.

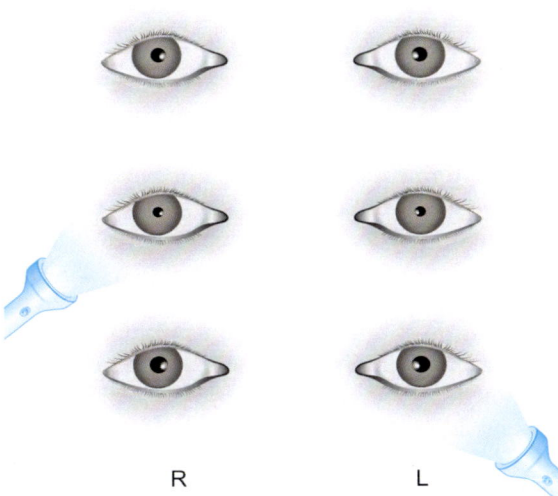

FIG. 3: Illustration of left afferent pupillary defect (RAPD).

TABLE 1: Characteristics of pupils encountered in neuro-ophthalmology

Condition	General characteristic	Response to light and near stimuli	Room condition in which anisocoria is greater	Response to mydriatics	Response to miotics	Response to pharmacologic agents
Essential anisocoria	Round, regular	Both brisk	No change	Dilates	Constricts	Normal and rarely needed
Horner's syndrome	Small, round, unilateral	Both brisk	Darkness	Dilates	Constricts	Cocaine 4% poor dilatation
Tonic pupil syndrome	Usually lager in bright light; sector pupil palsy, vermiform movement unilateral or less often bilateral	Absent to light, tonic to near; tonic redilation	Light	Dilates	Constricts	Pilocarpine 0.1% constrict
Argyll Robertson pupils	Small, irregular, bilateral	Poor to light, better to near	No change	Poor	Constricts	–
Midbrain pupils	Mid dilated; may be oval; bilateral	Poor to light, better to near	No change	Dilates	Constricts	–
Oculomotor palsy	Mid dilated, unilateral (rarely bilateral)	Fixed	Light	Dilates	Constricts	–
Pharmacologically dilated pupils	Very large round, unilateral	Fixed	Light	–	No	Pilocarpine 1% does not constrict.

Dilated Pupil (Anisocoria That Increases in Bright Illumination)

The patient has anisocoria that increase in bright light. Differential diagnoses of a dilated pupil include Adie's tonic pupil, third cranial nerve palsy, and pharmacologic blockade.

Adie's Tonic Pupil

Adie's tonic pupil predominately occurs in females aged 20–50 years. Patient may complain of photophobia, episodes of blurred near vision or blurred vision when switching from near to far viewing and may even complain of unequal pupils. Typically, the involved pupil displays a poor response to light, with a relatively preserved response to sustained near fixation but an abnormally slow or tonic contraction. Slit lamp examination often reveals sector palsies of the iris. The parasympathetic defect in Adie's pupil is believed to occur after the fibers leave the ciliary ganglion. As a result of denervation supersensitivity, the affected eye displays an abnormally brisk response to dilute (1/8%) pilocarpine and this test has been suggested as a way of differentiating preganglionic and postganglionic parasympathetic lesions. Recent literature reports, many patients who have mydriasis due to oculomotor nerve compression and have displayed reactivity to dilute pilocarpine, but these patients should show other signs of third nerve dysfunction.

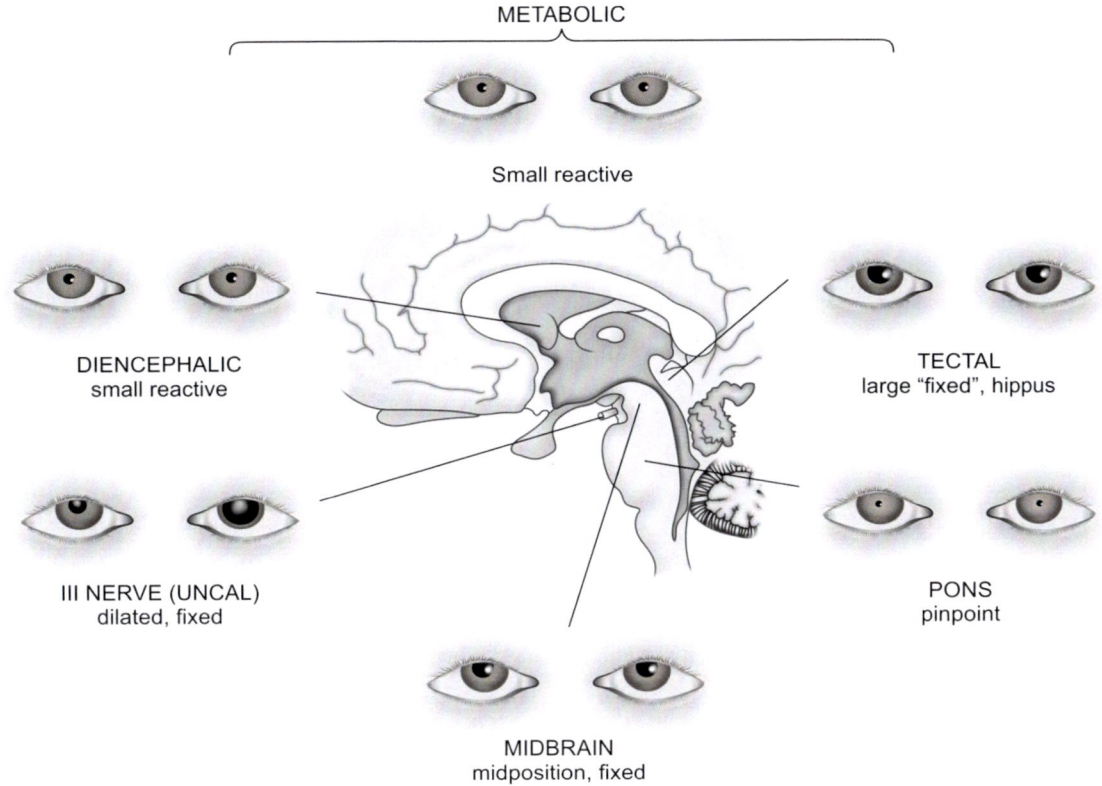

FIG. 4: Sites of lesions in pupillary abnormalities.

The combination of an idiopathic tonic pupil with decreased deep tendon reflexes and/or orthostatic hypotension is termed Holmes-Adie syndrome. The condition is commoner in young women. Adie's pupil is commonly unilateral, but may become bilateral in 10% cases. The symptoms of a tonic pupil tend to be self-limited. Adie pupil is believed to be of uncertain etiology. Other causes include neurosyphilis, diabetes, herpes zoster, giant cell arteritis, and alcoholism. A closely related rare condition is the Ross syndrome characterized by the triad of segmental anhidrosis, hyporeflexia, and tonic pupils. Only a handful of cases have been described in the world literature so far.

Harlequin syndrome refers to segmental anhidrosis only without any ocular manifestation. In fact, it is reasonable to assume that all these dysautonomic syndrome (Horner's, Adie's, Ross, and Harlequin) represent clinical manifestations of generalized autonomic injury with or without somatic nervous system involvement (e.g., areflexia) (Figs 5 and 6).

Oculomotor Nerve Dysfunction

Pupillary abnormalities due to third cranial nerve dysfunction may occur in a conscious or an unconscious subject. As the parasympathetic fibers to the pupil lie superficially they are apt to external compression. Hence, papillary involvement along with other features of third cranial nerve dysfunction in a conscious subject generally indicates a compressive lesion commonly a posterior communicating artery aneurysm and needs full neuroimaging studies. In an unconscious patient unilateral papillary dilatation generally indicates ipsilateral uncal herniation over the free margin of the tentorium. At a later stage, with progressive brain shift occurring, the opposite pupil may be dilated due to pressure on the opposite third nerve against the opposite

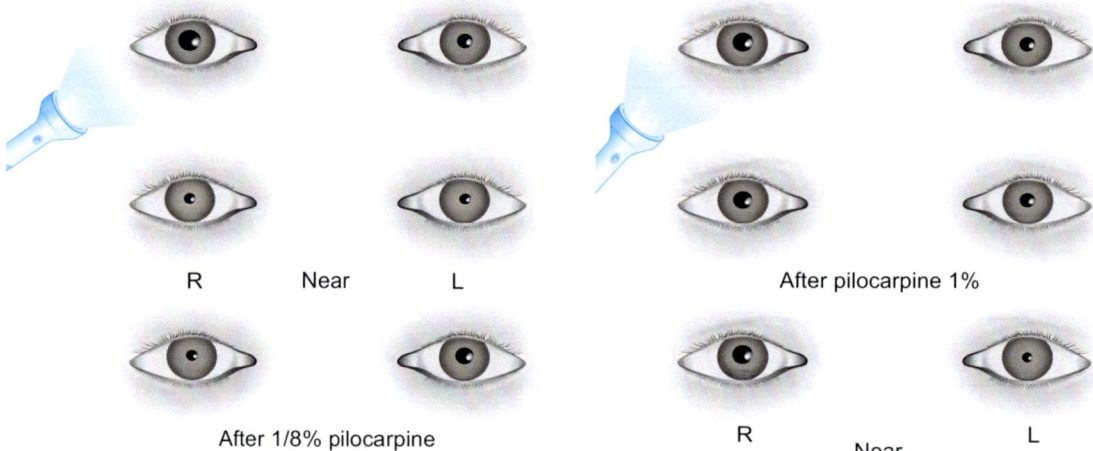

FIG. 5: Illustration of right Adie's pupil.

FIG. 6: Illustration of right pharmacologic pupil.

tentorial margin. Early recognition and prompt decompressive measures need to be instituted.

Other causes include strokes cranial neuropathies associated with Lyme disease, ophthalmoplegic migraine and alcoholism. Detailed evaluation of third cranial nerve palsy would be discussed in a subsequent chapter. Some points need to be highlighted:

Isolated Large Poorly Reactive Pupil in Conscious Patient: Neurologic or Pharmacologic?

- Full dose (1–4%) pilocarpine test positive (third cranial nerve trunk lesion)
- Cholinergic denervation supersensitivity: Lesion of third cranial nerve at or beyond ciliary ganglion—Intense contraction to weak (0.125%) pilocarpine
- Causes: Trauma, aberrant reinnervation.

Aberrant reinnervation of third cranial nerve (occurs only in traumatic cases):

- On attempting near gaze: Bell's phenomenon without NVII palsy at rest–levator inhibition, superior rectus stimulation, miosis.
  Westphal-Piltz reaction: Orbicularis spasm with miosis
- Reversed anisocoria
- Pseudo Graefe lid sign: Lid elevation on down gaze or adduction

- Pseudo-Argyll Robertson pupil
- Segmental iris contraction on external ocular movement on slit lamp examination (Czarnecki syndrome).

Hutchinson's Pupil

There are four stages during uncal herniation. In the first stage, the ipsilateral pupil to the site of pathology is small due to irritation and hyper function of the third nerve. In the second stage, the ipsilateral pupil is large because of third nerve compression and dysfunction. In the third stage, the contralateral pupil is constricted due to irritation against the free margin of the contralateral tentorium cerebelli. In the fourth and last stage, the contralateral pupil is large due to compression of opposite third nerve by opposite tentorium. Hence, in the last stage both pupils are fixed and dilated.

One important point needs to be mentioned in this context. Contrary to common belief, the earliest MRI sign is widening of the quadrigeminal cistern on the ipsilateral side of a mass lesion before the uncus actually slides through the gap between midbrain and the temporal lobe. This is due to pushing of the brainstem by the expanding mass on the ipsilateral side. It is only after that the uncus slides through (herniates) that the gap becomes a chink like or disappears.

Optic Nerve Pathology

The commonest condition is optic neuritis and in fact any other lesion of optic nerve might cause pupillary dilatation.

Pharmacologic Mydriasis

Another common condition causing an isolated dilated pupil is pharmacologic mydriasis caused by use of anticholinergic dilating drops. Instillation of 1% pilocarpine in the affected eye quickly resolves the issue. Sympathomimetics that are commonly used to facilitate nasotracheal intubation or ocular examination also cause mydriasis. Dilute pilocarpine (1/8%) can be used to differentiate between pathologic and sympathomimetic induced mydriasis, failing which 1% pilocarpine may be used. Patients using scopolamine patches for seasickness often develop mydriasis, "cruise ship anisocoria", which again can be sorted with use of weak pilocarpine solution. Small pupil (anisocoria that increase in dim illumination) apart from inflammatory eye disease with concomitant miosis, the differential lies between physiologic anisocoria and Horner's syndrome. Some eye drops for glaucoma cause miosis (e.g., pilocarpine).

Horner's Syndrome (Table 2)

Hallmark features include: (i) Unilateral miosis; (ii) ptosis; (iii) anhidrosis; (iv) loss of ciliospinal reflex; (v) enophthalmos. In ciliospinal reflex, there is ipsilateral dilatation of the pupil by pinching the skin of neck upto T2 dermatome under normal conditions. It is absent in sympathetic affection and is popularly known as the ciliospinal reflex. This reflex has a complex multineuron pathway and is lost in Horner's syndrome.

It is the result of disruption of the sympathetic innervation to the eye at any place along the pathway. The small pupil exhibits a dilatation lag, dilating several seconds after entering a dark room, causing anisocoria to be more apparent immediately after entering. Instillation of 4–10% cocaine solution is often helpful in confirming diagnosis. Cocaine inhibits the reuptake of norepinephrine, causing more norepinephrine made available at the neuromuscular junction of the iris dilator muscle. A normal pupil would dilate, but a sympathetically denervated pupil of Horner's syndrome would not.

The next step is to differentiate between a preganglionic and a postganglionic Horner's syndrome. Preganglionic ones are often associated with myelopathy or malignancy. Most postganglionic causes except carotid dissection are benign and recover. Absence of sweating in the face and arm points towards a preganglionic lesion. Central preganglionic conditions like lateral medullary syndrome or even transtentorial herniation leave tell-tale signs for recognition. Of the postganglionic lesions, carotid dissection is serious and painful. Hence all painful Horner's syndrome should be investigated angiographically.

TABLE 2: Common causes of Horner's syndrome

Central	Dorsolateral medullary infarct (Wallenberg's syndrome)
	Hypothalamic, thalamic, or mesencephalic infarct, hemorrhage, tumor, or demyelination
	Multiple system atrophy
	Cervicothoracic spinal cord lesion
Preganglionic	Cervicothoracic paraspinal mass (including neuroblastoma)
	Cervical disc herniation
	Apical lung cancer
	Cervical sympathectomy
	Neck during forceps delivery
	Internal carotid artery dissection
	Cervical adenopathy
	Cervical tumors
	Neck trauma
Postganglionic	Neck injury during forceps delivery
	Internal carotid artery dissection
	Cervical adeonopathy
	Cervical tumors
	Neck trauma
	Otitis media
	Cavernous sinus lesion
	Cluster headache

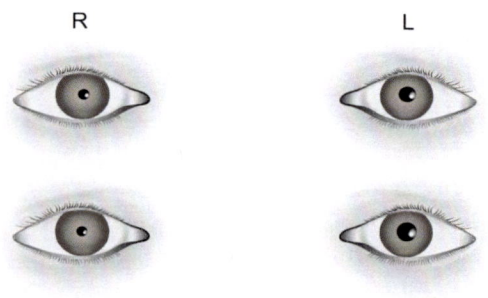

FIG. 7: Illustration of right Horner's syndrome.

Horner's syndrome may also present as a complication of inferior alveolar nerve block due to close proximity to the carotid sheath (Fig. 7).

Hydroxyamphetamine (HAMPH) Test

This test is employed to differentiate between a preganglionic and a postganglionic Horner's syndrome. The importance of such distinction has already been mentioned. Hydroxyamphetamine enhances the release of norepinephrine from the third order terminal. Thus, if the postganglionic neuron is injured the pupil will not dilate or will dilate poorly. Cremer et al. found that a 1 mm increase in the amount of anisocoria is associated with 85% probability that the lesion is postganglionic. A 2 mm increase is associated with a probability of 99% that postganglionic defect exists. However, the hydoxyamphetamine test is not perfect. Cremer et al. found that anisocoria increased in 93% of postganglionic cases. The anisocoria did not change in 90% preganglionic cases. Thus, one has to assume an approximately 10% error rate with this test.

In case of nonavailability of hydroxyamphetamine, one may substitute with adrenaline. Instillation of adrenaline (1:1000) in a case of postganglionic Horner pupil would cause pupillary dilatation due to the phenomenon of denervation supersensitivity. This test has its limitations.

Some Key Points in Differentiating Preganglionic from Post-ganglionic Horner's Syndrome

- Most cases of Horner's syndrome seen in practice are postganglionic
- Important preganglionic conditions: Posterior inferior cerebellar artery stroke; syringomyelia with chiari malformation; cervical tumor; Pancoast's tumor: Neck trauma/surgery
- Important postganglionic conditions: Carotid dissection (CC/IC: Common Carotid/ Internal Carotid)
- Preganglionic lesion anywhere: Sweating lost on ipsilateral face, neck, upper trunk, and upper limb
- Postganglionic common carotid dissection: Facial sweating lost
- Postganglionic internal carotid dissection: Facial sweat retained (sweat fibers to face leave through branches of external carotid artery)

(In Vertebral Artery dissection → PICA stroke → Preganglionic Horner's syndrome)

7. Sympathetic denervation supersensitivity (postganglionic): HAMPH, adrenaline, and tropicamide.

Simple Anisocoria

Simple anisocoria may be found in up to 20% of the general population and often is variable from day to day. In most patients, the degree of anisocoria is less than 1 mm, and no ptosis, dilation lag, or vasomotor dysfunction is present. Medication use to be excluded. Installation of 4–10% cocaine solution causes dilation of both eyes. Comparison with old photographs may reveal that the anisocoria had been present for some time.

Bilateral Constricted Pupil (Partial Horner's Syndrome)

The constricted pupil indicates lesion in the various circuitous pathway taken by the sympathetic supply to the dilator muscle. The lesion may be in the hypothalamus, brainstem, lateral aspect of the spinal cord, the sympathetic chain, the cervical sympathetic ganglia, the pericarotid plexus, or in the sympathetic fibers, which run to the orbit by accompanying the branches of the internal carotid artery. The common causes for constricted pupils include pontine hemorrhage, primary or secondary tumors involving the cervical sympathetic chain, vascular lesions of the carotid artery or its sheath, or toxins. Bilateral spontaneous miosis means almost invariably an upper brain steam lesion.

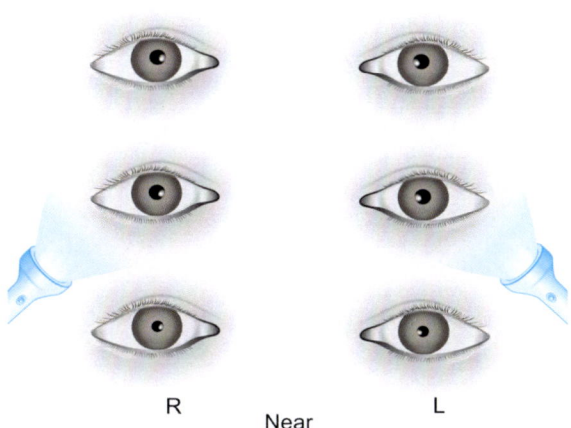

FIG. 8: Illustration of Argyll Robertson pupil.

Argyll Robertson Pupils (Fig. 8)

These pupils are classically associated with neurosyphilis. The exact location of the pathologic lesion is hotly debated. Consensus places the lesion in the dorsal midbrain interrupting fibers serving the light reflex with sparing of the ventral accommodative pathways. Clinical features include: (i) small pupils unreactive to light stimulation with an intact near response; (b) irregular pupils; (c) pupils that dilate poorly in the dark and to mydriatic agents. Similar pupillary findings may be seen in diabetic patients. Other causes of light near dissociation are:

- Dorsal midbrain syndrome. These patients have other clinical features besides light near dissociation like eyelid retraction, convergence, retraction nystagmus, and decreased upgaze
- Severe bilateral visual loss of optic nerve or retinal origin. These patients would have dilated pupils unreactive to light, but near convergence reaction with pupillary construction may be preserved by proprioceptive input to the brain
- Reverse light near dissociation: Cortical blindness.

Bilateral Dilated Pupil

Differential diagnosis of the dilated pupil is relatively small. Once angle-closure glaucoma and a mechanically damaged sphincter muscle are eliminated from the possible etiologies, dysfunction of the parasympathetic nervous system clearly has occurred. Such pupils are dilated and show poor reactivity. Dilated pupils are caused by the paralysis of the parasympathetic fibers either at their origin from the pretectal nuclei and the Edinger–Westphal nucleus in the midbrain, during their course with the oculomotor nerve or at the ciliary ganglion in the orbit. The common causes of the dilation include vascular accidents in the midbrain, tentorial herniation or aneurysms of the carotid artery.

CONCLUSION

Examination of the pupil must form an integral part of every neurological examination.

It requires minimum equipment, but can yield a host of useful information. For proper and relevant information a correct examination technique is important. In all cases both the eyes must be seen together and in isolation. The information gathered from the pupillary examination must be supplemented with relevant pharmacological and biochemical tests and imaging. If used judiciously a properly conducted pupillary examination can yield a lot of valuable clinical information which can help in proper diagnosis and management.

Almost all pupillary conditions would be diagnosed with the above approaches delineated. Further workup will depend on the specific diagnosis and requires investigations like chest X-ray, CT/MRI scan of the head and cervical spine. Episodic conditions may be difficult to diagnose at first evaluation and requires repeated evaluation to make a diagnosis.

The management of pupillary abnormalities will depend upon the cause of asymmetry, which may include the management of raised intracranial pressure, removal of irritative cause local or distant.

SUGGESTED READINGS

1. Adler FW, Scheie HG. The site of disturbance in tonic pupils. Trans Am Ophthalmol Soc. 1940;38:183-8.
2. Burde RW, Savino PJ, Trobe JD. Clinical decision in Neuro-Ophthalmology. St. Louis: Mosby, 2nd edn. 1998:221-45.
3. Chakravarty A, Mukherjee A, Roy D. Ross syndrome – a case documentation. Acta Neurol Scand. 2003;107:72.

4. Cremer SA, Thompson HS, Digre KB, et al. Hydroxy-amphetamine mydriasis in normal subjects. Am J Ophthalmol. 1990;100:66-70.
5. Johnson IN, Hill RA, Bartholomew MJ. Correlation of afferent pupillary defect with visual loss on automated perimetry. Ophthalmology 1988;95:1649-55.
6. Kordon RH, Thompson HS. The pupil. In: Rosen ES, Thompson HS, Cumming WJ, Eustace P. Eds. Neuro-ophthlmology, 1st edn. London. Mosby 1998:13.1–13.19.
7. Lowenfeld IE. The pupil: Anatomy, physiology and clinical application. Ames: Iowa State University Press. 1993.
8. Malmey WF, Younge BR, Mayer NJ. Evaluation of the causes and accurary of pharmacological localisation in Horner's syndrome. Am J Ophthalmol. 1980;90:394-420.
9. Muller NR, Newtron NJ. In: Walsh and Hoyt's Clinical Neuro-ophthalmology, 5th edn. Vol 1. Baltimore. William and Wilkins 1998. P. 827-1042.
10. Thompson HS, Corbett JJ. Spasms of the iris sphincter. Ann Neurol. 1980;8:547-9.
11. Tompson HS. Diagnosing Horner's Syndrome. Trans Am Acad Ophthalmol Otolaryngel 1977;820:840-8.
12. Thompson HS, Montague P, Cox TA, et al. The relationship between visual acuity, pupillary defects and visual field loss. Am J Ophthalmol. 1982;93:681-6.

6 Unexplained Visual Loss

Ambar Chakravarty

INTRODUCTION

One of the most vexing problems in neuro-ophthalmic diagnosis is subnormal visual acuity (VA) in the absence of obvious structural abnormalities in the eye to account for it. The cause may be optical, neural, or psychogenic. The clinician's task is to separate optical from neural causes and when neither seems plausible, to consider psychogenic causes. Optical disturbances include refractive errors and abnormalities of the ocular media, principally the cornea and lens. Neural disturbances involve the visual pathway from retina to visual cortex.

When visual loss is a patient's primary complaint, symptoms vary depending on whether one or both eyes are affected, whether the visual loss is abrupt in onset, gradual in onset, or suddenly discovered long after its onset; whether the visual loss is complete or partial; and, finally, whether the visual loss is manifested as visual hallucinations or illusions. The probable causes of visual loss are narrowed down to a very few possibilities on the basis of the patient's symptoms, the patient's age and sex, and the presumed anatomic location of the lesions (Table 1).

The visual pathway consists of elements easily examined directly at the bedside, such as the pupils, retina, and optic disk, and those that are indirectly examined using subjective tests, such as the more posterior elements of the optic nerve, chiasm, optic tract, lateral geniculate body, geniculocalcarine tract, and visual cortex. Damage to visual association cortices, parietal and inferior temporal, will produce symptoms with preservation of VA and sometimes normal visual fields.

Table 1: Visual loss by anatomical location

Retina	Detachment, ischemia, infections (cytomegalovirus, histoplasmosis, toxoplasmosis), toxic (ethambutol), degenerative (aging-macular degeneration, retinitis, pigmentosa, carcinomatous retinopathy
Optic disk	Ischemia, optic neuritis, papilledema, glaucoma, coloboma, tumors, sarcoid
Optic nerve	Demyelination, tumors (meningioma, glioma, mucocele, pituitary tumors, craniopharyngioma, Rathke's cleft cyst, aneurysm), thyroid opthalmopathy, inflammation, trauma
Chiasm/Tract	Tumors (pituitary, craniopharyngioma, glioma, meningioma, Rathke's cleft cyst), aneurysm, trauma, vascular
Retrochiasmal	Tumors (glioma, meningioma, metastases), vascular, demyelination, Alzheimer's disease, Cruetzfeldt-Jakob disease (Heidenhain variety)

VISUAL ACUITY

The first test is of course to quantify the VA and then to differentiate between acuity loss due to media abnormality (e.g., refractive error) and that caused by a more posterior pathology like in the retina or the neural pathway.

Although it is best to examine VA using a distance chart, the neurologist almost always examines VA using a near card. This should be done with a hand-held Snellen's chart or a Jaeger print card. If a near card is being used, be sure that patients are using their reading glasses. Push patients to give you the very best acuity possible.

Do not rush them. Do not start with the largest type; rather, ask patients to read the 20/25 line and then the 20/20 line. If this fails, gradually work your way up. Three fingers held up are the equivalent of the big E on the distance acuity chart, and a patient who can count fingers at 20 feet has 20/200 acuity. Thus, counting fingers at 5 feet would be equivalent to 20/800 acuity.

The pinhole test is an effective but imperfect means of sorting out visual dysfunction caused by aberrations of the ocular media. It improves acuity in persons with uncorrected refractive errors and with most corneal and lenticular abnormalities by selecting a narrow light path that produces a limited blur circle on the retina. Unfortunately, many patients seem unable to position or steady the pinhole well enough to find a hole to look through. Children younger than 6 years and elderly, infirm patients nearly always fail. Furthermore, if the media are sufficiently disrupted, as with an extremely dense cataract or vitreous hemorrhage, no clear optical path may exist. On the other hand, a two-line improvement on the Snellen's chart with pinhole vision is a reliable sign of an optical imperfection. The ideal pinhole device is one that has multiple holes with diameters between 2 and 2.5 mm, which minimizes the degradation from deafferanation (<2 mm) and surface aberrations (>2.5 mm).

Because the pinhole test is not failsafe, two other tests may be used before dismissing an optical cause of subnormal VA. These are the potential acuity meter (PAM) and the laser interferometer. The laser interferometer has not received wide clinical use because of its high cost. The PAM is more readily available, and justifiably so. Many patients whose acuity does not improve with pinhole demonstrate surprising improvement with PAM. The patient views a miniaturized Snellen's chart projected onto the retina from a box mounted on the slit-lamp biomicroscope. By projecting such a small image, the PAM is often able to bypass the eye's refractive and media aberrations. Its advantage over the pinhole test is that it does not require a steady hand from the patient. Its drawback is that the instrument is expensive and requires examiner expertise. Results generally have been accurate, except in the case of cystoid macular edema, where the PAM may overestimate the patient's maximum VA.

What's next?

Using the pinhole test acuity may improve or does not improve.

Acuity Improved

If the pinhole test shows improvement in VA, an optical problem is likely to be the basis of subnormal acuity. The first concern is that an uncorrected refractive error, has been overlooked. If repeat refraction does not solve the problem, slit-lamp examination (biomicroscopy) is performed to look for a subtle cornea or lens defect. Actually both these steps must be performed even if the pinhole test fails to improve acuity, because the pinhole test is not always perfectly reliable.

A minor disturbance in the integrity of the corneal epithelium can have a marked effect on VA. A fluorescein stain examination is essential. Keratoconus may be detected by an irregular retinoscopic reflex. Advanced cataract is rarely overlooked. However, early lens changes (nuclear sclerosis, mildly opacified posterior lens capsule) can degrade to a remarkable degree without causing obvious biomicroscopic abnormalities. The patient often reports seeing "ghost" images, which may be misinterpreted as diplopia. Irregular retinoscopic reflexes are a useful sign of subtle lenticular abnormalities.

Acuity Not Improved

A retinal or neural pathway lesion is likely. At this stage it is essential to establish whether the visual loss is uniocular or binocular, the nature of onset and progression (transient or persisting or progressive) and whether, the visual failure is due to fall in acuity/field defect or to a disturbance of visual recognizing process (cortical pathology of visual association areas). Transient visual loss has been discussed elsewhere in this volume. In clinical practice, differentiation between uniocular and binocular visual loss at times poses as a problem as many patients with a homonymous hemianopic field defect only points to loss of vision in the eye corresponding to the side of the homonymous defect (e.g., right homonymous hemianopic patients may complain of only right eye visual loss).

Two bedside tests are essential at this stage:
1. Swinging-light pupil test
2. Visual field testing by confrontation.

Swinging-Light Pupil Test

The swinging-light pupil test is a rapid, low cost, accurate, and objective method of identifying asymmetric optic nerve disease but it is useless unless proper technique is used. The idea is to look for a relative afferent pupillary defect (RAPD) in one eye compared to the other by alternate projection of light over each eye.

Technique

1. Dim the room illumination. Unless the test is performed in darkness, the amplitude of pupil constriction will be too low
2. Have the patient fixate on a distant target. This provides maximal relaxation of the iris sphincter muscle. A near target would evoke miosis associated with the synkinetic near reflex
3. Use a bright light stimulus. Dim lights do not produce enough pupil constriction. If neither pupil constricts very much to flashlight illumination, use a more potent light source, such as the indirect ophthalmoscope. Avoid a light so bright that it causes photophobia or extreme miosis
4. Direct the light from below the level of the patient's eyes. This is done so as not to provoke miosis from the patient's fixing on the light
5. Move the light briskly and rhythmically from eye-to-eye several times. If you move the light across the nose too slowly, you will evoke too much constriction and miss a subtle relative afferent pupil defect. Make about five swings. This repetition is necessary to be sure that any pupil dilation on one side does not reflect merely the adventitious sphincter movement of physiologic pupillary unrest.

Interpretation

A RAPD is a sensitive indicator of unilateral or asymmetric injury to the afferent pupillary pathway. If a RAPD is found, it needs to be investigated. In general, the size of the RAPD correlates with the asymmetry of visual field loss and the resultant asymmetry of pupillomotor input. It also tends to vary with the location of the lesion within the afferent pathway.

- Retina:
  - Large unilateral retinal lesions produce a clear RAPD (i.e., retinal detachment or central retinal artery occlusion). Acuity might be good if the macula is spared. A careful dilated fundoscopic examination is usually diagnostic, and so an ophthalmology consultation is important
  - Cataracts and corneal opacities are not causes of afferent pupillary defects.
- Optic nerve:
  Damage to the optic nerve almost always produces an RAPD. Visual acuity loss may be mild or severe, but a visual field abnormality can almost invariably be detected by formal perimetry testing. The optic disk may appear normal or acutely swollen but will later develop pallor. Examples of optic nerve disorders include optic neuritis, ischemic optic neuropathy, hereditary optic neuropathy, compressive lesions, toxins, trauma, and cellular infiltration.
  - The largest afferent defects occur in association with unilateral optic nerve disorders
  - "Resolved" optic neuritis may result in optic disc pallor and RAPD despite recovery to normal VA and normal visual field
  - The extent of damage in bilateral optic nerve disorders is rarely perfectly symmetrical. Therefore, a RAPD will be found on the side with greater damage. Look carefully.
- Optic chiasm:
  - Compressive lesions of the optic chiasm can produce asymmetric visual loss and, therefore, a RAPD. Commonly, a junctional scotoma is found
  - Symmetric bitemporal hemianopsia is not associated with a RAPD, because injury to the visual and pupillary pathways is symmetric.
- Optic tract:
  Slightly more nerve fibers decussate at the chiasm than do not. A pure optic tract lesion will produce a small RAPD in the contralateral eye.

Thus, a complete homonymous hemianopsia with an afferent defect in the eye with the temporal field loss should raise the possibility of a tract lesion as the cause of visual loss.
- Pretectal nucleus:
  - The pretectal nucleus in the dorsal midbrain is the final synapse site of pupillary fibers coming from tract via brachium of the superior colliculus. Visual fibers however have separated off to go on to the lateral geniculate nucleus. Therefore, a dorsal midbrain lesion can produce a small contralateral RAPD and no visual loss
  - Afferent pupillary defects from optic tract or midbrain injury are usually small and are fairly rare.

Further Observations

The intensity of RAPD, which is related more closely to differences in visual field loss than VA loss in the two eyes, can be quantitatively measured by placing progressively higher neutral-density filters over the normal eye until the RAPD is eliminated. The filters are particularly useful when the diagnosis of RAPD is equivocal. The examiner places the 0.3-log unit filter over each eye consecutively and performs the swinging-light test. If no RAPD is present, the pupil of the eye covered by the filter dilates slightly as the light is swung toward it. When RAPD is minimal, the filter placed over the affected eye makes the pupil dilation in that eye more obvious.

The swinging-light pupil test is useful even when only one iris sphincter muscle is operational. Constriction of the pupil in the unaffected eye as the light is swung toward it is equivalent to pupillary dilatation in the eye with the suspected RAPD. This phenomenon is called (misleadingly) a "reverse RAPD"; it is merely a different way to elicit a standard RAPD.

Visual Field Testing

Interpretations of visual field tests has been discussed elsewhere in this volume. Correct interpretation is essential for anatomical localization of any lesion in the optic pathway. At the bedside, field is generally tested using the confrontation method whereby the patient's fields are compared to that of the examiner's (assuming that the examiner has a normal field and normal acuity).

The ideal confrontation technique is one that reveals areas of differential visual sensitivity across a well-defined line. Instead of comparing the two eyes, as is done in the swinging-light, quadrants of the visual field in each eye are compared, with the vertical and horizontal fixation meridians serving as the dividing lines:

1. Fingers in single quadrants: With the patient positioned comfortably 3 feet away from you, close your right eye and have the patient occlude his or her left eye. Present one or two stationary fingers randomly in each visual field quadrant of the right eye, well within 30 degrees of fixation. Instruct the patient to count the number of fingers. Children and illiterate, demented, or very poorly sighted adults, are instructed to mimic the number of fingers presented. Alternatively, you should look for eye movements elicited by the stimulus.

   If some fingers are not identified correctly, display a single finger in the defective quadrant, move it towards the vertical meridian, and instruct the patient to identify it as soon as it is visible. Note whether the border of the defect is aligned to the vertical meridian. Now move the finger towards the horizontal meridian, and again note whether the border of the defect is aligned to the horizontal meridian. Repeat these steps in testing the patient's left eye
2. Fingers in double quadrants: If all the fingers are counted correctly and yet the index of suspicion of a quadrant defect is high, display one or two fingers of both hands simultaneously in two quadrants. The patient is instructed to total the number of fingers seen. If this is done correctly, yet the index of suspicion for a quadrant or hemianopic defect remains high, go to step 3
3. Brightness or clarity comparison: Ask the patient to compare the brightness of single fingers or whole hands presented simultaneously in two quadrants. Now go to step 4
4. Color saturation comparison: Display large, static, red stimuli in two quadrants and ask the patient if the color appears brighter or truer in one quadrant than in the other. Move the

target from the relatively defective quadrant towards the vertical meridian. If color marked by brightens or normalizes as the target crosses the meridian, a true hemianopic defect exists. Perform the same maneuver with respect to the horizontal meridian.

Performed correctly, these confrontation tests are helpful predictors of the results of formal perimetry. Although they seem crude, they may sometimes detect hemianopic defects not found even with the most precise formal methods. However, even if they are applied by the most experienced examiners, these techniques produce so many false-positive and false-negative results that they should not be considered a substitute for formal testing.

Interpreting the Results and Further Workup

Having established unilaterality or bilaterality of the visual problem and testing for acuity, RAPD, and field, a patient with visual loss may have the following combination of defects:
1. Relative afferent pupillary defect with nonhemianopic field defect
2. Relative afferent pupillary defect with hemianopic field defect
3. Relative afferent pupillary defect not present.

Relative Afferent Pupillary Defect with Nonhemianopic Field Defect

Nonhemianopic field defects are caused by an optic neuropathy or retinopathy. When the lesion affects the optic nerve or the retinal ganglion cells/axons (inner retina), the field abnormalities are called "nerve fiber bundle defects". When the deeper retinal layers are damaged, the abnormalities are termed "nonspecific nonhemianopic defects".

Nerve fiber bundle defects have a shape that is based on the organization of the nerve fiber layer of the retina. Optic neuropathies and inner retinal disorders may produce one of the following nerve bundle defects or a combination of them:
1. Central scotoma: Damage to papillomacular fibers emanating from the macular region
2. Centrocecal scotoma: Damage to papillomacular fibers emanating from the macula and the zone between the macula and the optic disc
3. Arcuate scotoma: Damage to temporal retinal fibers that bend around the papillomacular bundle and course into the optic nerve
4. Temporal wedge-shaped scotoma: Damage to nasal retinal fibers

In some cases, optic neuropathies do not produce nerve fiber bundle defects, but rather general elevation of all static thresholds or inward displacement of central isopters derived from kinetic perimetry. Such nonspecific defects are more common in optic neuritis than in other optic neuropathies.

The finding of a nonhemianopic defect in a patient with a normal looking fundus forces presumption of a retrobulbar optic neuropathy or a retinopathy without obvious ophthalmoscopic features that is nevertheless capable of causing an RAPD. The most likely candidate would be an old retinal artery or vein occlusion whose edema phase has passed.

Imaging centered on the orbit and orbitocranial junction is indicated to exclude compressive optic neuropathy. The rest of the brain should also be imaged, lest evidence of disseminated lesions, like those in multiple sclerosis or vasculitis, be overlooked.

Relative Afferent Pupillary Defect with Hemianopic Field Defect

The finding of a hemianopic defect in one or both eyes points to a chiasmal lesion. Loss of the entire hemifield is not necessary to diagnose a hemianopic defect. Instead, it is defined as any field defect whose border is aligned to the vertical fixation meridian. Although the classic pattern of visual field defects produced by disease at the optic chiasm is the bitemporal hemianopia, rarely is the visual loss total or even symmetrically depressed in the two temporal fields. In fact, the disease process usually extends to involve one optic nerve, and sometimes both, but usually asymmetrically. The result is that the patient often has subnormal acuity in at least one eye and a RAPD.

Some patients who have chiasmal lesions manifest a temporal hemianopia in the field of only one eye. The visual field of the other eye may be normal or have a mixture of hemianopic and nonhemianopic defects.

Visual field examinations performed in patients with subnormal VA and an RAPD may also disclose a homonymous hemianopia, a finding that would suggest a lesion involving both the optic nerve and the optic tract.

If high-resolution dedicated neuroimaging fails to disclose a lesion in a patient with an RAPD and a hemianopic visual field defect, the visual fields are checked again to determine whether defects that initially appeared hemianopic might actually be non hemianopic. If repeated testing still suggests hemianopia, MRI must be performed with fine section and ample contrast before a chiasmal lesion is ruled out.

Relative Afferent Pupillary Defect Not Present

If subnormal VA is not accompanied by an RAPD, the examiner must rule out an occult retinopathy. The causes include "Cystoid edema, serious macular detachment, vitreoretinal interface disorders, inflammatory outer retinopathies, photoreceptor and macular dystrophies, retinochoroidal ischemia, ocular trauma, phototoxicity, medication toxicity, neurolipidoses, paraneoplastic retinopathy, and age related macular degeneration".

Such patients need evaluation by an expert ophthalmologist by means of high magnification ophthalmoscopy, the Amsler grid test, the photostress test, fluorescein angiography and electroretinography.

Details of these would be beyond the scope of this chapter. (Chapter-4).
Note: If ophthalmological evaluation and the aforementioned tests exclude presence of occult retinopathy, evidence for presence of amblyopia to be sought.

AMBLYOPIA

Amblyopia is defined as subnormal VA associated with persistently unfocused imagery at the retina, or suppression of the fovea in a deviating eye. Occurring within the first years of life, amblyopic loss of VA results from failure of optic nerve axons coming from the affected eye to compete with those of the unaffected eye for synaptic connections in the lateral geniculate body and primary visual cortex.

Amblyopia usually arises in the setting of strabismus (ocular misalignment) but may also be associated with anisometropia (unequal refractive error in the two eyes), profound media opacities, or occluding ptosis in early childhood. If amblyopia is to develop, it does so well within the 1st decade of life, when the developing visual system is still vulnerable to deprivation.

Evidence for the diagnosis of amblyopia is entirely circumstantial. There are no distinctive physical makers or inclusionary tests. Thus, the diagnosis is always presumptive, made only if proper signs are present and other causes of visual loss have been carefully excluded. Compressive optic neuropathy by a slow growing lesion may closely mimic amblyopia.

If amblyopia not present?

If there is no RAPD, no occult retinopathy and no evidence of amblyopia, the only remaining possibilities for a subnormal VA are bilateral old partial retinal artery or vein occlusions (without fundus signs), symmetric optic neuropathy, a chiasmal lesion or psychogenic visual loss. Fundoscopy, formal field testing, electrophysiologic evaluation of visual pathway (evoked potential techniques) and high resolution neuroimaging would help. Essentially normal results in all these parameters, may suggest presence of psychogenic visual loss.

Unexplained Visual Disturbance with Normal Acuity and Fields

The final variant on the theme of unexplained visual loss is the patient who complains of disturbed vision, yet VA and field testing findings are certifiably normal. Four explanations are possible:

1. Inadequate testing methods: Standard automated threshold perimetry protocols sample the visual field within 30 degrees of fixation. They do not detect abnormalities in the peripheral field and may miss defects confined to the central 5 degrees because test points in that region are too few
2. Subclinical optic nerve or retinal disorders: Visual acuity and fields may be degraded so slightly that conventional measures do not

detect the abnormalities. Such cases are rare, given the sensitivity of modern static threshold perimetry. Visual evoked potential testing can be used in this context as a sensitive and objective measure of visual dysfunction

3. Spatial, attentional, or visual recognition disorders: Patients with these higher-order disorders of vision often score normal on tests of elementary vision (VA and fields). They have lost the ability to locate objects in space and to recognize whether they are familiar. The lesions lie in vision-related parietal, temporal, or occipital lobes and are caused by stroke, bihemispheric leukoencephalopathy (tumor, multiple sclerosis, malignant hypertension, progressive multifocal leukoencephalopathy, and adrenoleukodystrophy), or polioencephalopathies (Alzheimer's disease, Creutzfeldt-Jakob disease). Many patients have other prominent neurologic symptoms; others have primarily visual complaints

Patients with these cerebral disorders complain of blurred vision, objects "popping out of sight", and difficulty in reading and judging distances, especially when driving or picking up objects. Unless the standard ophthalmologic and screening mental status examinations include tasks that challenge spatial and recognition skills, the diagnosis will be missed

4. Illusions and hallucinations: Patients who describe altered shape, position, size, movement, or color of objects, and hallucinations of dots and lines, complicated geometric shapes, and animate objects often have a disorder that does not cause VA or visual field defects. The approach to these disorders has been discussed elsewhere in this volume.

SUGGESTED READINGS

1. Bauer RM, Heilman KM, Valenstein E (eds). Clinical Neuropsychology, 3rd ed. New York: Oxford University Press; 1993. 215-78.
2. Cogan DG. Visual disturbances with focal progressive dementing disease. Am J Ophthalmol. 1985;100: 68-72.
3. Damasio AR. Disorders of complex visual processing: Agnosias, achromatopsia, Balint's syndrome and related difficulties of orientation and construction. In: Mesulam MM (ed). Principles of Behavioral Neurology. Philadelphia: F.A. Davis. 1985: 259-88.
4. Daw NW. Visual Development, New York: Plenum Press; 1995. 123-38.
5. Fineberg E, Thompson HS. Quantitation of the afferent pupillary defect. In: Smith JL (ed). Neuro-ophthalmology Focus. New York: Masson; 1979: 25-30.
6. Guyton DL. Misleading prediction of postoperative visual acuity [Editorial]. Arch Ophthalmol. 1986;104: 189-90.
7. Johnson LN, Hill RA, Bartholomew MJ. Correlation of afferent pupillary defect with visual loss on automated perimetry. Ophthalmology. 1988;95:1649-55.
8. Keltner JL, Johnson CA, Spurr JO, Beck RW for the Optic Neuritis Study Group. Visual field profile of optic neuritis: One-year follow-up in the Optic Neuritis Treatment Trial. Arch Ophthalmol. 1994;112:946-53.
9. Minkowaski JS, Palese M, Guyton DL. Potential acuity meter using a minute aerial pinhole aperture. Ophthalmology. 1983;90:1360-8.
10. Rubin ML, Optics for Clinicians, Gainesville, Fla : Triad, 1971:185.
11. Savino PJ, Paris M, Schatz NJ, et al. Optic tract syndrome: A review of 21 patients. Arch Ophthalmol. 1978;96:656-63.
12. Spurny RC, Zaldivar R, Belcher CD 3rd, et al. Instruments for predicting visual acuity: A clinical comparison. Arch Ophthalmol. 1986;104:196-200.
13. Thompson HS. Montague P, Cox TA, et al. The relationship between visual acuity, pupillary defect, and visual field loss. Am J Ophthalmol. 1982;93:681-6.
14. Trobe JD. Visual distress in patients with Alzheimer's disease. In: Smith JL, Katz RS (eds). Neuro-ophthalmology Enters the Nineties. Miami: Dutton Press; 1989:277-83.

CHAPTER 7

Transient Visual Loss

Jayanta Roy

INTRODUCTION

Transient visual loss (TVL) is characterized by sudden onset and reversible deficit of visual function lasting less than 24 hours. It can be monocular or binocular. Numbers of causes have been described, but three mechanisms are considered to be important for all practical purposes: ischemia, migraine, and seizure. The term amaurosis fugax [amauros (Greek) = dim/dark; fugax (Latin) = transitory, flying swiftly] is commonly reserved for transient monocular blindness (TMB) due to emboli in the retinal circulation from carotid vessels or heart. Amaurosis fugax (AF) remains a therapeutic challenge, because of the difficulty in differentiating between these and other causes. Many a times, the patient seeks medical attention when the deficit has already reversed, and the physician is left with a description of the event and a negative neuro-ophthalmic examination. A thorough history with detailed ocular and systemic examination supplemented with relevant investigation remains the key to the diagnosis.

APPROACH TO DIAGNOSIS

History

Following questions are pertinent:
- *Is it monocular or binocular?*
  This distinction is important because binocular symptoms usually localizes to primary visual cortex. The causes of monocular and binocular TVL have been listed in Boxes 1 and 2, respectively. Sometimes, patients cannot make the distinctions reliably and often a hemianopsic defect is described as a deficit of the eye with the temporal field defect.

Box 1: Causes of mononuclear transient visual loss

1. Occlusive arterial disease
   - Atherosclerosis and other lesions of internal carotid artery (e.g., dissection)
   - Thromboemboli from heart/aortic arch atheroma
   - Arteritis (Takayasu's/giant cell/Wegener's granulomatosis, etc.)
2. Migraine
3. Vasospastic
4. Low perfusion pressure
   - Postural hypotension
   - Multiple occlusions of extracranial cerebral arteries
5. Transient visual obscuration
   - Papilledema
   - Orbital mass (gaze-evoked obscuration)
6. Macular photostress phenomenon
7. Ocular causes
   - Angle-closure glaucoma
   - Partial retinal vein occlusion
   - Hyphema
8. Hyperviscosity syndrome
9. Demyelinating disease (Uhthoff's phenomenon)
10. Miscellaneous causes
    - Phencyclidine toxicity
    - Dural arteriovenous fistula
    - Pulmonary arteriovenous fistula
    - Paranasal sinus mucositis
    - Metastasis at tuberculum sellae
    - Paraneoplastic retinopathy
    - Interleukin-2 therapy
    - Sickle cell disease
    - Essential thrombocythemia
    - Psychogenic

- *Did any particular maneuver provoke the TVL?*
  Transient visual loss are mostly spontaneous, but sometimes they are triggered like assuming upright posture, bright light, head trauma, and cerebral angiography (Flowchart 1)
- *Was there any associated scintillation?*
  Flickering, zigzag lines that march across a hemifield and build up over 20–30 minutes, is typical of migraine. Vitreoretinal diseases may cause brief temporal flashes in one eye.
- *What was the duration of the visual disturbance?*

Box 2: Causes of binocular transient visual loss

- Migraine
- Posterior circulation thromboembolism
- Systemic hypotension
- Head trauma
- Seizures
- Malignant hypertension
- Eclampsia
- Papilledema
- Psychogenic

Duration for 1 second is typical of a visual obscuration due to optic disc edema. In migraine, it usually lasts 20–30 minutes. In AF, the attacks are sudden in onset, lasting seconds to minutes. Blindness is complete, although it is sometimes limited to a sector of the field of vision. Often the blindness develops as if a shade were drawn upward or downward over the eye, rarely sideways. Attacks can be single or multiple. Some patients have hundreds or even thousands of episodes. Pain, scintillations, and diplopia are typically absent. In most patients the prognosis for recovery of the retina is good; in a few, retinal infarction occurs.

Physical Examination

The physical examination includes a detailed general and systemic examination with particular attention to any ocular abnormality, measurement blood pressure with postural changes, palpation of

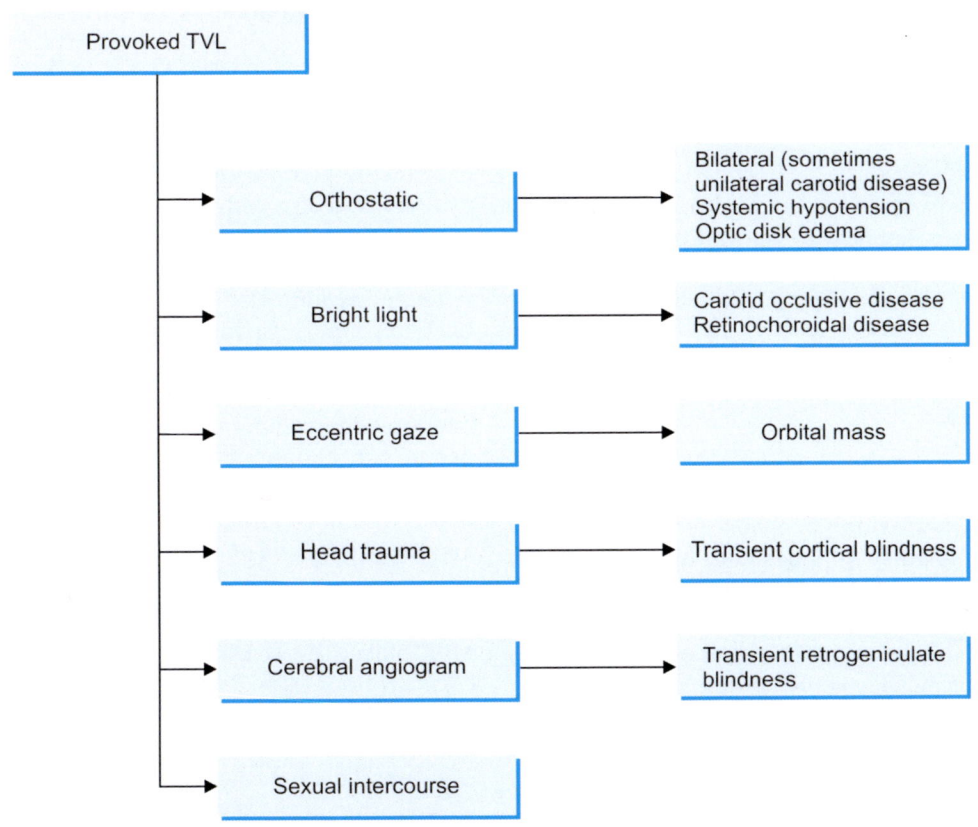

FLOWCHART 1: Provoked transient visual loss.

> **Box 3: Investigations for transient vision loss**
> - Complete blood count
> - Erythrocyte sedimentation rate
> - Coagulation profile
> - Antinuclear antibody
> - Antiphospholipid antibody
> - Protein electrophoresis
> - Serum electrolytes, creatinine
> - Liver function test
> - Urinalysis
> - Chest radiography
> - Carotid ultrasound
> - Transcranial Doppler study
> - Computed tomography/magnetic resonance angiogram of neck and intracranial vessels (when indicated)
> - Echocardiogram
> - Electroencephalography
> - Fasting homocysteine
> - Protein C, protein S, antithrombin III
> - Factor V Leiden
> - Prothrombin G20210A mutation

> **Box 4: Photostress test**
> - After measuring baseline visual acuity, shine a bright light into symptomatic eye for 10 s
> - Measure the delay in patient's ability to correctly identify the letters on the next larger line on the acuity chart
> - Perform the same step on the fellow eye
> - Full recovery normally occurs within 50 s. Doubling of the latency in the affected eye is considered a positive result for outer retinal dysfunction

superficial temporal and peripheral arteries, and auscultation of carotids/heart/renal arteries.

Investigations

The investigations for a TVL are listed in Box 3. They should be ordered with relevance to the history and clinical findings. They have been discussed separately in the later part of this chapter.

PROVOKED TRANSIENT VISION LOSS

Orthostatic

In case of marginal ocular perfusion, upright posture induces symptoms of visual loss. The reduced perfusion is probably in the ciliary circulation which supplies both outer retina and optic nerve head. The choroidal vessels are well collateralized compared to the vessels supplying optic nerve head and with reduced perfusion, optic nerve head becomes ischemic.

With anterior circulation stenosis, standing up causes ocular ischemia and results in abrupt dimness or loss of vision. Chronically, low perfusion is evident as retinal microaneurysm, dilated veins, hemorrhage, and neovascularization. With optic disc edema, transient visual obscuration typically lasts a second or two. Sometimes can be induced by straining.

Bright Light

Exposure to strong light causes delayed recovery of vision. The presumed mechanism is impaired regeneration of photopigments of retina due to ocular ischemia. It is also seen in hereditary or inflammatory retinochoroidal diseases. Photostress test can reliably assess this abnormality (Box 4).

Eccentric Gaze

Monocular TVL may be caused by eccentric gaze due to compression of the optic nerve by an orbital mass situated within extraocular muscle cone. It takes 1020 seconds for complete loss of vision once eyes are taken into extreme gaze and recovers in almost the same time when taken back to primary position. Usually a hemangioma or optic sheath meningioma is the cause. Orbital schwannoma had also been reported. Very rarely, eye movement induced visual obscuration may occur with idiopathic intracranial hypertension. The presumed mechanism is cessation of blood flow (which is already compromised) due to kinking of the optic nerve head.

Head Trauma

Mild closed head trauma may cause transient cortical blindness in a setting of intact neurological function. Early recognition and understanding of this syndrome can lead to a decreased anxiety level, not only for the patient, but also for the parents as well. The mechanism is not clearly known, but it is presumed to be cortical. Ophthalmologic examination is normal including fully reactive pupil. Brain imaging is normal; sometimes, the electroencephalography shows posterior slow waves. The blindness usually reverses within a few hours. The patients with this transient blindness are thought to be vulnerable to migraine and seizures.

Cerebral Angiography

Transient visual loss following cerebral angiogram has been reported. One possible cause of this complication is an adverse reaction to contrast agent, resulting in an osmotic disruption of the blood–brain barrier that seems to be selective for the occipital cortex. It is also reported after coronary angiogram and contrast-enhanced computed tomography scan of brain.

Sexual Intercourse

Teman et al. have reported a case of stereotyped monocular TVL during sexual intercourse where all relevant investigations were normal, and the patient improved with nifedipine taken before the act.

UNPROVOKED TRANSIENT VISION LOSS (FLOWCHART 2)

When scintillation is present, four causes should be considered in the differential diagnosis.

Migraine

Visual scintillation is the most common type of migraine aura. Headache usually follows the aura, but sometimes may not (called "migraine equivalent" or "acephalgic migraine"). Migraineurs often report gradual lessening of the severity of headache with age and the aura remains the predominant symptom. In children, the aura often accompanies the headache or may precede it.

The features suggesting migraine are described in Box 5.

Ischemia

Scintillation may occur with ischemia of the calcarine cortex. It may affect hemifield or entire vision depending on involvement of one or both posterior cerebral artery territories. It may look like a snowflake, sparkle, soap flakes, tadpole or

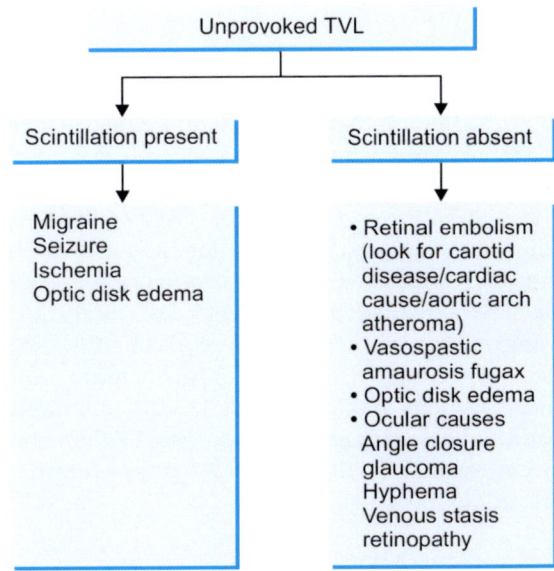

FLOWCHART 2: Unprovoked transient visual loss.

Box 5: Features of migraine

- Scintillation is binocular, often confined to one hemifield, but may affect the other hemifield is subsequent attacks
- Patients usually describe the same pattern in every attack
- It typically expands or build up across the hemifield over 20–30 min
- The visual aura may march as a paresthesia or numbness to face, lips, or fingertips. It may happen without a visual aura
- The most common pattern of scintillation is the "scintillating scotoma". The term "teichopsia" [teichos (Greek) = city wall] is also used as it looks like the outline of a medieval fortress. Being an evanescent phenomenon, the scintillating scotoma is also called "fortification spectrum" (spectral or ghost like)

glowing lights. In posterior circulation transient ischemic attack, the typical fortification spectrum doesn't occur and they never march over 20–30 minutes typical of migraine. Other features of vertebrobasilar ischemia like vertigo, nausea, vomiting, ataxia, diplopia, dysarthria, weakness/numbness of extremity should be looked into. Headache rarely accompanies ischemia, but infarction of posterior visual cortex may cause referred pain to the ipsilateral eye, originating from trigeminal innervations of occipital meninges.

Seizure

Scintillation along with TVL may occur from an occipital lesion often detected in imaging studies. It is also seen in benign childhood epilepsy with occipital paroxysm affecting mostly preadolescent girls. The scintillation usually lasts several minutes, never march across hemifield and consists of lines, stars, squares, sparkling dots, and very rarely zigzags. Associated features of seizure like gaze deviation, frequent blinking, neck deviation, tonic-clinic movements and alteration of consciousness are important in diagnosis. In occipital lobe arteriovenous malformations (AVM), marching scintillations with hemianopsic visual defect may occur repeatedly. Removal of AVM may improve this condition.

Optic Disc Edema

Transient visual obscuration may be associated with brief scintillation.

When scintillation is absent, following causes should be considered in the differential diagnosis:

Retinal Embolism

Three main types of endogenous emboli may arrive at retina:
- Cholesterol emboli (Hollenhorst): They are small, yellow, refractile particles derived from carotids or aortic arch atheroma and lodge at bifurcations. They may be found in patient who complain of a recent TVL, but may be asymptomatic and detected incidentally. Asymptomatic patients with Hollenhorst plaques have a 50% risk of myocardial infarction within 7 years.
- Platelet-fibrin emboli: They are white particles originating from cervical carotid atheroma of heart valves, mold themselves to distal retinal vessels and usually breakup and disappear. They rarely cause retinal infarct.
- Calcium emboli: They are large, white, nonrefractile, originating from heart valves or calcified atheroma. Being large and stiff, they lodge at large retinal vessels and may cause infarct.

Vasospastic Amaurosis Fugax

Repeated attacks of monocular TVL have been reported in patients where extensive investigations could not reveal any carotid/cardiac cause of retinal embolism. Each attack lasts around 10–15 minutes in average, the severity ranging from graying out of vision to complete blindness, rarely associated with periorbital ache. Some patients may experience several attacks a day. Ophthalmic examination during attacks revealed pale optic disc, narrowed and threadlike arteries; the veins were segmentally constricted with discontinuous blood columns (described as boxcarring or rouleaux formation), indicating sluggish or absent blood flow. Visual acuity, color vision, visual fields, pupils, ocular motility, intraocular pressure, ophthalmodynamometric findings, and ophthalmoscopic appearance were normal between attacks. No emboli were visualized at any time. Nifedipine 60 mg/day or verapamil 120 mg/day improved the condition in these patients. Exercised induced vasospastic AF has also been reported.

Optic Disc Edema

Transient visual obscuration for seconds without scintillations may occur.

Ocular Causes

- Angle closure glaucoma: It may raise intraocular pressure to the point of compromising retinal and optic nerve perfusion. The angle reopens spontaneously and circulation re-establishes. Presence of periocular pain with TVL and an occludable angle detected by gonioscopy helps in the diagnosis.
- Hyphema: Episodic bleeding from a cataract wound or iris root may cause TVL.
- Venous stasis retinopathy: It is caused by chronically reduced arterial perfusion or impaired venous drainage like hyperviscosity syndrome, congestive orbitopathy, etc.

Other Uncommon Causes of Transient Visual Loss

Many other causes of TVL have been reported in the literature which are relatively rare. Vasculitis syndromes like giant cell arteritis, Wegener's granulomatosis, and Takayasu arteritis have been reported to cause TVL. In a series of 78 patients with Takayasu arteritis, amaurosis fugax has been reported in 25.6% cases. Other reported causes of TVL include phencyclidine inhalation, interleukin-2 therapy, paraneoplastic retinopathy, dural arteriovenous fistula from ophthalmic artery, pulmonary arteriovenous fistula, Paranasal sinus mucositis and metastatic deposits at tuberculum sellae. Hematological conditions like sickle cell disease and essential thrombocythemia have been reported to cause TVL. Other rare vascular causes like fibromuscular dysplasia anomalous origin of ophthalmic artery with atherosclerotic narrowing of external carotid and carotid dysplasia.

INVESTIGATIONS

Box 3 shows the list of the investigations usually performed in a case of TVL. Some of them deserve mention because of their importance in management and prognostication.

Carotid Ultrasound

Duplex doppler of carotid has become a routine baseline investigation in diagnosis of carotid disease. It can reliably measure the severity of stenosis based on Doppler frequency shift or calculated flow velocities, expressed as a percentage of area reduction commonly reported in the range of 0–15%, 16–49%, 50–69%, 70–99%, and occlusion. Information regarding the plaque morphology may be assessed by B-mode ultrasonography. In laboratories with high quality standards, carotid duplex is capable of high degree accuracy compared to angiography. Addition of color flow imaging enhances the diagnostic accuracy. Ultrasound may produce a false-positive impression of carotid occlusion. In ACAS trial, careful standardization and training of sonographers produced a 93% positive predictive value for ultrasound compared with angiography.

Computed Tomography Angiography of Carotids

Differentiation between total and near occlusion of internal carotid artery is important because patients with total occlusion do not benefit from surgery. Color-coded carotid duplex ultrasonography has a sensitivity of 86–94% in diagnosing near occlusion. Multislice CT angiography of the neck vessels showed an excellent correlation with catheter angiogram in diagnosis of total and near occlusion. It may be considered as a substitute of catheter angiogram to confirm sonographic findings in diagnosing total and near occlusion. Computed tomography angiography is of particular importance to diagnose disease at the petrous or cavernous part of carotid which can also cause retinal ischemia, more commonly in Asian patients. In a Taiwanese study, 16% of patients with AF had carotid siphon stenosis. Both carotid duplex and MR angiography has limitation to detect these lesions.

Magnetic Resonance Angiography of Carotids

Nederkoorn et al. have reviewed and compared the published data on the diagnostic value of duplex ultrasonography (DUS), MR angiography (MRA), and digital subtraction angiography. For the diagnosis of 70–99% stenosis versus <70% stenosis, MRA had a pooled sensitivity of 95% and pooled specificity of 90%. These numbers were 86% versus 87% respectively for DUS. For recognizing occlusion, MRA showed a sensitivity of 98% and specificity of 100% and DUS has a sensitivity of 96% and specificity of 100%. So, MRA has a better discriminatory power to diagnose 70%-99% stenosis. Both 3D-time of flight (TOF) and contrast enhanced MRA can effectively diagnose carotid stenosis of occlusion.

Transcranial Doppler

In a hemodynamically significant carotid stenosis, transcranial Doppler (TCD) may contribute to the assessment of the collateral flow through the anterior circulation. For the transorbital approach, the strongest indicators of a residual lumen diameter less than 1.5 mm were reversal of flow in the ipsilateral ophthalmic artery and a more than 50% peak systolic velocity difference between the carotid siphons [distal internal carotid artery (ICA)] in patients with unilateral ICA origin stenosis. They were 100% specific and 31% and 26% sensitive, respectively. For the transtemporal approach in patients with a unilateral stenosis, a more than 35% difference in ipsilateral middle cerebral artery (MCA) peak systolic velocity relative to the contralateral MCA or a more than 50% difference in contralateral anterior cerebral artery (ACA) peak systolic velocity relative to the ipsilateral ACA were 100% specific for identifying a residual lumen diameter of less than 1.5 mm. Sensitivities were 32% and 43%, respectively. Irrespective of contralateral stenosis, a more than 35% difference in ipsilateral MCA peak systolic velocity relative to the ipsilateral posterior cerebral artery had a 100% specificity and a 23% sensitivity for detecting a less than 1.5 mm minimal residual lumen diameter. Although the TCD sensitivity for detecting a clinically and hemodynamically significant stenosis is relatively low, it can be highly specific (up to 100%) and could enhance the diagnostic accuracy of highly sensitive DUS criteria for detecting a hemodynamically significant ICA stenosis.

Echocardiography

Transthoracic echocardiography (TTE) should be performed in a suspected case of AF. Transesophageal echocardiogram is an invasive procedure and should be ordered if indicated. Atherosclerotic plaque at the arch of the aorta has been identified as a potential source for atheroembolic stroke. Imaging of aortic arch plaque can be performed with transesophageal echocardiography. Magnetic resonance study of aortic plaques with T1, proton density, T2-weighed images and MR-angiography allows a comprehensive study of the aorta as well.

MANAGEMENT OF TRANSIENT VISION LOSS

It varies with the cause of the TVL. Management of carotid disease and a retinal embolism will be discussed here because they constitute the majority cases of AF.

Management of Carotid Stenosis

1. Symptomatic carotid stenosis <50%: Symptoms were defined as a retinal or hemispheric transient ischemic attack (TIA) or a nondisabling stroke (modified Rankin score <3). For them, medical treatment is recommended.
2. Symptomatic stenosis 70–99% as documented by noninvasive imaging: This group benefit from carotid endarterectomy (CEA) along with medical therapy if the perioperative morbidity and mortality risk is estimated to be less than 6%.
3. Symptomatic carotid occlusion: They do not benefit from CEA because of high percentage of perioperative complication rate. So, medical therapy is recommended.
4. Symptomatic stenosis 50–69% detected by angiography or noninvasive imaging: CEA is recommended depending on patient-specific factors, such as age, sex, and comorbidities, if the perioperative morbidity and mortality risk is estimated to be less than 6%.
5. When revascularization is indicated for patients with TIA or minor, nondisabling stroke, it is reasonable to perform the procedure within 2 weeks of the index event rather than delay surgery if there are no contraindications to early revascularization.
    - Carotid angioplasty and stenting (CAS) is indicated as an alternative to CEA for symptomatic patients at average or low risk of complications associated with endovascular intervention when the diameter of lumen of ICA is reduced by more than 70% by noninvasive imaging or more than 50% by catheter-based imaging or noninvasive imaging with corroboration and the anticipated rate of periprocedural stroke or death is less than 6%.
    - It is reasonable to consider patient age in choosing between CAS and CEA. For older patients (i.e., older than ≈70 years), CEA may be associated with improved outcome compared with CAS, particularly when arterial anatomy is unfavorable for endovascular intervention. For younger patients, CAS is equivalent to CEA in terms of risk for periprocedural complications (ie, stroke, MI, or death) and long-term risk for ipsilateral stroke.
    - Among patients with symptomatic severe stenosis (>70%) in whom anatomic or medical conditions are present that greatly increase the risk for surgery
    - or when other specific circumstances exist, such as radiation-induced stenosis or restenosis after CEA, CAS is reasonable
    - For patients with a recent (within 6 months) TIA or ischemic stroke ipsilateral to a stenosis or occlusion of the middle cerebral or carotid artery, extracranial-intracranial bypass surgery is not recommended

Surgery in Asymptomatic Carotid Disease

Carotid endarterectomy in asymptomatic carotid stenosis has marginal benefit and questionable safety. Large number of patients must be treated to prevent a stroke. With the available evidence, medical therapy and risk factor stratification remains the best option. There may be a subgroup which clearly benefits from surgery, but that group cannot be identified with the available evidence.

Treatment of Intracranial Stenosis

Atherosclerotic lesion at petrous or cavernous ICA can cause TVL. Those lesions are surgically inaccessible and can be treated through endovascular technique only. However, angioplasty and stenting of intracranial lesions do not provide clear benefit over best medical management due to the high percentage of procedural risk involved. The largest body of evidence comes from SAMMPRIS trial which was a randomized controlled trial comparing intracranial stenting and best medical management. The recommendations are:

- For patients with recent stroke or TIA (within 30 days) attributable to severe stenosis (70–99%) of a major intracranial artery, the addition of clopidogrel 75 mg/d to aspirin for 90 days might be reasonable
- For patients with a stroke or TIA attributable to moderate stenosis (50–69%) of a major intracranial artery, angioplasty or stenting is not recommended given the low rate of stroke with medical management and the inherent periprocedural risk of endovascular treatment
- For patients with severe stenosis (70–99%) of a major intracranial artery and recurrent TIA or stroke after institution of aspirin and clopidogrel therapy, achievement of systolic blood pressure more than 140 mm Hg, and high-intensity statin therapy, the usefulness of angioplasty alone or placement of a Wingspan stent or other stent is unknown and is considered investigational.

Thrombolytic Therapy in Retinal Embolism

Intravenous thrombolytics (recombinant tissue plasminogen activator) has been tried in central retinal artery and retinal vein occlusion on a few patients in a pilot study. Large scale data is not available. Selective intra-arterial infusion of fibrinolytic agents achieved a good prognosis in a few studies, but it is always not very effective.

CONCLUSION

In conclusion, among the many causes of TVL, retinal artery embolism from a carotid disease remains the most important one. Careful history and appropriate investigations help in determining the underlying cause of the visual loss. Judicious use of CEA combined with medical therapy may prevent recurrence of visual loss and reduce the chance of future stroke as well.

SUGGESTED READINGS

1. Barnett HJM, Meldrum HE, Eliasziw M for the North American Symptomatic Carotid Endarterectomy Trial (NASCET) Collaborators. The appropriate use of carotid endarterectomy. Can Med Assoc J. 2002;166(9):1169-79.
2. Bernard JT, Ameriso S, Kempf R, et al. Transient focal neurologic deficits complicating interleukin-2 therapy. Neurology. 1990;40(1).
3. Burde RM. Amaurosis fugax: An overview. J Clin Neuro-ophthalmology 1989;9:185-9.
4. Butz B, Strotzer M, Manke C, et al. Selective intraarterial fibrinolysis of acute central retinal artery occlusion. Acta Radiol. 2003;44(6):680-4.
5. Cackett P, Weir C. Wegener's granulomatosis presenting with amaurosis fugax. Eye. 2002;16(5):676.
6. Can U, Furie KL, Suwanwela N, et al. Transcranial Doppler ultrasound criteria for hemodynamically significant internal carotid artery stenosis based on residual lumen diameter calculated from en bloc endarterectomy specimens. Stroke. 1997;28:1966-71.
7. Chen CJ, Lee TH, Hsu HL, et al. Multi-slice CT angiography in diagnosing total versus near occlusions of the internal carotid artery: Comparison with catheter angiography. Stroke. 2004;35:83-5.
8. Chun YS, Park SJ, Park IK, et al. The clinical and ocular manifestations of Takayasu arteritis. Retina. 2001;21(2):132-40.
9. Davidoff RA. Migraine: Manifestations, Pathogenesis and Management. Philadelphia F.A. Davis, 1995.
10. Ernest JT. Choroidal circulation. In: Ryan SJ (ed). Retina, Vol 1. St. Louis: C.V. Mosby;1989. p. 67-8.
11. Finelli PF. Sickle cell trait and transient monocular blindness. Am J Ophthalmol. 1976;81(6):850-1.
12. Fisher CM. Late-life migraine accompaniments as a cause of unexplained transient ischemic attacks. Can J Neurol Sci. 1980;7:9-17.
13. Fisher CM. The posterior cerebral artery syndrome. Can J Neurol Sci. 1986;13:232-9.

14. Furlan AJ, Whisnant JP, Kearns TP. Unilateral visual loss in bright light: An unusual symptom of carotid occlusive disease. Arch Neurol. 1979;36:675-6.
15. Gastaut H, Zifkin BG. Benign epilepsy of childhood with occipital spike and wave complexes. In: Andermann F, Lugaresi E (eds). Migraine and Epilepsy. An overview. Boston: Butterworth, 1987.
16. Gautier JC. Amaurosis fugax. N Engl J Med. 1993;329:426-8.
17. Glaser JS, Savino PJ, Sumers KD, et al. The photostress recovery test: A practical adjunct in the clinical assessment of visual function. Am J Ophthalmol. 1977;83:255-60.
18. Glaser JS. Neuro-ophthalmology, 2nd ed. Philadelphia: J.B. Lippincoat, 1990. p. 18-20.
19. Greenblatt SH. Posttraumatic transient cerebral blindness. Association with migraine and seizure diathesis. JAMA. 1973;225:1073-6.
20. Griffith JF, Dodge PR. Transient blindness following head injury in children. N Eng J Med. 1968;278: 648-51.
21. Hachinski VC, Porchawka J, Steele JC. Visual symptoms in migraine syndrome. Neurology. 1973;23: 570-9.
22. Hamard H, Couderc JL, d'Esperey-Fougeres R, Bregeat MP. Transient monocular blindness and carotid dysplasia. Bull Soc Ophtalmol Fr. 1973;73(12):1161-4.
23. Hathout GM, Duh MJ, El-Saden SM. Accuracy of contrast-enhanced MR angiography in predicting angiographic stenosis of the internal carotid artery: Linear regression analysis. Am J Neuroradiol. 2003;24(9):1747-56.
24. Hattenbach LO. Systemic lysis therapy in retinal vascular occlusions. Ophthalmologe. 1998;95(8): 568-75.
25. Heckenlively JR, Arden GB. Principles and Practices of Clinical Electrophysiology of Vision. St Louis, Mosby-year Book, 1991.
26. Hedges TR. The terminology of transient visual loss due to vascular insufficiency. Stroke. 1984;15:907-8.
27. Hochstetler K, Beal S. Transient cortical blindness in a child. Ann Emerg Med 1987;16:218-9.
28. Howard G, Cambless LE, Baker WH, et al. A multicenter validation study of Doppler ultrasound versus angiogram. J Stroke Cerebrovasc Dis. 1991;1:1421-8.
29. Hoyt WF. Transient bilateral blurring of vision. Consideration of an episodic ischemic symptom of vertebro-basilar insufficiency. Arch Ophthalmol. 1963;70:746-51.
30. Hsu HY, Yang FY, Chao AC, et al. Distribution of carotid arterial lesions in Chinese patients with transient monocular blindness. Stroke. 2006;37(2):531-3.
31. Hupp SL, Kline LB, Corbett JJ. Visual disturbances of migraine. Surv Ophthalmol. 1989;33:221-36.
32. Jacobson DM, Thirkill CE, Tipping SJ. A clinical triad to diagnose paraneoplastic retinopathy. Ann Neurol. 1990;28:162-7.
33. Jehn A, Frank Dettwiler B, Fleischhauer J, et al. Exercise-induced vasospastic amaurosis fugax. Arch Ophthalmol. 2002;120(2):220-2.
34. Kaiboriboon K, Piriyawat P, Selhorst JB. Light-induced amaurosis fugax. Am J Ophthalmol. 2001;131(5): 674-6.
35. Kattah JC, Lussenhop AJ. Resolustion of classic migraine after removal of an occipital lobe AVM. Ann Neurol. 1980;7:93.
36. Kernan WN, Ovbiagele B, Black HR, et al; American Heart Association Stroke Council, Council on Cardiovascular and Stroke Nursing, Council on Clinical Cardiology, and Council on Peripheral Vascular Disease. Guidelines for the prevention of stroke in patients with stroke and transient ischemic attack: A guideline for healthcare professionals from the American Heart Association/ American Stroke Association. Stroke. 2014;45(7): 2160-236.
37. Kinn RM, Breisblatt WM. Cortical blindness after coronary angiography: A rare but reversible complication. Cathet Cardiovasc Diagn. 1991; 22(3):177-9.
38. Koudstaal PJ, Koudstaal A. Neurologic and visual symptoms in essential thrombocythemia: Efficacy of low-dose aspirin. Semin Thromb Hemost. 1997; 23(4):365-70.
39. Krill AE, Deutman AF, Fishman G. The cone degenerations. Doc Ophthalmol 1973;35:1-80.
40. Krzanowski M. Fibromuscular dysplasia of the internal carotid artery as a cause of transient cerebral ischemia episodes. Pol Arch Med Wewn. 1997;98(12):546-50
41. Lantos G. Cortical blindness due to osmotic disruption of the blood-brain barrier by angiographic contrast material: CT and MRI studies. Neurology 1989;1989:567-71.
42. Luchtenberg M, Berkefeld J, May A, et al. Transient unilateral amaurosis. Optic nerve compression in paranasal sinus mucositis. Ophthalmologe. 2002;99(5):390-1.
43. Ludwig BI, Ajmone C. Clinical ictal patterns in epileptic patients with occipital electroencephalographic foci. Neurology. 1975;25:463-71.
44. Manor RS, Bensira I. Amaurosis fugax in downward gaze. Surv Ophthalmol. 1987;31:411-6.
45. Meduri A, Natale L, Marano P. Imaging of aortic atherosclerosis. Rays. 2001;26(4):237-45.
46. Mentzel HJ, Blume J, Malich A, et al. Cortical blindness after contrast-enhanced CT: Complication in a patient with diabetes insipidus. Am J Neuroradiol. 2003;24(6):1114-6.
47. Minor RH, Kearns TP, Millikan CH, et al. Ocular manifestations of occlusive diseases of the vertebro-basilar arterial system. Arch Ophthalmol. 1959;62:112-24.
48. Nederkoorn PJ, van der Graaf Y, Hunink MGM. Duplex ultrasound and magnetic resonance angiography compared with digital subtraction angiography

48. in carotid stenosis: A systematic review. Stroke. 2003;34:1324-32.
49. Nederkoorn PJ, van der Graaf Y, Eikelboom BC, et al. Time-of-flight MR angiography of carotid artery stenosis: does a flow void represent severe stenosis? Am J Neuroradiol. 2002;23(10):1779-84.
50. Orcutt JC, Tucker WM, Millis RP, et al. Gaze-evoked amaurosis. Ophthalmology. 1987;94:213-8.
51. Padolecchia R, Puglioli M, Ragone MC, et al. Superselective intraarterial fibrinolysis in central retinal artery occlusion. Am J Neuroradiol. 1999; 20:565-7.
52. Panayiotopolous CP. Benign childhood epilepsy with occipital paroxysms: A 15-year prospective study. Ann Neurol. 1989;26:51-6.
53. Panayiotopolous CP. Difficulties in differentiating migraine and epilepsy based on clinical and EEG findings. In: Andermann F, Lugaresi E (eds). Migraine and Epilepsy. Boston: Butterworth, 1987. p. 31-46.
54. Pascual J, Combarros O, Berciano J. Gaze-evoked amaurosis in pseuotumor cerebri. Neurology. 1988;38:1654-5.
55. Peris Martinez C, Espana Gregori E, Risueno Reguillo P, et al. Amaurosis fugax as the early manifestation of orbital schwannoma. Arch Soc Esp Oftalmol. 2000;75(12):831-4.
56. Pfaffenbach DD, Hollenhorst RW. Mortality and survivorship of patients with embolic cholesterol crystals in the ocular fundus. Am J Ophthalmol. 1973;75:66.
57. Plant GT. The fortification spectra of migraine. BMJ. 1986;293:1613-7.
58. Polak JF, Bajakian RL, O'Leary DH, et al. Detection of internal carotid artery stenosis: Comparison of MR angiography, color Doppler ultrasonography and arteriography. Radiology. 1992;182:35-40.
59. Riaz G, Hennessey JJ. Meningeal lesions mimicking migraine. Neuro-ophthalmology. 1991;11:41-8.
60. Robison JE, Okun MS. Amaurosis fugax from metastatic prostate cancer to the Tuberculum sellae. South Med J. 2001;94(10):1043-4.
61. Ron A, Meisel S, Shapiro-Feinberg M, et al. Cortical blindness following coronary angiography. Harefuah. 2000;138(4):279-81, 342.
62. Ronchetto F. Transient monocular blindness in a patient with giant-cell arteritis. Pathogenetic and therapeutic considerations. Recenti Prog Med. 1992;83(4):241-2.
63. Rowe SE, Trobe JD, Sieving PA. Idiopathic photoreceptor dysfunction causes unexplained visual acuity loss in later adulthood. Ophthalmology. 1990;97:1632-7.
64. Sawamura Y, Nakagawa Y, Sakuragi M, et al. A case of amaurosis fugax with anomalous origin of the ophthalmic artery and atheromatous stenosis of the external carotid artery. No Shinkei Geka. 1984;12(3 Suppl):377-81.
65. Schmidt DP, Schulte-Monting J, Schumacher M. Prognosis of central retinal artery occlusion: Local intraarterial fibrinolysis versus conservative treatment. Am J Neuroradiol. 2002;23(8):1301-7.
66. Sommer JB, Tomandl BF. Vertigo and amaurosis fugax secondary to Takayasu's arteritis. J Neurol Neurosurg Psychiatry. 2001;71(2):276-7.
67. Stoddard WE, Davis DO, Young SW. Cortical blindness after cerebral angiography. Case report. J Neurosurg. 1981;54:240-4.
68. Teman AJ, Winterkorn JM, Weiner D. Transient monocular blindness associated with sexual intercourse. N Engl J Med. 1995;333(6):393.
69. Troost BT, Mark LE, Maroon JC. Resolution of classic migraine after removal of an occipital lobe AVM. Ann Neurol. 1979;5:199-201.
70. Ubogu E. Amaurosis fugax associated with phencyclidine inhalation. Eur Neurol. 2001;46(2):98-9.
71. Weinberger J. Noninvasive imaging of atherosclerotic plaque in the arch of the aorta with transcutaneous B-mode ultrasonography. Neuroimaging Clin N Am. 2002;12(3):373-80, v-vi.
72. Weiskrantz L, Warrington EK, Sanders MD, et al. Visual capacity in the hemianopsic field following a restricted occipital ablation. Brain. 1974;97:709-28
73. Williams D, Wilson TG. The diagnosis of the major and minor syndrome of basilar insufficiency. Brain. 1962;85:741-74.
74. Winterkorn JMS, Kupersmith MJ, Wirtschafter JD, et al. Treatment of vasospastic amaurosis fugax with calcium-channel blockers. N Engl J Med. 1993;329:396-8.
75. Woodward GA. Posttraumatic cortical blindness: Are we missing the diagnosis in children? Pediatr Emerg Care. 1990;6(4):289-92.
76. Xiong L, Li J, Jinkins JR. Amaurosis fugax caused by a dural arteriovenous fistula from the ophthalmic artery. Am J Neuroradiol. 1993;14(1):191-2.
77. Yamakuchi M, Tanaka S, Tomosugi T, et al. Pulmonary arteriovenous fistula manifesting as amaurosis fugax--case report. Neurol Med Chir (Tokyo). 2000;40(5):264-7.
78. Young LH, Appen RE. Ischemic oculopathy: A manifestation of carotid disease. Arch Neurol. 1981;38:358-60.

CHAPTER 8

Optic Neuritis

Debasish Roy, Ambar Chakravarty

INTRODUCTION

The eyes and the optic nerves are accessible, easy to study sensory systems within the brain. The retina can be viewed directly as a specialized part of the brain's gray matter and the optic nerve is a simplified central nervous system white matter tract. The peripheral nerves are myelinated by the Schwann cells, whereas the optic nerve is myelinated by the oligodendrocytes. So, rather than being a peripheral nerve, the optic nerve can be thought of as an extension of the brain's white matter. Therefore, it is not surprising that diseases which affect the white matter of the brain would also affect the optic nerve. Hence, the optic nerve is preferentially involved in multiple sclerosis, a disease of the white matter. It is clinically manifested as a demyelinating self-limiting inflammatory condition of the optic nerve called "optic neuritis". The present chapter would primarily discuss demyelinating neuropathy (optic neuritis) and then briefly highlight on other not so common inflammatory optic neuropathies. Neuromyelitis optica will be discussed in a separate chapter.

Optic nerve disorders were first reliably diagnosed in the late 19th century when ophthalmoscopy became the part of ophthalmic examination. In the early 1900s, salient clinical features of optic neuritis and its relationship to "systemic sclerosis" were recognized. During the course of twentieth century, optic neuritis could be differentiated from infectious, toxic, nutritional, and other causes. The advent of magnetic resonance imaging (MRI) and results of recent clinical trials have highlighted on the relationship between optic neuritis and multiple sclerosis.

FUNCTIONAL ANATOMY

The retina is a specialized CNS gray matter within the eye. This is where the neuronal organization of the visual sensory system begins. The retina is a transparent structure and specialized ganglion cells are arranged within the layers of the retina. Parvocellular ganglion cells (X cells) detect contrast and dominate central retinal areas. Magnocellular ganglion cells (Y cells) detect motion and are peripherally located. All the ganglion cells join at the optic nerve head as they exit the globe.

The optic nerve head (papilla) is a flat disc with a central depression called the optic cup. The retinal ganglion cells exit from the papilla and it is 1.5–2 mm in diameter. The optic cup to disc ratio is 0.39 horizontally and 0.34 vertically. Retinal sensory receptors (rods and cones) are absent in the optic disc.

The optic nerve has four parts: (i) intraocular (1 mm); (ii) intraorbital (25–30 mm); (iii) intracanalicular (10 mm); (iv) intracranial (15–20 mm). The nerve is 50–60 mm long. In the globe it is about 1.5–2 mm in diameter. After it exits from the lamina cribrosa it increases in size to 3.5 mm as oligodendrocytes have formed the myelin along axons. The nerve sheath adds 1.5 mm more to its diameter to make the total width to about 5 mm. In the orbit the nerve is about 25 mm long although the orbit is only 20 mm long. Then the optic nerve enters the optic canal which is 4–10 mm long. The canal runs through the sphenoid bone and contains the optic nerve, the ophthalmic artery, branches of the sympathetic plexus, and meninges that form the optic nerve sheath. The subarachnoid space of the optic nerve communicates freely with the intracranial subarachnoid space. The inferior portion of the frontal lobes are placed above the intracranial portion of the optic nerve. The two optic nerves join at the optic chiasma at the floor of the third ventricle. The intracranial length of the nerve is about 15–20 mm and it rises at an angle of 45° from the anterior clinoid.

About 10 mm behind the globe a large branch of the ophthalmic artery enters the inferior portion of the optic nerve and becomes the central retinal artery. The artery supplies blood to most of the optic nerve and the retina except the optic nerve head. The optic nerve head is supplied by the circle of Zinn–Haller which is a collection of anastomotic arteries arising from the posterior ciliary arteries as well as the pial and peripapillary choroidal arterial circulation.

CLINICAL FEATURES

Optic neuritis is the most common acute optic neuropathy in people aged 18–45 years in high risk populations. The high-risk incidence is 3 per 100,000 and in lower risk groups the incidence is 1 per 100,000 individuals. The exact incidence of the disease in India is not known, but would be expected to be similar to the low-risk group.

In acute optic neuritis, there is often pain in the affected eye which is increased by ocular movement or pressure on the eyeball. There is rapid decline in visual acuity, often causing total blindness, within hours or days. Many patients first notice the visual loss on waking or after accidentally closing one eye. Some notice selective impairment of central vision with preservation of the peripheral field on movement. The extent of visual loss varies from slight blurring of vision to total blindness. Some patients notice selective impairment of colors particularly in the red range. There are other disturbances in visual perception like persistence of images or flashes of light (phosphenes) provoked by eye movement. The pain disappears over a few days, vision improves rapidly at first and slowly afterward and full recovery may take several months. Approximately 90% of patients make an almost full visual recovery.

In the acute phase, optic neuritis is associated with visual field defects (central or centrocecal scotomas), abnormal visual evoked potentials, afferent pupillary defects, decreased color vision and reduced visual acuity. Ophthalmoscopy may reveal swelling of the optic nerve head (papillitis) if the lesion is anterior, but may reveal nothing in posteriorly located lesions. Hence, the common adage "the patient does not see a thing, and you don't either."

The afferent pupillary defect is clinically manifested by the "swinging flashlight sign". In a normal pupil with intact sensory pathways there is constriction of both pupils when light is shown on one eye. In a deafferented pupil the ipsilateral and contralateral constriction is absent when light is shown on the affected eye and pupillary constriction occurs in both eyes when light is shown on the healthy eye. When light is flashed from one eye to the other at regular intervals there may be apparent dilatation of the pupils when light is flashed on the affected eye. This is called the Marcus–Gunn pupil or the swinging flashlight phenomenon or relative afferent pupillary defect. It is found in optic neuritis, but may be found in any other clinical condition which causes deafferentation of the pupil. The classical features of monosymptomatic optic neuritis are summarized in box 1.

CLINICAL EVALUATION

History

Any person with visual loss should be evaluated promptly as many conditions of visual loss represents medical emergencies. Previous history

---

Box 1: Classical features of optic neuritis

- Visual symptoms of recent onset
- Progressive loss of vision over several days
- Periocular pain particularly with eye movement
- Abnormal color vision, visual acuity and/or visual field consistent with optic neuropathy
- Afferent pupillary defect in the eye with the abnormal function
- Optic disc edema (due to papillitis) or a normal optic nerve without atrophy
- Age in the later teens to mid forties
- No evidence of a contributory systemic illness associated with optic neuropathy with the exception of multiple sclerosis

of lazy eye, ocular trauma, or family history of visual loss should be taken. Onset of visual loss is very important. It is equally important to differentiate between sudden visual loss and sudden awareness of a visual loss that may have been existent for an indefinite period. History of systemic illnesses like, diabetes and hypertension must be taken. History of previous ocular or neurologic involvement suggestive of multiple sclerosis must be taken. Carotid stenosis or other related cardiovascular conditions must be looked for. One must be sure whether the visual dysfunction is unilateral or bilateral; the tempo of visual loss must be ascertained and presence or absence of pain on ocular movement must be specifically asked for.

Clinical Examination

The first step is to determine whether actual visual loss exists and to rule out refractive errors. The visual acuity of a patient must be assessed by help of a Snellen's chart at 6 meters or a near vision card at an appropriate distance. The patient should wear his or her spectacles during testing. If the visual loss is due to refractive error, the vision will improve if asked to look through a pin hole. Visual fields by the confrontation method must be done on every patient. Each eye should be tested separately and each of the four quadrants of vision should be assessed. The pupils should be examined for size, shape, and reactivity to light and near. The swinging flash light test can elicit an afferent pupillary defect.

Ophthalmoscopic examination is an essential part of the neurological examination. If the fundus cannot be seen, the anterior segment of the eye must be examined to exclude common obstacles like corneal abnormalities, lens opacities, blood in the anterior chamber, and vitreous abnormalities.

If the latter conditions are suspected an ophthalmological referral is mandatory. The optic disc should be seen and the macula and peripheral portions of the retina should also be examined. The blood vessels should also be studied in detail. Peripheral retinal venous sheathing suggests multiple sclerosis. Other sophisticated methods for examining the fundus and other parts of the eye are usually in domain of the ophthalmologist. This includes slit lamp microscopy which provides a three-dimensional cross-sectional magnified view of the cornea, anterior chamber, lens, and vitreous. Slit lamp examination with a 90 diopters, 60 diopters or Ruby lens allows for a three-dimensional view of the posterior pole. Indirect ophthalmoscopy gives a three-dimensional view of the fundus, with a wider view including the peripheral retina. These methods may be employed where the initial examination by the neurologist is negative or there are clues in the initial examination which suggests a more detailed examination of the other ocular structures.

Classical features of the optic neuropathy are:
- Central visual loss
- Clear view through to the optic nerve
- A relative afferent pupillary defect
- A normal, swollen, or pale appearing optic nerve head.

Two interesting phenomena are associated with optic neuritis. In the Pulfrich phenomenon, an object swinging front and back in the plane of vision is perceived as if moving in a circle. This phenomenon also arises in normal persons when one eye is covered with a gray filter, it is thus nonspecific. In the Uhthoff phenomenon, vision worsens when the body temperature rises as after a hot bath or after a sustained physical activity or athletic activity. This tends to occur mainly when optic neuritis is already wearing off, or when it takes a chromic course. The Uhthoff phenomenon is multiple sclerosis specific, but arises in only half of the patients. One-third have mild deficits on the opposite side as well, which one might be tempted to attribute to inattentiveness during perimetry; however, the Optic Neuritis Treatment Trial (ONTT) showed that the "solitary" deficit in the opposite optic nerve is real and quite typical.

INVESTIGATIONS

Routine blood tests and standard CSF studies are of no help in a classical case of demyelinating optic neuritis. Presence of IgG oligoclonal band in the CSF gives additional corroborative evidence to suggest that it is a part of multiple sclerosis but such studies are not mandatory in all patients. Among the blood tests, a high ESR and positive antinuclear factor may suggest autoimmune optic neuritis. Serological tests for syphilis, AIDS, cryptococcus, cytomegalovirus, varicella etc. may be indicated in specific situations.

The visual evoked potential is abnormal in acute optic neuritis. There is marked attenuation or loss of the PI00 amplitude following pattern reversal stimulation of the affected eye. Following the acute attack, the VEP may show some recovery but the PI00 latency remains prolonged even after normal vision is restored. In patients with past history of optic neuritis the PI00 latency is typically prolonged but wave form morphology and amplitude may remain well preserved. Pattern shift VEPs are abnormal in nearly 100% of cases of definite optic neuritis.

Imaging is now recommended in all cases of optic isritisisallallptic neuritis. MRI is certainly a very major ancillary test; it can directly reveal inflammation of the optic nerve, typically as contrast uptake in a contrast enhanced T1 sequence. It cannot, however, be used as a substitute for clinical diagnosis. An optic nerve sheath meningioma can be a major differential on MRI and should be suspected if the enhancement does not subside within 3 months.

Contrast enhancement involving more than half of the length of the optic nerve or continuing into the chiasm should arouse the suspicion of neuromyelitis optica spectrum disorder. Any foci of demyelination in the brain must be carefully looked for; those most commonly appear in the undersurface of the corpus callosum and periventricular white matter and are best seen on T2 FLAIR images including sagittal sections. Active foci of multiple sclerosis take up contrast medium. The number of inactive typical white matter lesions is the most important criterion for estimating the risk that the patient will develop multiple sclerosis.

Optic neuritis with two or more white matter lesions is the most important criterion for estimating the risk that the patient will develop multiple sclerosis. Optic neuritis with two or more white matter lesions and no other symptoms except visual loss may be designated as "Clinically Isolated Syndrome". According to the new McDonald criteria (2011), multiple sclerosis can be diagnosed when MRI in a patient with optic neuritis reveals two or more typical lesions at least one of which is contrast enhancing.

There are certain "red flags" in the history and clinical examination where imaging should be mandatory:
- A poor historian—where exact timing of visual loss is uncertain
- Patient with an abnormal external examination like unilateral proptosis
- Any patient who does not improve within 3 months of onset of symptoms
- Evidence of compression in the examination like optic atrophy or optociliary shunt vessels
- Any patient with evidence of a junctional syndrome, i.e., a superior temporal field defect in the contralateral eye, needs imaging to exclude any compressive lesion at the chiasma.

Role of Optical Coherence Tomography

Optical coherence tomography is now an increasingly used tool in research on the pathogenesis and treatment of multiple sclerosis. Thinning of the peripapillary retinal nerve fiber layer is correlated with other parameters for assessing the course of multiple sclerosis. Optical coherence tomography thus reflects the severity of damage in optic neuritis and in related conditions like neuromyelitis optica. The best parameter is probably the peripapillary nerve fiber layer thickness in ring scan that is centered on the optic disc. However, in routine clinical practice its utility is limited as the retinal nerve fiber layer thickness is variable amongst normal subjects and in those with glaucoma.

Differential Diagnosis: What Is Not Optic Neuritis?

Many ocular conditions can cause sudden visual loss and many of these may be confused with optic neuritis. Important clinical conditions and clinical clues which suggest anything other than optic neuritis are highlighted in this section.

Anterior Ischemic Optic Neuropathy

Older people usually above 50 years of age have AION. It is associated with disc elevation due to ischemia. Patients usually have a small cup to disc ratio in the opposite eye. Pain is usually absent. The patients often have risk factors for cerebrovascular disease. The visual loss does not recover in most of the cases.

Giant Cell Arteritis
Usually affects individuals over the age of 70 years. Systemic features often associated include jaw and tongue claudication, scalp tenderness, headache, fever, malaise, weight loss, anorexia, anemia, and joint aches. Erythrocyte sedimentation rate is very high, visual loss is severe and disc has a pallid or milky swelling which is characteristic. It responds to high dose of corticosteroids.

Hereditary Optic Neuropathy (Leber's)
Onset usually between 15 and 35 years of age. Painless visual loss starts in one eye but becomes bilateral. Optic disc may have edema; blood vessels are typically tortuous and hemorrhages and exudates may be present.

Toxic and Deficiency Optic Neuropathy
Usually has a gradual onset and slow decline. Usually found in undernourished individuals. Exposure to a known toxin may be elicited from the history. This does not recover spontaneously unless the cause is corrected.

Traumatic Optic Neuropathy
It can be a complication of both direct and indirect trauma to the brain or orbit. There may not be evidence of severe head trauma. Imaging is needed to look for fracture and acute bleeding.

Optic Nerve Drusen
Autosomal dominant inherited hyaline bodies in optic nerves can be seen on ophthalmoscopic examination. Usually causes peripheral field loss and rarely central visual loss.

Neuroretinitis
Seen more in children than adults. Disc edema present, but lots of exudates are present around the macula (macular star appearance). It is usually associated with a viral disease.

Big Blind Spot Syndrome
May be associated with unilateral swollen optic nerve. There is little loss of visual acuity and visual testing reveals an enlarged blind spot.

Angle-closure Glaucoma
Acute painful condition associated with nausea as part of vagal reflex, painful eye from elevated pressure, red eye from vascular congestion, large and nonreactive pupil due to ischemia in the iris and decreased vision due to corneal haze.

Central Serous Retinopathy
Occurs mostly in males (10:1) in the 4th and 5th decades of life in people under increased stress. Sudden painless blurred and dim central vision usually with morphopsia. There may be spontaneous improvement in 1–6 months. The afferent pupillary defect is absent. Indeed, the absence of a relative afferent pupillary defect distinguishes most forms of maculopathy from optic neuritis.

Central Retinal Artery Occlusion
Sudden in onset with central and severe visual loss which is painless and often without warning, some patients experience transient monocular blindness prior to visual loss. Ophthalmoscopically, the retina is white in which the macula appears as a cherry red spot. This is because the retina is very thin at the level of the macula and the choroidal circulation appears red in the white background. Initially the optic nerve head may appear normal, but with progression it may become pale. In ophthalmic artery occlusion both the central retinal artery circulation and the ciliary circulation are compromised resulting in ischemia to the inner and outer retina and the optic nerve. Fundoscopic appearance is that of both retinal and optic nerve swelling with no cherry red spot (the choroidal circulation is also compromised).

Central Retinal Vein Occlusion
Visual loss may be minimal, but fundoscopic appearance is dramatic. Veins are markedly dilated with diffuse hemorrhage involving the superficial and deep layers of the retina. Cotton-wool spots are present due to infarction of the nerve fiber layer with swelling of the optic nerve head.

Multiple Sclerosis and Optic Neuritis
Several studies give conflicting reports as to the relationship between optic neuritis and

subsequent development of multiple sclerosis. The incidence varies from 10% in certain studies to 80–90% in others. This may depend on the patient population studied as well as the study designs and criteria for diagnosis of multiple sclerosis. There are certain points which favor a subsequent development of multiple sclerosis:
- Presence of three or more white matter signals in the MRI
- Immunoglobulin G oligoclonal bands in the CSF
- Abnormal evoked potentials
- Demographic characters - female gender, white race, temperate climates, age 15–45 years.

Three clinical features are associated with less risk of multiple sclerosis, they are: (i) Lack of pain on ocular movement; (ii) marked optic disc swelling at presentation; (iii) mild visual acuity loss at presentation. Brain MRI should be considered for all patients in relevant ethnic groups for subsequent risk assessment of multiple sclerosis. The 5-year risk of development of multiple sclerosis after optic neuritis is about 30%. The risk increases substantially with MR signal abnormalities in white matter. One to two MR lesions confer a risk of 20% at 2 years and 37% at 5 years. Greater than three lesions carry a risk of 32% at 2 years and 51% at 5 years. A normal MRI carried a risk of only 16% for progression to multiple sclerosis over 5 years. A more recent study suggested that patients with three or more MRI detected lesions presented a shorter first interattack interval and a higher relapse rate as compared to subjects with only 1–2 lesions. The predictive value of CSF examination and or visual evoked potential is poor.

The 10 years follow-up data of patients enrolled in the ONTT is now available. The overall 10 years risk was 38%. Those who had one or more MR brain lesions had a lower risk of 22%. Male gender and optic disc swelling were associated with a lower risk. Other factors favoring a lower risk of MS include no light perception, absence of pain, severe disc edema, peripapillary hemorrhages and/or exudates. Interestingly, higher number of MR brain lesions at baseline was not associated with higher risk of clinically definite multiple sclerosis (CDMS) at 10 years.

According to a current study, optic neuritis accounts for 43% of the cases of clinically isolated neurological syndromes that are considered potential precursors of multiple sclerosis. The ophthalmologist is thus often confronted with an otherwise healthy young woman whom he must tell that she might one day develop multiple sclerosis or might already have the disease.

Simultaneous bilateral involvement points to a monophasic illness and chance of subsequent development of multiple sclerosis is less. It is usually a form of encephalomyelitis—a variant form of neuromyelitis optica. This is discussed later in a subsequent chapter.

Pediatric Optic Neuritis

Optic neuritis in the pediatric age group has several distinguishing features. It can occur in association with viral infections like mumps, chickenpox, or influenza and also after vaccinations. Children usually have bilateral involvement; disc edema is a prominent feature. Recovery is usually excellent and subsequent rate of development of multiple sclerosis is low. A study by Luechinetti et al. revealed that only 19% of patients with childhood optic neuritis developed multiple sclerosis during the follow-up period. Association with viral infection may be protective for subsequent development of multiple sclerosis.

Optic Perineuritis

This is also an orbital inflammatory disease, but it is distinct from demyelinating optic neuritis. Patients with optic perineuritis are older at onset and they usually show sparing of central vision. MRI reveals circumferential involvement around the optic nerve rather than within the nerve. Response to steroids is more dramatic than in optic neuritis, but recurrence is also higher.

MANAGEMENT

Several workers have undertaken different trials for standardizing the best treatment option in optic neuritis and some of these are enumerated in Table 1. These studies date back from 1952 to 1999 and have given conflicting and varying evidence as to what should constitute optimum therapy in this self-limiting condition.

The Optic Neuritis Treatment Trial (ONTT) analyzed, in a prospective fashion, the role of high dose intravenous corticosteroids is the management of optic neuritis. A total of 457 patients (77% female and 85% white) were enrolled between 1988 and 1991. Mean age was 33 years. The major objective of this trial was to test the efficacy of corticosteroid treatment in optic neuritis and relationship of optic neuritis to subsequent development of multiple sclerosis.

Patients were divided into three groups—oral steroids, 3 days of intravenous methyl prednisolone followed by 11 days of oral steroids, and placebo.

Most clinics nowadays modified initial intravenous regime to 1000 mg daily for 3 days to allow single day dosing and facilitate treatment on an outpatient basis.

Results

The patients receiving intravenous methyl prednisolone sodium succinate started to recover vision sooner than patients in the other two groups. After 30 days however the 3 groups were essentially the same. At 6 months and 12 months there was no significant difference between the three treatment groups. There was an increased rate of recurrence in the group of patients treated with oral steroids. Within the first two years of follow-up, a neurologic event sufficient to diagnose a patient as having CDMS developed at a slower rate in the group of patients taking intravenous methyl prednisolone. After two years this benefit did not persist. A meta-analysis done in 2012 concluded that faster recovery was the sole benefit of high dose intravenous corticosteroids (Flowchart 1).

There is no consensus of opinion as to what to do in those in whom visual acuity fails to improve significantly. Most tend to use the original therapy at double the dose or for a longer period. The other option is plasmapheresis which is sometimes very effective. However, late spontaneous recovery may also occur. Plasmapheresis is particularly useful in cases of neuromyelitis optica.

Ten years follow-up data of visual outcome for patients in the ONTT is now available. Most patients retained good to excellent vision 10 years after optic neuritis. Recurrences were more frequent in patients with multiple sclerosis.

Newer Modes of Therapy (Immune Prophylaxis)

Immunomodulatory therapies have become one of the mainstays in the treatment for multiple sclerosis. The Food and Drug Administration (FDA) has approved three agents: Interferon beta-la, interferon beta-lb, and glatiramer acetate.

A double blind, randomized multicenter study called the Controlled High Risk Avonex Multiple Sclerosis Prevention Study (CHAMPS) has tested the efficacy of interferon beta-la with placebo in patients who had a monosymptomatic demyelinating event (optic neuritis, spinal cord, brainstem or cerebellar involvement). Patients had at least two white matter abnormalities on MR imaging. Analysis of CHAMPS data suggests that interferon beta-1a delays the onset of multiple sclerosis. The clinical and brain MRI results of the trial support initiating interferon beta-la treatment at the time of the first episode of optic neuritis occurring in patients at high risk of multiple sclerosis based on the presence of subclinical brain MRI lesions.

Newer oral drugs for multiple sclerosis like teriflunomide and dimethyl fumerate are not yet approved for this condition.

A study of intravenous immunoglobulin in optic neuritis has failed to show any statistical benefit and intravenous immunoglobulin is not recommended for routine use for patients with monosymptomatic optic neuritis. However, occasional cases, who did not respond to steroid

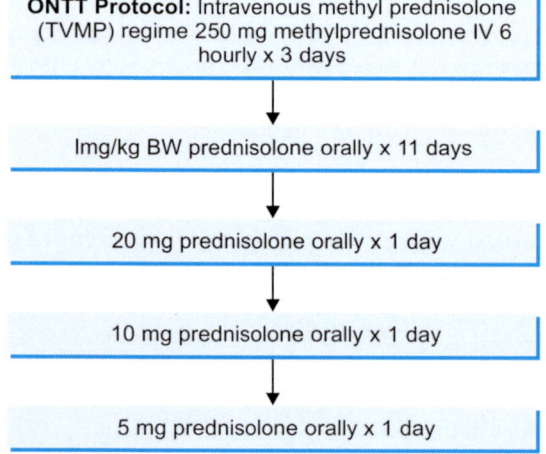

FLOWCHART 1: ONTT Protocol: Intravenous methyl prednisolone regime.

therapy may benefit from this agent and hence in such cases, the agent may be worth trying.

Can Any Drug Promote Optic Nerve Regeneration?

No current treatment can restore the function of a damaged optic nerve. In a phase II trial, an antibody against LINGO-1 (leucine-rich repeat and IgG domain containing a protein inhibitor of axonal growth) was found to diminish the latency of visual evoked potentials; this may be interpreted as optic nerve regeneration. The results of another phase II trial of anti-LINGO-1 are expected soon (the SYNERGY trial). Pilot trials have shown benefit from erythropoitin and simvastatin. A controlled trial of erythropoetin is in progress.

Chronic Recurrent Immune Optic Neuropathy

Chronic recurrent immune optic neuropathy begins like typical optic neuritis and improves rapidly under steroid treatment. However, recurs when the steroid dose is tapered. The disease often affects one eye first, then the other. If untreated, it leaves marked residual damage behind. In one-third of all affected eyes, visual acuity remains low. Prednisolone for at least 3 months at a dose below the threshold for producing Cushing syndrome (7.5 mg/day), or at the lowest dose that prevents recurrences to be continued. If this proves insufficient, then azathioprine or methotrexate can be considered as the second line of treatment

Other Inflammatory Optic Neuropathies (Other than Neuromyelitis Optica)

These are relatively uncommon, but need recognition for appropriate treatment. Inflammatory diseases of the choroid and retina may involve the optic nerves. Distinction from classic optic neuritis is important and is aided by the finding of vitreous cells during slit lamp examination. Neurologists should seek help from their ophthalmological colleagues in all cases where the presentation of optic neuritis may appear even slightly atypical. Inflammatory optic neuropathies may be infective or immune-mediated.

Infective Optic Neuropathies

Infectious meningitis and encephalitis, syphilis, toxoplasmosis, herpes simplex and zoster, tuberculous (part of basal meningitis), Lyme disease, bacterial sinusitis, fungal sinusitis.

Immune Optic Neuropathies

Postviral, postvaccinal, acute disseminated encephalomyelitis, *Guillain–Barré syndrome*, posterior uveitis, retinitis, Crohn's disease, ulcerative colitis, Reiter's syndrome, Sjogren's syndrome, *Behçet's disease*, Wegener's granulomatosis, lupus erythematosus.

Sarcoid optic neuropathy is well documented. Vision deterioration occurs with or without swelling of the disc, but systemic symptoms may be minimal. The optic nerve involvement is generally secondary to basal meningeal involvement. Response to corticosteroid is usually dramatic, but relapses with discontinuation is common. Hence, the need for maintenance therapy for several months or even years.

SUGGESTED READINGS

1. Alejandro PM, Castandon-Gonzalez JA, Miranda-Ruiz R, et al. Comparative treatment of acute optic neuritis with boluses of intravenous methyl prednisolone or oral prednisone. Gac Med de Mex. 1994;130:227-30.
2. Amiga J, Sanders MD. Ophthalmologic findings in 70 patients with evidence of retinal embolism. Ophthalmology. 1982;89:1336-47.
3. Beck RW, Cleary PA, Anderson MA, et al. A randomized, controlled trial of corticosteroid in the treatment of acute optic neuritis. N Engl J Med. 1992;326:581-8.
4. Beck RW, Cleary PA, Trobe JD, et al. The effect of corticosteroid for acute optic neuritis on the subsequent development of multiple sclerosis. N Engl J Med. 1993;329:1764-9.
5. Beck RW, Gal RL, Bhatti MT, et al. Visual function more than 10 years after optic neuritis: experience of the optic neuritis treatment trial. Am J Ophthalmol. 2004;137:77-83.
6. Beck RW, Trobe JD, Moke PS, et al. High and low risk profiles for the development of multiple sclerosis within 10 years after optic neuritis; experience of die optic neuritis treatment trial. Arch Ophthalmol. 2003;121:944-9.
7. Bowden AN, Bowden PMA, Friedman AL, et al. A trial of corticotrophin gelatin injection in acute optic neuritis. J Neurol Neurosurg Psychiatry. 1974;37:859-79.

8. Bradley WG, Wittey WM. Acute optic neuritis: Its clinical features and their relation to prognosis for recovery of vision. J Neurol Neurosurg Psychiatry. 1967;30:531-8.
9. CHAMPS study group. Interferon beta-la for optic neuritis patients at high risk for multiple sclerosis. Am J Ophthalmol. 2001;132:463-71.
10. Curro Dossi B, Amadoti A, Cirafisi C, et al. New therapeutic perspectives for demyelinating retrobulbar optic neuritis. Ital J Neurol Sci. 1998;19:45-8.
11. Ebers GC. Optic neuritis and multiple sclerosis. Arch Neurol. 1985;42:702-4.
12. Fletcher WA. The big blind spot syndromes. Ophthalmol Clin NA. 1991;4:531-46.
13. Galwan MJ, Kellen RI, Burde RM, et al. Sarcoidosis of the anterior visual pathway: Success and failures. J Neurol Neurosurg Psychiat. 1980;51:1381-6.
14. Garling J, Kommerell G. Short term effect of megadose steroid therapy in optic neuritis. Klin Monatsbi Augenheilkd. 1992;201:375-80.
15. Ghessi A, Martinelli V, Rodegher M, et al. The prognosis of idiopathic optic neuritis. Neurol Sci. 2000;21(4 suppl 2):S865-9.
16. Giles CL, Isaacson JD. The treatment of acute optic neuritis. Arch Ophthalmol 1961;66:52-5.
17. Glaser GH, Meritt HH. Effects of corticotrophin (ACTH) and cortisone on disorders of the nervous system. JAMA. 1952;148:898-904.
18. Glaser JS. Neuro-ophthalmology, 2nd ed. JB Lippincott Company: Philadelphia; 1990.
19. Gould ES, Bird AC, Leaver PK. McDonald WI Treatment of optic neuritis by retrobulbar injection of triamcinolone. BMJ. 1977;1:1485-97.
20. Hayrch SS. Anterior ischaemic optic neuropathy. Arch Neurol. 1981;38:675-8.
21. Heley MA, Mc Manis PG, Dovan TJ, et al. Acute optic neuritis: A prospective study of risk factors for multiple sclerosis. J Neurol Neurosurg Psychiatry. 1986;498:1125-30.
22. Herishanu YO, Badarna S, Sarov B, et al. A possible harmful late effect of methylprednisolone therapy on a time cluster of optic neuritis. Acta Neurol Scand. 1989;80:569-74.
23. Jacobs L, Munschauer FE, Kaba SE. Clinical and magnetic resonance imaging in optic neuritis. Neurology. 1991;41:15-9.
24. Jacobs LD, Beck RW, Simon JH, et al. Intramuscular interferon beta-la therapy initiated during a first demyelinating event in multiple sclerosis. CHAMPS study group. N Engl J Med. 2000;343:898-904.
25. Kapoor R, Miller DA Jones SJ et al. Effects of intravenous methylprednisolone on outcome in MRI - based prognostic subgroups in acute optic neuritis. Neurology. 1998;50:230-7.
26. Keltner JL. Giant cell arteritis. Signs and symptoms. Ophthalmology. 1982;89:1101-10.
27. Kitazava Y. Primary angle closure glaucoma. In: Fraunfelder FT, Ray FH. Current ocular therapy 3. WB Saunders Co., Philadelphia; 1990. p. 577-9.
28. Kurtzke JE. Optic neuritis or multiple sclerosis. Arch Neurol. 1985;42:704-10.
29. Lona-Pexoto MA, Andrade GC. Arq Neuropsiquiar. 2001;59:311-7.
30. Luechinett CF, Kieis L, O'Duffy A, et al. Risk factors for developing multiple sclerosis after childhood optic neuritis. Neurology. 1997;49:1413-8.
31. Miller NR, Newmann W. Walsh and Hoyt's Clinical Neuro-Ophthalmology, 4th ed. Williams & Wilkins, Baltimore; 1997.
32. Newman NJ. Hereditary optic neuropathies. In: Clinical Neuro Ophthalmology; Ed: Miller NR, Newman NJ 5th Ed. 1998. p. 649-62.
33. Newmann NJ. Optic neuropathy. Neurology. 1996;46:315-22.
34. Noseworthy JH, O'Brien PC, Patterson TM, et al. A randomized trial of intravenous immunoglobulin in inflammatory demyelinating optic neuritis. Neurology. 2001;56:1514-22.
35. Okasala A. Cortisone therapy in fasculitis optica. Ophthalmoplegica. 1964;148:13-24.
36. Optic Neuritis Study Group. The 5 year risk of multiple sclerosis after optic neuritis. Neurology. 1997;49:1404-18.
37. Petzold A, Plant GT. Chronic relapsing inflammatory optic neuropathy: A systemic review of 122 cases reported. J Neurol. 2013;261:17-26
38. Purvin V, Kawasaki A, Jacobson DM. Optic perineuritis: Clinical and radiographic features. Arch Ophthalmol. 2001;119:1299-306.
39. Rawson MD, Liversedge LA, Goldfarb G. Treatment of retrobulbar neuritis with corticotrophin. Lancet. 1966;2(7472):1044-6.
40. Rilkorsen R, Kelowen L, Sippessen J. Magnetic resonance imaging, evoked responses and cerebrospinal fluid studies in a follow up study of children with optic neuritis. Acta Neurol Scand. 1988;77:44-9.
41. Rizzo JF, Lersell S. Risk of developing multiple sclerosis after uncomplicated optic neuritis. A long term prospective study. Neurology. 1988;38:185-90.
42. Rucker CW. Optic neuritis of unknown etiology. Trans Am Acad Opthalmol Otolaryngol. 1956;60:93-6.
43. Sellebjerg F, Nielsen AS, Frederiksen JL, et al. A randomized controlled trial of high dose methylprednisolone in acute optic neuritis. Neurology. 1999;52:1479-84.
44. Spoor TC, Rockwell DL. Treatment of optic neuritis and intravenous megadose corticosteroid. A consecutive series. Ophthalmology. 1988;95:131-4.
45. Steinsapir KP, Goldberg RA. Traumatic optic neuropathies. In: Clinical Neuro-Ophthalmology; Ed Miller WR, Newman NJ, 5th ed, 1998. P. 719-39.

46. Toczolowski J, Lewandowska-Furmanik M, Stelmasiak Z, et al. Treatment of acute optic neuritis with large doses of corticosteroids. Klin Oczna 1995;97:122-5.
47. Trauzettel-Keosinski S, Aulhorn E, Diener HD, et al. Effect of prednisolone on the course of optic neuritis. Results of a double-blind study. Fortschor Ophthalmol. 1991;88:490-501.
48. Van Engelen BG, Hommes OR, Pinckers A, et al. Improved vision after intravenous immunoglobulin in stable demyelinating optic neuritis. Ann Neurol 1992;32:834-5.
49. Volpe NJ. Optic neuritis: Historical aspects. J Neuro Ophthalmol. 2001;21:302-9.
50. Wakakura M, Mashimok, Oono S, et al., Multicenter clinical trial for evaluating methylprednisolone pulse treatment for idiopathic optic neuritis in Japan. Optic Neuritis Treatment Trial Multicenter Cooperative Research Group (ONMRG). Jpn J Ophthalmal. 1999;43:133-8.

9 Neuromyelitis Optica Spectrum Disorders

Debasish Roy, Ambar Chakravarty

INTRODUCTION

Neuromyelitis optica (NMO) (previously known as Devic's disease) and neuromyelitis optica spectrum disorders (NMOSDs) are a heterogeneous group of disorders characterized by severe immune-mediated demyelination and axonal loss involving mainly the optic nerves and the spinal cord. It is now known that it involves other areas of the nervous system and has extra neurological manifestations as well. It is characterized by the presence of a disease-specific antibody which binds to aquaporin-4 (AQP4) located at the foot process of astrocytes. It is a unique biomarker for this disease and may be present in about 80% of cases using proper assay methods.

Neuromyelitis optica spectrum disorder causes significant morbidity and mortality and is prone to relapse in about 90% of the cases. It needs tailored therapy for the initial acute attack and relapses and also requires long-term immunotherapy to prevent relapses.

HISTORICAL ASPECTS

The first clinical account of presumed NMO is often attributed to Sir Clifford Allbutt, a pioneering physician who promoted the adoption of the direct ophthalmoscope in clinical practice. However, even before Allbutt's seminal publication, "On the Ophthalmoscopic Signs of Spinal Disease", clinicopathologic reports of individuals with concurrent vision loss and myelitis by Antoine Portal in 1804, Giovanni Pescetto in 1844, and Jacob Clarke in 1865 likely represent the earliest accounts of NMO in the literature. The term "neuromyélite optique aiguë" was originally coined in 1894 by Eugène Devic and his student Fernand Gault when they presented a case of concurrent optic neuritis (ON) and transverse myelitis (TM) and reviewed 16 additional cases from the literature. Although their initial article included patients with simultaneous and relapsing episodes of ON and TM, NMO was initially defined as a monophasic disorder. Interestingly, in the early 1900s, more than 100 cases had been reviewed in the literature, and an increasing number of relapsing cases were reported. Wingerchuk and his coworkers performed the first systematic evaluation of the demographics, clinical presentation, neuroimaging, and cerebrospinal fluid (CSF) in cases of monophasic and relapsing NMO. "Strict" NMO was defined as bilateral ON and TM occurring within a 2-year interval, whereas NMO "not meeting strict criteria" included cases of unilateral ON or recurrent demyelinating events occurring over greater than a 2-year period. Relapsing cases of NMO, which outnumbered monophasic cases by two-fold, were defined by the occurrence of additional clinical attacks outside the incident event. Although demographics distinguished monophasic and relapsing patients with NMO, common clinical, imaging, and CSF findings allowed the first modern diagnostic criteria to be proposed (Table 1). Several tenets of the 1999 NMO criteria persist in subsequent criteria including the clinical hallmarks of ON and TM, and also spinal cord magnetic resonance imaging (MRI) demonstrating a signal abnormality extending over three vertebral segments longitudinally. Neuromyelitis optica was initially believed to be a variant of multiple sclerosis (MS). Later it was found that the natural history, clinical course, and response to therapy were different from the common relapsing remitting form of MS.

TABLE 1: Historical classification of neuromyelitis optica (NMO) and neuromyelitis optica spectrum disorder (NMOSD).

Wingerchuk 1999 NMO criteria	Wingerchuk 2006 NMO criteria	IPND 2015 NMOSD criteria

All absolute criteria and one major or two minor supportive criteria.
Absolute criteria:
• Optic neuritis
• Acute myelitis
• No evidence of clinical disease outside optic nerve or spinal cord
Supportive criteria:
• Major
  ○ Negative brain MRI at onset
  ○ Spinal cord MRI with lesion extension over three vertebral segments
  ○ CSF pleocytosis of 50 WBC
• Minor
  ○ Bilateral optic neuritis
  ○ Severe optic neuritis with fixed visual acuity worse than 20/200 in at least one eye
  ○ Severe, fixed, and attack-related weakness (MRC grade 2) in one or more limbs
	All absolute criteria and two supportive criteria.
	Absolute criteria:
	• Optic neuritis
	• Acute myelitis
	Supportive criteria:
	• Contiguous spinal cord MRI lesion extending over three vertebral segments
	• Brain MRI not meeting diagnostic criteria for MS
	• AQP4-IgG–seropositive status
		NMOSD with AQP4-IgG:
		• At least one core clinical characteristic
		• Positive test for AQP4-IgG using best available detection method
		• Exclusion of alternative diagnoses
		NMOSD without AQP4-IgG:
		• At least two core clinical characteristics occurring as a result of one or more clinical attacks and meeting all of the following requirements
		• At least one core clinical characteristic must be optic neuritis, acute myelitis with LETM, or area postrema syndrome
		• Dissemination in space (two or more different core clinical characteristics)
		• Additional MRI requirements, as applicable
		• Negative tests for AQP4-IgG using best available detection method or testing unavailable
		• Exclusion of alternative diagnoses
		Core clinical characteristics:
		• Optic neuritis, acute myelitis, area postrema syndrome (hiccups, nausea, and vomiting), acute brainstem syndrome, symptomatic narcolepsy or acute diencephalic clinical syndrome with NMOSD-typical diencephalic MRI, and symptomatic cerebral syndrome with NMOSD-typical brain AQP4-IgG serology. Cell-based assay is strongly recommended

AQP4-IgG, aquaporin-4 immunoglobulin G; CSF, cerebrospinal fluid; IPND, International Panel for NMO Diagnosis; LETM, longitudinally extensive transverse myelitis; MRI, magnetic resonance imaging; WBC, white blood cell; MRC, Medical Research Council; MS, multiple sclerosis.

A set of diagnostic criteria was devised in 1999. In 2004, the novel biomarker, the AQP4 antibody was detected. A new set of criteria was devised in 2006 by Wingerchuk and his coworkers. Later it was realized that the disease was not restricted to the optic nerves and spinal cord and a new set of diagnostic criteria was devised in 2015 and the universal term of NMOSDs was introduced. This enabled a diverse group of disorders to be grouped together sharing some common pathological features and characterized by the presence of AQP4 antibody.

EPIDEMIOLOGY

In India, there is insufficient data for demyelinating disorders and NMO and NMOSD. A population-based survey in urban Mangalore has shown a prevalence of 2.6/100,000 for NMO and 8.3/100,000 for MS. Neuromyelitis optica represents about 20% of all demyelinating disorders in India. In African-Americans, Hispanics, and Asians, the ratio of NMO and NMOSD to MS is higher than that of Caucasians. Women and men are equally represented in the monophasic form of the illness whereas females out number males in a ratio of about 9–10:1 in the relapsing form. The mean age of onset (32.6–45.7 years) and mean time to first lapse (8–12 months) are same across different population groups and it is about a decade older than MS populations.

CLINICAL FEATURES

The core clinical features of NMOSDs include ON, acute long segment myelitis, area postrema syndrome, acute brainstem syndrome, symptomatic narcolepsy, acute diencephalic syndrome, and symptomatic cerebral syndrome.

Optic Neuritis

Optic neuritis presents with severe visual loss, loss of color vision, and pain on eye movements. In NMOSD, the involvement is usually severe and bilateral or rapidly sequential with poor recovery. Usually, a long segment of the nerve is involved and posterior extension to involve the optic chiasma is fairly common. In addition to central and centrocecal scotomas, altitudinal field defects, or meridian defects are common.

Acute Myelitis

Myelitis in NMOSD is usually longitudinally extensive involving more than three vertebral segments. The cord may be swollen and edematous in the acute phase. Usually, the central part of the cord and the gray matter are involved and more than 50% of the cross-sectional area is affected. In MS, the cord is involved in a restricted fashion and the dorsolateral regions are commonly affected. Long segment myelitis usually results in complete paralysis below the level of the lesion with complete sensory loss and bladder and bowel involvement. In an acute attack, the symptoms progress in a time frame of more than 4 hours to less than 21 days. The thoracic and cervical cords are commonly involved and the lesion may extend cranially to involve the medulla which may cause respiratory dysfunction. Myelitis is often characterized by the presence of Lhermitte's sign (electric shock-like sensation on neck flexion) and painful tonic spasms. Recovery from a long segment myelitis is usually incomplete and patients are left with significant residual neurological deficit after an acute attack.

Area Postrema Syndrome

Area postrema syndrome is characterized by intractable nausea, vomiting, and hiccups either occurring together or in isolation. They can be treated by gastroenterologists and the etiology may be unknown unless there is clinical suspicion and a brain MRI is performed. The area postrema is believed to be the site of entry of the AQP4 antibody. These symptoms usually respond well to corticosteroids.

Acute Brainstem Syndrome

Brainstem syndromes are frequent in NMOSD. Vomiting and hiccups are very common. Ocular motor abnormalities, pruritus, facial palsy, and trigeminal neuralgia have also been recorded. Vertigo and vestibular ataxia may also be present.

Symptomatic Narcolepsy and Acute Diencephalic Syndrome

A syndrome of narcolepsy and excessive daytime somnolence has been observed in this group of patients with hypothalamic involvement. These patients usually have low hypocretin or orexin levels. Some patients may have disorders of temperature regulation like hypo- or hyperthermia or even poikilothermia. Anorexia, obesity, and other types of feeding disorders may be present. Bilateral thalamic lesions may present with altered sensorium or an acute confusional state.

Symptomatic Cerebral Syndrome

Large cerebral lesions may present with encephalopathy, focal motor deficits, or seizures. Sometimes, symptoms may resemble posterior reversible encephalopathy syndrome (PRES) and such patients may have typical imaging findings.

EXTRACEREBRAL MANIFESTATIONS

Neuromyelitis optica spectrum disorder may involve structures outside the central nervous system (CNS). Patients may present with myalgia and raised creatine phosphokinase (CPK) levels. The placenta may be involved resulting in abortion. Internal otitis and gastritis have also been reported.

DISEASE ASSOCIATIONS

Neuromyelitis optica spectrum disorder can be associated with systemic lupus erythematosus (SLE), Sjögren syndrome, rheumatoid arthritis, Behçet's disease, and other connective tissue or autoimmune disorders. There may be associations with autoimmune thyroid disorders, pernicious anemia, gastritis, inflammatory bowel disease, and other organ-specific autoimmune disorders. Several types of autoantibodies may be present. Paraneoplastic autoantibodies like CRMP5 have been detected in a small number of cases. N-methyl-D-aspartate (NMDA) receptor antibodies have also been described. These antibodies are not considered pathogenic unless they are associated with relevant clinical features.

MAGNETIC RESONANCE IMAGING IN NEUROMYELITIS OPTICA SPECTRUM DISORDER

Brain

Brain findings in NMOSD are different from what we find in MS. Juxtacortical and periventricular lesions are conspicuously absent. Dawson's fingers, lesions perpendicular to the ventricular margin are not found.

The most common finding is the presence of widespread T2 abnormalities and periependymal lesions adjacent to the ventricular system including the diencephalic area and callosal and brainstem regions. In MS, the callosal lesions are small, oval shaped, and discrete with clear cut margins. In NMOSD, the lesions are larger. They usually do not have clear cut margins. Corpus callosal lesions may have a lot of edema showing a heterogeneous marbled appearance when the entire thickness of the corpus callosum is involved. It may give an arch bridge appearance on occasions. Large hemispheric lesions may also be seen and lesions may be visualized along the line of the corticospinal tracts.

The lesions may enhance with gadolinium if imaging is done in the acute phase. Sometimes, there may be a thin rim of enhancement along the line of the ventricles (pencil thin enhancement).

When in regression, these lesions may disappear but there may be persistent T1 hypointensity and cavitary lesions may be found.

Spinal Cord

Spinal cord lesions are long, often involving more than three vertebral segments. They occupy the central position of the cord. In the acute phase, the cord may be swollen and takes up contrast. After treatment, the long segment of contrast-enhanced cord may break up into smaller fragments. In later stages, the cord may be atrophied and thin and may not take up any more contrast.

Optic Nerves

Orbital sections are needed for proper evaluation of NMOSD. Optic nerves show gadolinium enhancement in the acute phase. A long segment of the optic nerve may be involved. More posterior extension up to the level of the optic chiasm may be seen. During remission, there is no contrast enhancement.

AQUAPORIN-4 IMMUNOGLOBULIN G ANTIBODY

In 2004, Lennon made the groundbreaking observation that most patients with NMO express serum autoantibodies [aquaporin-4 immunoglobulin G (AQP4-IgG)] against the AQP4 water channel. Subsequently, multiple investigators devised a variety of assays to detect AQP4-IgG in serum and CSF. Although the sensitivity and specificity of individual assays vary, AQP4-IgG seropositivity is generally considered to have 75% sensitivity and 99% specificity for disease. Importantly, AQP4 autoantibodies are typically undetected in clinically definite MS.

The AQP4 also known as NMO-IgG is a stable marker for this disease. It is detected in the severe phase in about 80% of cases. There are different methods of detection. The reliable and accurate method is a cell-based assay which may be live antigen or prefixed antigen based. A cell-based assay is the gold standard for the detection of AQP4 antibody. It is positive in about 80% of cases and is highly specific. Titers rise during acute attacks and relapse and fall during remission.

Because of increased sensitivity, cell-based serum assays using microscopy-based or flow cytometry-based detection are recommended for AQP4-IgG serologic testing. Enzyme-linked immunosorbent assay (ELISA) and indirect immunofluorescence (IIF) of tissue sections are typically less sensitive and often yield lower-titer and false-positive tests. Therefore, caution is recommended in making a diagnosis of NMOSD with AQP4-IgG in cases where low-titer AQP4-IgG is detected by ELISA or IIF, and symptoms are outside the three most common core clinical presentations: (1) ON, (2) TM, or (3) area postrema syndrome. Confirmatory testing using more than one assay is generally recommended.

ANTIMYELIN OLIGODENDROCYTE GLYCOPROTEIN ANTIBODY

Anti-myelin oligodendrocyte glycoprotein (MOG) is present in a subset of patients with NMOSD who are AQP4 negative. As the name suggests, the antibody is directed against the oligodendrocytes. The disease pattern may be different from the classic form. It is more common in males and children. Bilateral ON is more common. It is a monophasic illness and runs a benign course. If the cord is involved, the caudal portion, i.e., conus is more frequently involved and there is a lot of bladder, bowel, and sexual dysfunction.

CEREBROSPINAL FLUID STUDIES

Examination of the CSF is not mandatory for the diagnosis of NMOSD but it may yield valuable information. During an acute episode or relapse, the CSF is cellular with about 300–500 cells. In addition to lymphocytes, eosinophils and neutrophils may be found. Oligoclonal bands are found in only 20% of cases in contrast to MS where it is a common association. During an acute attack, the CSF may show acute phase reactants like glial fibrillary acidic protein (GFAP), interleukin-6 (IL-6), and other complement products.

OPTICAL COHERENCE TOMOGRAPHY

Optical coherence tomography (OCT) is not routinely used in the work up of NMOSD. It shows a greater retinal nerve fiber layer thinning than MS and this is associated with worse prognosis. Microcystic macular edema may be found and is characteristic.

DIAGNOSTIC CRITERIA

The International Panel for NMO Diagnosis (IPND) was convened in 2011 and tasked with developing new diagnostic criteria based on clinical, laboratory, and neuroimaging data. In recognition of accumulating data that the clinical behavior, treatment, and pathology of AQP4-IgG–seropositive patients with incomplete or atypical presentations of NMO are not different from patients fulfilling previous diagnostic criteria, the term NMOSD was chosen as a new diagnostic marker. Because approximately 25% of patients meeting previous NMO criteria were seronegative for AQP4-IgG, separate diagnostic criteria for seronegative NMOSD were formulated using a mixture of clinical and radiologic criteria. The result was the generation of two new diagnoses: (1) NMOSD with AQP4-IgG and (2) NMOSD with negative or unknown AQP4-IgG.

Six core characteristics were identified:
1. Optic neuritis
2. Acute long segment myelitis
3. Area postrema syndrome
4. Acute brainstem syndrome
5. Symptomatic narcolepsy or acute diencephalic syndrome
6. Symptomatic cerebral syndrome.

Diagnosis of Neuromyelitis Optica Spectrum Disorder in the Presence of Aquaporin-4 Antibodies

- At least one core clinical characteristic must be present
- A positive test for AQP4-IgG antibody using the best available assay (cell-based assay is strongly recommended)
- Exclusion of alternative diagnosis.

Diagnosis of Neuromyelitis Optica Spectrum Disorder with Negative or Unknown Aquaporin-4 Antibody Status

- At least two core clinical characteristics must be present occurring as a result of one or more clinical attacks and meeting the following requirements:

- At least one core characteristic must be ON, longitudinally extensive transverse myelitis (LETM), or area postrema syndrome
- Dissemination in spare (two or more core clinical characteristics)
- Fulfillment of additional MRI requirement as applicable.

Additional Magnetic Resonance Imaging Requirements for Neuromyelitis Optica Spectrum Disorder with Negative or Unknown Aquaporin-4 Status

- Acute ON requires brain MRI to be normal or showing only nonspecific white matter lesions.
  Optic nerve MRI with T2 hyperintense lesions or T1 gadolinium-enhancing lesions extending over more than one-half of optic nerve length or involving optic chiasma
- Acute myelitis—Required associated intramedullary MRI lesion extending over more than three contiguous segments or segments of total spinal cord atrophy in patients with prior history compatible with myelitis
- Area postrema syndrome—Requires additional dorsal medulla and pontine lesions
- Acute brainstem syndrome—Required associated periependymal lesions.
  This diagnostic criteria has helped in bringing a range of neurological disorders under one broad diagnostic umbrella.

FUTURE CLASSIFICATIONS

The ultimate classification of NMOSD may be molecular, using multiple discrete biomarkers to combine seemingly diverse demyelinating disorders into a common nosologic category based on shared immunopathology and histopathology. The most notable has been AQP4-IgG, a serum biomarker of humoral immunopathology that is highly specific for NMOSD and has important prognostic and therapeutic implications. Unfortunately, additional biomarkers of NMOSD immunopathology and CNS injury lack the sensitivity and specificity to provide successful categorization of all cases of seronegative NMOSD. In addition, it remains unclear which cases of clinically defined AQP4-IgG–seronegative NMOSD show NMO-specific lesional histopathology.

Approximately 20% of AQP4-IgG–seronegative patients are seropositive for MOG-IgG. Multiple immunologic and histopathologic features of MOG-IgG–seropositive NMOSD indicate that this condition is nosologically distinct from AQP4-IgG–seropositive NMOSD despite its overlapping clinical presentation. The combined clinical and experimental data indicate that MOG-IgG–seropositive patients with TM and ON should be classified outside NMOSD and may represent a subgroup of patients with MS or acute disseminated encephalomyelitis.

A molecular classification of demyelinating disorders may ultimately require substantial advances in technology to reach fruition. Improvement in serologic, radiologic, and immunologic assays is likely to be required to reach levels of sensitivity and specificity necessary to delineate closely aligned demyelinating disorders with overlapping clinical presentations and immunopathologies.

PATHOGENESIS

Neuromyelitis optica and NMOSD are characterized by focal demyelination of optic nerves and spinal cord. There are widespread axonal changes in addition to demyelination. There is vascular proliferation and cellular infiltration not only with lymphocytes but also with neutrophil and eosinophils. The complement cascade and various mediators of inflammation are incorporated. As a result, there is severe inflammation at the site of injury. The AQP4 antibody is directly pathogenic and is directed against the foot processes of the astrocytes. The astrocytes involved result in the breach of the blood–brain barrier. Increasing titers of AQP4 antibody is associated with increasing severity of the disease. This disease is an autoimmune disease which is primarily antibody-mediated. As a result of this, anti-inflammatory agents and immunosuppressives form the basis of therapy.

In the connective tissue diseases, myelitis is often associated with the presence of AQP4 antibody and the myelitis should be regarded as a NMOSD rather than a manifestation of the autoimmune disease.

How Does Neuromyelitis Optica Spectrum Disorder Differs from Multiple Sclerosis?

- Neuromyelitis optica spectrum disorder patients are generally older than MS patients
- Neuromyelitis optica spectrum disorders are more common than MS in nonwhite populations
- Female preponderance is higher in NMOSD
- Compared to MS, NMOSD myelitic lesions are longitudinally more extensive, complete spinal cord involvement is more common, central cord involvement is more common, more than half cross-sectional area involvement is more common, T1 hypointensity may be present, and poor recovery is more common
- Compared to multiple sclerosis: In NMOSD, simultaneous bilateral ON is more common, posterior extension even up to chiasm is more common, and poor recovery is more common
- Area postrema syndrome and diencephalic syndrome occurs exclusively in NMOSD
- In brain magnetic resonance imaging: Both Dawson's finger lesions and juxtacortical lesions are uncommon in NMOSD whereas, extensive hemispheric lesions are more common
- Aquaporin IgG antibody always absent in MS but present in 80% of NMOSD cases
- Cerebrospinal fluid oligoclonal band is found more commonly in MS (about 90%) than NMOSD (<25%)
- Cerebrospinal fluid GFAP often very elevated in NMOSD but not in MS.

TREATMENT

Acute attacks of NMOSD and relapses are immediately treated with intravenous (IV) methylprednisolone and are followed by plasma exchange (PLEX) if symptoms progress or are refractory to initial therapy. As about 90% of the patients tend to relapse long-term immune suppression is needed.

Acute Treatment

- Acute attacks should be treated with utmost urgency. The widely used and accepted regimen is IV methylprednisolone IgG daily for 3–5 days. This is the preferred initial therapeutic option as it is cheap and widely available, safe, and easy to administer
- A large majority of patients do not respond to initial IV methylprednisolone therapy or are left with significant residual neurodeficit. In such cases, the initial pulse glucocorticoid therapy is usually followed by therapeutic PLEX. Plasma exchange is a process where the patient's blood cells are separated from the serum by centrifugation and transfused back. The plasma is replaced by appropriate fluids and proteins. The body gets rid of the circulating antibodies and by this method, PLEX creates a therapeutic response. Normally about five to seven such exchanges are made over a 7–10 days period. Plasma exchange requires a setup with trained personnel experienced with the procedure. Plasma Exchange has complications in the form of central venous access, bleeding, volume overload and coagulation abnormalities, and hypocalcemia
- It has been seen that glucocorticoids followed by PLEX usually gives a better therapeutic response than glucocorticoids alone
- Intravenous immunoglobulins have widespread use in other neuroimmunological disorders like acute inflammatory demyelinating polyneuropathy (AIDP) and myasthenic crisis. It is not found to be as effective in NMOSD. It is only used if patients do not show a response to glucocorticoids and facilities for PLEX are not available or it is contraindicated
- Intravenous cyclophosphamide can be tried in very refractory cases but because of its toxicity, many do not recommend its use.

Preventive Treatment

Neuromyelitis optica spectrum disorders are seen to relapse in about 90% of cases. Long-term immunosuppression is necessary for prevention of relapses.

There is scarcity of data which is mostly retrospective and no standard regime is recommended. The most commonly used agents are azathioprine, mycophenolate mofetil, and rituximab.

Azathioprine

This is a purine analog and prevents proliferation of lymphocytes. It is used along with steroids as it takes about 12 weeks to exert its full therapeutic effect. The normal therapeutic dose is 2–3 mg/kg of body weight. Therapy is started with 75 mg daily and dose is gradually titrated upward. It must be used very cautiously in patients with thiopurine methyltransferase deficiency. Common side effects include gastrointestinal and dermatological side effects, emergence of neoplasms, and depressed blood counts. Routine tests are done weekly for the 1st month, twice a month for the next 2 months, and monthly thereafter.

Mycophenolate Mofetil

It has been used as an immunosuppressant in different autoimmune disorders. Mycophenolate mofetil has shown promise in NMOSD. It is used in a dose of 2,000–3,000 mg orally usually in two divided doses. It has almost similar efficacy to azathioprine, is quicker acting, and somewhat less toxic. It is a known teratogen and is contradicted during pregnancy. Monitoring is similar to azathioprine.

Rituximab

- Rituximab is a chimeric monoclonal antibody which acts against CD20 cells and has been used in a large variety of autoimmune disorders and hematological malignancies. It has been found to be very effective in NMOSD. It is either used as 375 mg/m² in four doses 1 week apart or a fixed dose of 1,000 mg 2 weeks apart. Maintenance therapy is usually after 6 months or whenever there is rise in lymphocyte count or emergence of CD19 or CD27 T cells. Rituximab can cause emergence of hepatitis B and other opportunistic infections which may arise as a consequence of therapy. Because of anaphylaxis, it is usually coadministered with parenteral antihistaminic, analgesic, and glucocorticoids
- No consensus exists about the duration of therapy. Best practice parameters say that long-term immune suppression should continue for at least 5 years since the appearance of the last symptoms or until the AQP4 antibody is persistently negative. Sometimes, lifelong therapy may be necessary
- Some other agents like cyclophosphamide and methotrexate have been used but evidence is lacking
- Tocilizumab is a novel monoclonal antibody acting against the chemokine IL-6. It has shown promise in some therapeutic trials
- Eculizumab is also a monoclonal antibody and acts against some complement components and has also been found effective in a small subset of patients
- Bortezomib, a commonly used medication in multiple myeloma has also been used. It is known to produce severe painful neuropathy
- The agents used in MS like interferons, fingolimod, and alemtuzumab are not useful and may worsen the course of illness.

ADJUNCTIVE THERAPY

- Neuromyelitis optica spectrum disorder affects several areas of the neuraxis and causes severe disability and handicap. Generalized weakness and fatigue, gait dysfunction, depression, urinary discomfort, and sleep disturbances are found in a significant number of patients. These issues must be taken into account and addressed with appropriate therapeutic measures
- Pain is a common symptom and may respond to antiepileptic drugs like gabapentin or carbamazepine. Sometimes, antidepressants like amitriptyline or duloxetine may be needed in refractory cases. Tramadol and similar strong analgesia may be needed
- Painful tonic spasms often respond to low dose of long-acting carbamazepine (100–200 mg). Baclofen or tizanidine may be needed if spasms are persistent and do not respond to carbamazepine
- Poor visual conditions may be managed with physical measures like prisms and other devices with help of ophthalmologists
- A multidisciplinary approach may be needed for optimal management of this long-term debilitating disorder.

PROGNOSIS

- Neuromyelitis optica and NMOSD are very aggressive diseases and usually lead to long-

term disability and handicap. Because of relapses, there is accumulation of motor and sensory deficits and bladder and bowel dysfunction. Repeated attacks may leave a patient almost blind. Predictors of poor outcome are:
  - Number of relapses in the first 2 years
  - Increased severity of the first attack
  - Older age at onset
  - Poor response to initial therapy
  - Coassociation with other autoimmune disorders.
- Mortality rates may be high in patients who develop neurogenic respiratory failure with cranial extension of cervical lesions or primary brainstem lesions
- With advances in long-term immune therapy, the mortality rates have declined in recent years. Patients also have better intensive care support during periods of acute attacks or relapses. Although NMOSD is a severe debilitating disorder, the future holds some promise with development of newer immune suppressants, better intensive care management, and rehabilitative measures.

CONCLUDING REMARKS

- Neuromyelitis optica spectrum disorders are inflammatory diseases of the nervous system characterized by severe immune-mediated demyelination and axonal damage of the optic nerves and the spinal cord. Other areas of the nervous system may also be involved
- Hallmark features include unilateral or sequential ON causing visual loss, long segment TM causing limb weakness and bladder and bowel dysfunction, and area postrema syndrome presenting with intractable hiccups, nausea, and vomiting
- Neuromyelitis optica spectrum disorder has a relapsing course in 90% of cases and females out number males by a ratio of about 10:1
- In addition to a detailed history and comprehensive neurological examination, diagnosis requires the estimation of AQP4 status using a cell-based assay and MRI imaging of the brain and spinal cord with gadolinium contrast in all cases
- For an acute attack, initial therapy is with high dose IV methylprednisolone IgG daily for 3–5 days
- For patients with severe disease or who do not respond to IV methylprednisolone, PLEX is recommended
- Long-term immune suppression is needed and should be continued for at least 5 years since last relapse or for as long as patients remain seropositive
- Immunosuppressive therapy must be complemented with a multidisciplinary approach addressing the multiple needs of the patient for best outcome measures.

SUGGESTED READINGS

1. Abboud H, Petrak A, Mealy M, et al. Treatment of acute relapses in neuromyelitis optica: Steroids alone versus steroids plus plasma exchange. Mult Scler. 2016;22(2):185-92.
2. Bennett JL. Finding NMO: The evolving diagnostic criteria of neuromyelitis optica. J Neuroophthalmol. 2016;36(3):238-45.
3. Katz Sand I. Neuromyelitis optica spectrum disorders. Continuum (Minneap Minn). 2016;22(3):864-96.
4. Pandit L. Neuromyelitis optica spectrum disorders: An update. Ann Indian Acad Neurol. 2015;18(Suppl 1):S11-5.
5. Wingerchuk DM, Banwell B, Bennet JL, et al. International consensus diagnostic criteria for neuromyelitis optica spectrum disorders. Neurology. 2015;85(2):177-89.
6. Wingerchuk DM, Lennon VA, Pittock SJ, et al. Revised diagnostic criteria for neuromyelitis optica. Neurology. 2006;66(10):1485-9.

10 Noninflammatory Optic Neuropathies

Debasish Roy, Sandip Chatterjee, Ambar Chakravarty

INTRODUCTION

Several noninflammatory pathologies may involve the optic nerves to cause visual loss. To distinguish them from one another and from typical demyelinating optic neuritis, one must ascertain the course of the visual loss, whether the condition is monocular or binocular, the pattern of the visual field loss and the ophthalmoscopic findings. Ancillary tests, including brain imaging may be necessary to make a definitive diagnosis. The present chapter would briefly highlight the major forms of noninflammatory optic neuropathies— their recognition and management principles, when applicable.

ISCHEMIC OPTIC NEUROPATHIES

Ischemic optic neuropathy (ION) is a general term and includes all ischemic causes of optic neuropathy (Box 1). Anterior ischemic optic neuropathy (AION) indicates pathology in the optic disk—swelling with peripapillary hemorrhages. Posterior (or retrobulbar) ischemic optic neuropathy (PION) indicates that no disc swelling or abnormality is evident. The AION accounts for about 90% of the cases.

Blood Supply

The anterior portion of the optic nerve is supplied by a pial plexus derived from branches of the ophthalmic artery and the central retinal artery. The optic nerve head near the lamina cribrosa is supplied by a rich capillary network called the circle of Zinn-Haller which receives blood from three sources (Fig. 1):
- Choroidal feeder vessels
- Short posterior ciliary vessels
- Vessels derived from distal branches of the ophthalmic artery.

Box 1: Causes of anterior ischemic optic neuropathy (AION)

- Arteritic AION
  - Giant cell arteritis
  - Systemic vasculitis other than giant cell arteritis: Systemic lupus erythematosus, periarteritis nodosa, Chugh–Strauss syndrome
- Non-arteritic AION
  - Anatomical factors: Small crowded disk—"disk-at risk" Drusen
  - Anomalous disk, severe papilledema
  - Hypotension: Operative (spinal and cardiac surgery), systemic hemorrhage, local surgery (intraocular hypertension), cardiac arrest, renal dialysis
  - Anemia
  - Hypercoagulability disorders
  - Radiation optic neuropathy

The posterior segment of the nerve has a poorer blood supply. It is supplied by the pial capillary plexus that surrounds it. Only a small number of capillaries actually penetrate the nerve and extend to its central portion (Fig. 2).

Anterior Ischemic Optic Neuropathy (AION)

A common physiological variation involved in the pathogenesis of AION is the so-called "disk at risk". A small cup-to-disk ratio causes crowding of the vascular supply at the optic nerve head and makes it vulnerable to ischemia. Often in a patient suffering from AION the small cup-to-disk ratio is visible in the fellow eye (Fig. 3).

Clinical Characteristics and Pathophysiology

The average age of onset of AION ranges from 55 to 70 years but it has been recorded in as young as 11-year-old patients, especially when associated with a "disk at risk".

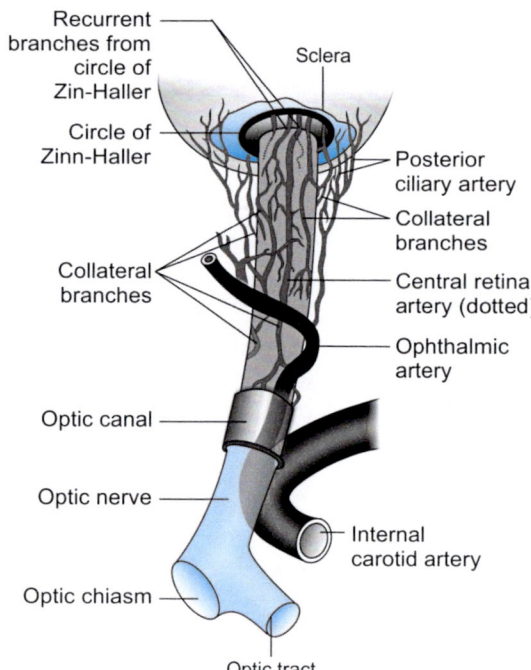

FIG. 1: Blood supply of the optic nerve and disk.

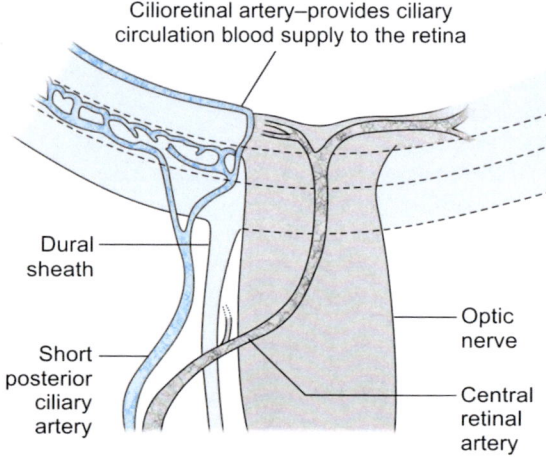

FIG. 2: A simplified scheme of blood supply to optic disk and retina. The importance of the cilioretinal artery is evident.

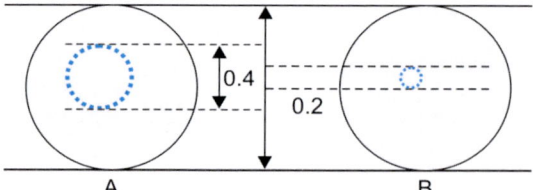

FIG. 3: Diagram to illustrate cup-to-disk ratio. A, Normal; B, Small cup favoring anterior ischemic optic neuropathy.

ratio. However, the present authors feel that the condition is on the whole underdiagnosed in Indians.

The AION is characterized by acute, painless monocular loss of vision. It may progress over several hours or days. Examination shows a relative afferent pupillary deficit and optic disk swelling (which may be focal or segmental) along with peripapillary hemorrhages. Gradually, the disk develops sectorial pallor and the edema resolves. The visual field defect is altitudinal and mainly inferior although the type of field defect is not specific enough to diagnose AION with certainty. Superior altitudinal defects, arcuate defects, ceco and ceco-central scotomas have all been described. The AION patients have relatively well-preserved visual acuity, compared to giant cell arteritis (GCA) with about 50–60% of patients having visual acuity of 20/60 or better. Recurrence is uncommon but fellow-eye involvement risk is about 15% at 5 years. Increased incidence of fellow eye involvement is associated with poor baseline visual acuity in the involved eye and diabetes. It is not related to age, sex, smoking or aspirin use.

Associated systemic diseases in AION include hypertension in about 51% of patients and diabetes in about 74%. Ischemic heart disease, dyslipidemia, cerebrovascular accidents, smoking, and systemic arteriosclerosis are often associated. In the Ischemic Optic Neuropathy Decompression Trial (IONDT) 60% of patients had risk factors for small vessel cerebrovascular disease. Anterior ischemic optic neuropathy can also be precipitated by hypotension or blood loss.

Some medicines have been implicated in the causation such as sumatriptan or other triptans, sildenafil, amiodarone, and nasal decongestants. Mechanical factor such as elevated intraocular pressure during ocular surgery (refractive or cataract surgery) may act as a triggering factor. The

Incidence of nonarteritic AION is about 2–3 per 100,000, persons over the age of 50 years and 0.54 per 100,000 for all ages. It is more common among Caucasians, and this may result from genetic differences including the cup-to-disk

AION is rarely associated with ipsilateral carotid artery stenosis.

Embolic AION is extremely rare. This is a disease of the small vessels supplying the optic nerve head. On a few occasions, optic nerve infarction results from reduced perfusion pressure secondary to severe carotid occlusive disease (especially dissections) and poor collateral blood supply.

It is not necessary to obtain a carotid ultrasound in all patients who develop AION. If there is a carotid bruit, if visual symptoms are suggestive of hypoperfusion of the eye (blurred vision with change of posture, bright light or exercise) or if AION was preceded by transient monocular visual loss, Horner's syndrome or orbital pain, noninvasive carotid imaging may be justified.

Rare cases of AION have been associated with congenital thrombotic tendencies. Anterior ischemic optic neuropathy have been reported with antiphospholipid antibodies, protein C, and protein S deficiency, factor V Leiden mutation, hyperhomocysteinemia, and *MTHFR* mutation. According to data published by Salomon et al. routine laboratory testing for hypercoagulable states in a patient without family or past medical history is not justified.

In all cases of AION, the arteritic form must be identified and treated as early treatment is essential to prevent permanent damage. Arteritic AION will be discussed later.

Classically, it was considered that AION presents with nonreversible severe visual loss. The IONDT has demonstrated that AION could present with mild or no visual loss and that about 31% of patients spontaneously regained three or more lines of visual acuity above baseline at 6 months of follow-up.

Recurrence in the same eye is reported in less than 5% of cases. Atrophy of impacted axons may relieve the crowding of nerve fibers at the vulnerable disk and create more space, and make it less vulnerable to subsequent attack of AION.

Treatment

There is no established treatment for nonarteritic AION. The clinician's primary role is to exclude giant cell arteritis and to control other factors that might affect visual outcome in the fellow eye.

Since some of the risk factors for nonarteritic AION and small vessel cerebrovascular disease are common, it would seem logical to take steps for modification of these risk factors. However, overzealous control of hypertension with risk of nocturnal hypotension may precipitate AION.

It would seem reasonable to use antiplatelet agents but the IONDT trial has failed to show a protective effect of aspirin in the fellow eye.

However, considering the low side effect, and cost of low dose aspirin therapy, it may be justified. Other antiplatelet agents may also be considered.

Other modes of therapy like anticoagulants, thrombolytics, vasodilators, vasopressors, phenytoin, corticosteroids, levodopa, and hyperbaric oxygen have all been tried and discarded.

Surgical treatment has been proved ineffective. In 1989, Sergott et al. suggested that optic nerve sheath decompression might improve vision. In progressive form of AION, surgery consists of making 2 or 3 slits or a window in the optic nerve sheath just behind the eyeball allowing cerebrospinal fluid to escape and thereby reducing pressure around optic nerve.

The IONDT study[5] was initiated in 1992 to test the safety and efficacy of optic nerve decompression surgery compared to careful follow-up in patients with nonarteritic AION in a randomized multicenter controlled trial. Inclusion criteria included nonarteritic unilateral AION over age of 50 years with no evidence of concurrent or past vasculitis, collagen vascular, or demyelinating disease. Total of 420 patients joined the study and 258 patients with visual acuity worse than 20/60 were randomized to surgery and follow-up. Patients who went for surgery did no better than patients with follow-up. Based on this, the trial was terminated earlier than planned.

Approximately, 32.6% of surgical group improved three or more lines of vision compared to 42.7% of the follow-up group. Around 23.9% of surgical group worsened by three or more lines of vision compared to 12.4% in the follow-up group. The IONDT concluded that optic nerve decompression surgery for nonarteritic AION is not effective, may be harmful and should be abandoned.

Giant Cell Arteritis

Giant cell arteritis (GCA) commonly produces visual loss. Anterior ischemic optic neuropathy accounts for 75% of GCA, related visual loss, while retinal artery occlusion or PION make up the rest. Approximately, 5% of cases with AION are related to GCA, but it is crucial to identify this subgroup as it has important therapeutic considerations.

Incidence of GCA increased with age from approximately 2.3/100,000 in the sixth decade to 33.7/100,000 in the ninth decade. Female to male ratio is 3.4:1 and there is a higher incidence in Caucasians of -northern European descent. Giant cell arteritis is relatively uncommon in India. In 1972, Wadia commented that he had not seen a single case in India. One of the present authors (AC) could collect only 38 cases over a period of 15 years. The sex bias was not that obvious as in the West. Interestingly, though all patients presented with headache, only one male patient had visual loss. It is possible that this condition is also underdiagnosed in India and a high index of suspicion is warranted.

Clinical Features

Arteritic AION may have a sudden onset or follow episodes of transient visual loss. Visual loss is more severe than with classical nonarteritic AION. The disk exhibits pallid edema and cotton wool spots

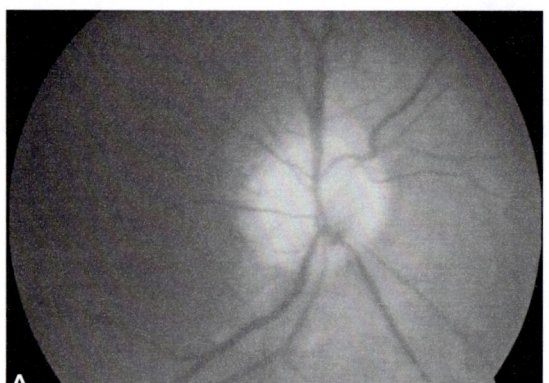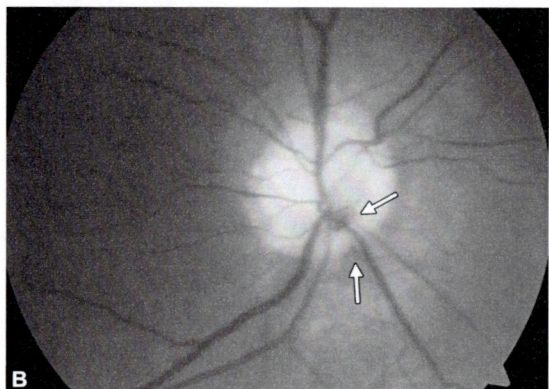

FIG. 4: Fundoscopy in a case of anterior ischemic optic neuropathy showing discal and peripapillary hemorrhages (Fundus anterior ischemic optic neuropathy). *(For color version, see Plate 1)*

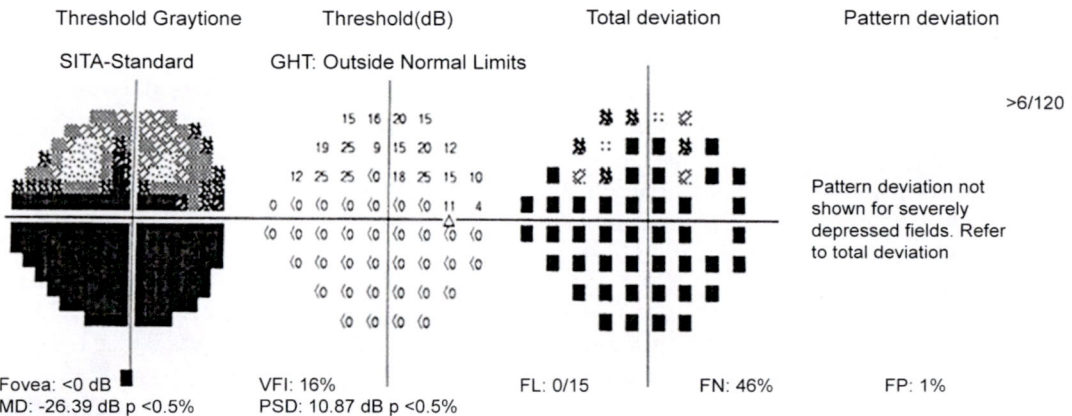

FIG. 5: Right eye visual field showing inferior altitudinal field defect.

(nerve fiber layer infarction) may be present. The presence of cotton wool spots and disk edema implies involvement of both central retinal artery and posterior ciliary arteries and indicates a widespread vascular process. The cup-to-disk ratio is not a risk factor and the cup may be of any size. Fellow eye may be involved in 20–50% of untreated cases. Bilateral simultaneous onset indicates GCA. Giant cell arteritis is a systemic disease and most patients have extravisual symptoms, which include headache, scalp tenderness, jaw claudication, myalgia (polymyalgia rheumatica), anorexia, weight loss, and fever.

Although headache is the most common extravisual symptom, jaw claudication is the most specific symptom. Jaw claudication should be considered a hallmark of GCA and treated as such until proved otherwise.

Laboratory Features

Include a raised erythrocyte sedimentation rate (ESR), high leukocyte count and a raised C-reactive protein (CRP). Most patients demonstrate an elevated ESR; some authorities believe that CRP is more sensitive and specific than ESR. However, ESR is also an important prognostic guide and generally used to monitor response to therapy.

Temporal artery biopsy is easy to perform and safe in experienced hands. It should be performed even with a low index of suspicion. Biopsies may remain positive even up to 3 weeks after initiation of therapy and so in cases with high index of suspicion, therapy should be initiated before the results become available.

Treatment

This should be prompt and aggressive. Therapy should be started with high index of clinical suspicion. Most authorities favor a high dose of intravenous steroids initially to be substituted later with high dose of oral prednisolone. Steroid tapering should be very slow and ESR/CRP can be used as a therapeutic guide to monitor the activity of inflammatory process. Some patients may have to remain on steroids for life.

The majority of patients do not regain visual loss from GCA once it has occurred and so the treatment aim would be to identify patients at risk and treat them before visual loss appears. Treatment protocol thus includes—"treat first, biopsy later, and treat aggressively from the start."

Distinguishing features of demyelinating optic neuritis (ON), nonarteritic and arteritic forms of AION are depicted in table 1.

Table 1: Comparative clinical features of optic neuritis and anterior ischemic optic neuropathy

	Optic neuritis	AION (Nonarteritic)	AION (Arteritic)
Age	Younger	Older >75 years	Older >65 years
Laterality	Unilateral	Unilateral	Unilateral or bilateral
Visual loss	Rapidly progressive; acuity rarely spared	Acute; acuity variable	Acute with severe visual loss
Pain	Orbital pain frequent with eye movements	Pain infrequent	Pain common
Color vision	Abnormal	Commonly spared	Spared if vision not totally lost
Visual field	Central defect	Altitudinal defect (inferior)	Any defect
Optic disk	Acute phase normal (2/3); disk edema (1/3); late temporal pallor	Acute phase: Segmental disk edema, small cup-disk ratio, late segmental pallor	Diffuse pallor, cotton wool spots, cupping late
Visual prognosis	Good; 25% recurrence	Variable; 15% second eye risk in 5 years	Poor; 75% second eye risk in 2 weeks
Systemic disease	Risk of multiple sclerosis	Hypertension (51%) Diabetes (24%)	Giant cell arteritis: 25% have isolated visual loss.

Posterior Ischemic Optic Neuropathy

This is much less common compared to AION. Diagnosis of PION is made only after other causes of retrobulbar optic nerve dysfunction (inflammatory, toxic, compressive) have been excluded. The posterior segment of the nerve is supplied by the pial capillary plexus that surrounds it and only a small number of capillaries actually penetrate the nerve and extend to its central portion along the pial septae. As a result, the center of the posterior portion of the optic nerve is much poorly vascularized compared with its anterior portion. No structural abnormalities of the optic disk has been identified as "disk at risk" seen in AION.

Patients with PION have sudden visual loss in one eye, typically painless. Examination reveals decreased visual acuity, visual field loss, relative afferent papillary defect and a normal-appearing optic disk. Optic disk pallor may ensue 4–6 weeks after acute visual loss.

Most cases of PION have been described in specific clinical setting including immediately following a variety of surgical procedures and in patients with a variety of systemic vascular disorders, including GCA, Takayasu arteritis, SLE, migraine, carotid dissection, and sickle cell hemoglobinopathy.

Sadda et al. reviewed 72 cases of PION from two large medical centers. Three distinct groups of patients emerged. One group consisted of patients with nonarteritic PION. This patients have some underlying vascular disorders and risk factors as patients who develop nonarteritic AION do not have the structural variation of "disk at risk".

The second group consists of patients with arteritic PION. These patients most commonly have GCA although other forms of vasculitis need to be excluded. These group patients are older, have worse initial visual acuity and have lesser tendency to improve than patients with nonarteritic PION.

The third group of patients are those who develop the disease in the perioperative setting. These patients tend to be younger and may have bilateral simultaneous involvement. Patients with perioperative PION have worse initial vision and worse ultimate vision than patients with nonarteritic PION.

Over 50% of patients with perioperative PION develop it after spinal surgery, typically of the lower back and typically after being kept in the prone position for many hours. Intraoperative risk factors include hypotension, anemia, hypovolemia, blood loss, hypoxia, and hemodilution. There may be an anatomical watershed region involving the vascular supply of posterior optic nerves in some individuals, rendering these patients more vulnerable to fluctuation in blood pressure and oxygen delivery compared to others.

Spinal surgeons and anesthetists should discuss the potential risk of visual loss in patients with prolonged spinal surgery in the prone position which may involve significant blood loss.

The course of nonarteritic PION is similar to that of AION with about one third of patients having some visual improvement.

Prognosis for visual recovery in patients with arteritic PION and those in the perioperative setting is poor.

Radiation Optic Neuropathy

Optic nerve and retinal toxicity may follow megavoltage irradiation of paranasal sinus, nasopharyngeal, or middle fossa neoplasms. If radiation doses of more than 4000 Gy reach the retina, the fundus may show microaneurysms, hemorrhages, exudates, cotton wool spots, and neovascularization, a picture similar to that seen in diabetes. The clinical course tends to be slowly progressive, leading to severe, or even total visual loss and to intractable neovascular glaucoma. Photocoagulation may be helpful, but reports are anecdotal.

If the optic nerves, rather than the eyes, lie within the irradiated field, optic neuropathy without retinopathy typically occurs at total tumor doses in excess of 6000 Gy and daily dose fractions greater than 180 Gy. The patient has acute loss of sight, but the optic fundi are normal. A relative afferent pupillary defect and nerve fiber bundle visual field defects localize the damage to the optic nerve. A bitemporal or junctional hemianopic defect indicates that the lesion also involves the optic chiasm. MRIs, which may be difficult to interpret because of postoperative changes, usually demonstrate enhancement of the involved region of the optic nerve or chiasm. Sometimes the tissue is swollen enough to falsely suggest a new tumor or tumor recurrence. Spinal fluid is generally normal.

Pathologic studies show changes similar to those of delayed radiation effects on the spinal cord and brain—vascular endothelial proliferation and fibrinoid necrosis, necrosis of white and gray matter, and reactive astrocytosis. Although direct toxicity to neuronal tissue is a possibility, more likely the principal target is the vascular endothelium; brain tissue is damaged by ischemia.

There is no effective treatment. Despite initial enthusiasm over hyperbaric oxygen and corticosteroids, neither has proved helpful. A regimen of heparin followed by warfarin anticoagulation produced a modest improvement in nonvisual neurologic signs in a small cohort, but there is no published experience with visual loss.

COMPRESSIVE OPTIC NEUROPATHY

In compressive optic neuropathy, visual loss may gradually worsen in the face of a slowly expanding intraorbital or intracranial mass or decline apoplectically in the face of a rapidly enlarging mass (pituitary), hemorrhage, aneurysm, mucocele, or craniopharyngiomatous cyst. Pain is a variable accompaniment. High-resolution imaging is essential in diagnosis. Corticosteroid treatment often produces rapid improvement in visual function, leading to a misimpression of optic neuritis.

Most masses that compress the optic nerve intracranially also affect the optic chiasm and cause hemianopic visual field defects. Intraorbital masses that compress the optic nerve usually cause proptosis or other congestive ocular adnexal signs.

INFILTRATIVE OPTIC NEUROPATHY

Infiltration of the optic nerve may be associated with lymphoma, leukemia, plasmacytoma, or carcinoma. Sudden, painless (usually monocular) loss of vision occurs with a normal or swollen optic disk. Optic neuritis is often mistakenly diagnosed at first.

Some evidence of a primary malignancy usually turns up, but it may be subclinical. Parenchymal central nervous system metastases need not be present, but magnetic resonance imaging (MRI) may show enhancement of the optic nerves and meninges. Cancer cells can be difficult to harvest even after several lumbar punctures.

Vision often improves dramatically in response to systemic steroid therapy and local irradiation. In fact, infiltrative optic neuropathy is quite often more steroid-responsive than is typical optic neuritis.

Thus, dramatic improvement in vision within 48 hours of commencing corticosteroid treatment should be regarded as suspicion for atypical optic neuritis or compressive/infiltrative optic neuropathy.

HEREDITARY OPTIC NEUROPATHY

The hereditary optic neuropathies may be divided into those in which the optic neuropathy is the predominant manifestation and those in which optic neuropathy is part of a systemic disorder. Among the disorders isolated to the eyes, two follow Mendelian inheritance pattern and one mitochondrial inheritance pattern.

Dominant Optic Neuropathy

This genetically dominant disorder accounts for most cases of inherited optic neuropathy. It depresses visual acuity within the first decade of life but so minimally and insidiously that diagnosis is often long delayed. Visual acuity loss is typically symmetric (within 2–3 Snellen lines) and ranges from 20/25 to 20/400 (median 20/80). Visual fields reveal central or cecocentral scotomas and there is a tritan axis of color blindness. Optic disks show a characteristic wedge-shaped temporal pallor. In some pedigrees, the degree of optic disk excavation is severe enough to suggest glaucoma. Because of the symmetric visual loss, there is no afferent pupil defect. In the early-onset cases, nystagmus is common.

There is so much intrafamilial variation in the degree of acuity loss that mildly affected family members do not suspect that they have the disease until their optic disks are discovered to be pale and when sensitive tests of visual function (contrast sensitivity, foveal thresholds, color vision, VEPs) show abnormalities. Pathologic examination reveals loss of retinal ganglion cells and their axons within the papillomacular bundle. The genetic defect has been located on the chromosome 3q region. There is no effective treatment.

When the familial nature of this disorder is not known, examiners may be misled by the bilateral cecocentral visual field defects, which often resemble bitemporal hemianopic defects, to believe that this slowly progressive disorder is caused by a mass lesion in the chiasmal region.

Recessive Optic Neuropathy

This extremely rare disorder presents at birth or within the first year of life with severe visual loss, pendular nystagmus, intensely pale but normally configured optic disks, and attenuation of retinal vessels. Parents are often consanguineous. The attenuated retinal vessels cause the diagnostician to suspect congenital photoreceptor dystrophy (Leber's congenital amaurosis), but electro-retinographic findings are normal. An imaging evaluation for a chiasmal region mass is inevitable.

Most of the genetically recessive optic neuropathies have associated systemic abnormalities. These should be sought whenever severe binocular optic neuropathy presents within the first years of life.

Leber's Hereditary Optic Neuropathy

Unlike dominant and recessive optic neuropathy, which are based on defects in nuclear DNA, Leber's hereditary optic neuropathy (LHON) is a disorder of mitochondrial DNA transmitted through females, mostly to their sons. The mitochondrial source accounts for the maternal transmission; mitochondria are passed to offspring exclusively through the mother's ovum. The preferential involvement of male is still unexplained.

The LHON has four mitochondrial genome mutation sites at DNA positions 11778, 3460, 14484, and 14459 (the latter causes dystonia in addition to optic neuropathy). The mutated mitochondrial DNA fails to code for the proper enzymes to mediate energy production (adenosine triphosphate) in the electron transport oxidative phosphorylation pathway of the mitochondria. Each mutation appears to affect different aspects of the energy chain, although most abnormalities involve the first step (complex I). Retinal ganglion cells succumb to energy failure, but why these cells are harmed selectively remains a mystery, since the mutation affects mitochondria in cells everywhere in the body.

The relative prevalence of the different mutations varies from country to country, but the 11778 mutation accounts for more than 50% of cases, the 14484 and 3460 are less common, and 14459, the rarest. The male preponderance varies from 8:1 for the 14484 mutation to 4:1 for the 11778 and 3460 mutations.

The diagnosis of LHON is confirmed biochemically by assessing the patient's whole blood for one of the recognized mutations. The absence of any of these mutations reasonably excludes LHON. On the other hand, an identified mutation does not necessarily mean that the patient will develop clinical signs of LHON. This discrepancy may be partially explained by "heteroplasmy", the phenomenon of having a mixture of mutant and normal (wild-type) mitochondrial DNA. Heteroplasmy has been discovered in as many as 14% of cases, principally at the 11778 site. Presumably, a greater proportion of normal DNA protects the cells against energy failure. The mutant signature in the person's blood gives no indication of the proportion of mutant DNA in the retinal ganglion cells. Other factors that could determine a genetically affected individual's chance of developing the disease include mutations at other mitochondrial DNA sites (secondary mutations) whose association with LHON is indeterminate.

The LHON has two clinical phases, presymptomatic and symptomatic. In the presymptomatic phase, which may last many years, ophthalmoscopy discloses thickening of the peripapillary retina and dilatation of fine retinal surface vessels. This telangiectasia does not leak with fluorescein injection. Visual function is normal. Many presymptomatic LHON patients never develop symptoms.

The symptomatic phase usually begins between ages 15 and 40 years (but ranges from age 6 to 80 years) with painless acute or subacute monocular visual acuity loss. An afferent pupil defect is usually present but may be subtle. Visual fields show a central or cecocentral scotoma. The peripapillary telangiectasis and nerve fiber layer thickening become more florid, but fluorescein angiography shows no leakage, an indication that the blood-retina barrier remains intact. In some cases, the fundus abnormalities are extremely subtle or even absent. Visual loss progresses over days to weeks to reach 20/200 or worse. Months after symptoms appear, the optic nerve turns diffusely pale and the succulent peripapillary changes give way to an atrophic nerve fiber layer. Within weeks to months after the attack in the first eye, the second eye begins to lose vision and the sequence is repeated. Some visual recovery, which may be delayed for years, occurs in 5% of patients with 11778 mutation, 22% with 3460, and 37% with 14484.

The LHON is frequently missed, at least initially. In young persons, swelling of the optic disk region is mistaken for optic neuritis and in older patients for AION. If the optic disk region appears normal, young persons receive a diagnosis of retrobulbar optic neuritis, and older ones are investigated for compressive or infiltrative diseases. In persons with LHON, MRI may further mislead by demonstrating optic nerve enlargement[56] or white matter signal abnormalities typical of MS. In the presymptomatic phase, binocular peripapillary plethora may be misinterpreted as papilledema.

Since LHON has been genetically typed, the clinical spectrum of the disorder is recognized as being much wider than was originally supposed. Some patients with bilateral visual loss and optic disk pallor, initially assumed to have optic neuropathy or a toxic-nutritional cause, have tested positive for a LHON mutation. Another important feature of LHON is that it may not be limited to the eyes. Some patients demonstrate features of MS, ataxia, peripheral neuropathy, and cardiac conduction abnormalities. This spectrum is reminiscent of other mitochondrial disorders.

There is yet no effective treatment. Because of the link to the oxidative phosphorylation pathway, patients have been prescribed antioxidants (vitamins C and E, coenzyme Q) and urged to avoid tobacco and foods containing cyanide.

TOXIC OPTIC NEUROPATHY

Toxins causing optic neuropathy target the maculopapillar bundle, causing visual acuity loss, central and cecocentral scotomas, and dyschromatopsia. This pattern is shared with most hereditary and nutritional deficiency optic neuropathies. The only hope of reversing toxic optic neuropathy is to remove the offending factor quickly, and even then it may be too late.

Many medications and substances has been linked to optic neuropathy, but cause-and-effect relationship have been conclusively established only for a few.

Methanol Optic Neuropathy

Methanol poisoning causes apoplectic, profound, and largely irreversible binocular optic neuropathy, usually in alcoholics seeking an ethyl alcohol substitute or in depressed persons attempting suicide. The methanol is metabolized to formic acid, which produces a severe metabolic acidosis that leads to vomiting, reduced consciousness, delirium, and parkinsonism. Vision is poor. Pupillary responses are symmetrically reduced, and ophthalmoscopy demonstrates either no abnormalities or mild optic disk edema, especially in the peripapillary region. The optic nerves eventually turn pale.

The MRI signal abnormalities are concentrated in the basal ganglia and in parieto-occipital white matter. Pathologic examination shows anoxic injury in these regions and in the retrobulbar optic nerve. The pattern of brain involvement is similar to that of asphyxiation or cardiopulmonary arrest. Treatment is aimed at correcting the acidosis, but when poisoning has been severe, blindness, parkinsonism, and memory loss persist.

Ethambutol Optic Neuropathy

Ethambutol, an antituberculosis agent, causes a slowly progressive binocular optic neuropathy. Like many toxins, it has a predilection for damaging the papillomacular fibers, causing cecocentral scotomas and poor color vision, but it may also involve the optic chiasm to produce bitemporal hemianopia. With currently recommended daily doses (15–25 mg/kg) the incidence of clinical optic neuropathy is less than 3%. Patients with renal failure may be at higher risk.

Visual loss and dyschromatopsia develop after 2–8 months of therapy. Because pupillary reactions are normal and no structural alterations are discernible in the globes at this stage, the complaint may be dismissed as psychogenic visual loss. The VEPs are useful to document whether the complaints are organic. If the medication is not discontinued, visual acuity continues to decline, and eventually temporal optic disk pallor appears.

Once disks are pale and visual loss is profound, withdrawing the medication may not restore any vision. In fact, vision may continue to deteriorate.

Isoniazid Optic Neuropathy

Because isoniazid is rarely administered without ethambutol, evidence for its independent optic nerve toxicity is less secure than for ethambutol. The damage pattern is similar to that of ethambutol except that optic disk edema may occur. Peripheral neuropathy is common, and pyridoxine may be protective against both peripheral and optic neuropathy.

Clioquinol Optic Neuropathy [Subacute Myelo-Optic Neuropathy (SMON)]

In the mid-fifties, there was described in Japan a new neurological disorder that, a decade later, achieved epidemic proportion with a peak annual incidence of 2300 cases in 1969. Cases had possibly been described earlier in 1938; however, clear clinical information was scanty. The clinical features consisted of myelopathy, optic atrophy, and peripheral neuropathy, in various combinations and of variable severity. These features gave the name SMON to the disease. Characteristically, the patient complained of symmetrical paresthesia and dysesthesia in the feet, ascending the legs and this was often preceded by abdominal pain. The subsequent evaluation was the development of other neurologic features, namely neuropathy, myelopathy, and unilateral visual disturbances including optic atrophy. This indeed was a novel clinical entity and reached epidemic proportion in Japan in the late 1960s.

In spite of detailed epidemiological studies, the cause of the syndrome remained unclear till 1970 when it was noted that some SMON patients had green tongues as well as green urine and feces. This green pigment was subsequently found to be an iron chelate of clioquinol (an antiamoebic drug) and hence SMON was attributed to a neurotoxic effect of clioquinol. The sale of the drug was banned in Japan and by one year there had been a dramatic fall in the incidence of SMON. The cause–effect relationship was thought to be clearly established; though doubted by some as a small proportion of patients with clinical picture similar to SMON never took the drug. The latter was later interpreted as misdiagnosis or as related to clioquinol ingestion unknowingly.

The clioquinol neurotoxicity appeared to be largely a Japanese problem; although a few cases were reported in the literature as also to the manufacturers from countries other than Japan. Since at one time clioquinol (Mexaform) was widely prescribed in India, a few cases mimicking SMON were probably encountered by some Indian neurologists as well but not given adequate attention in subsequent reviews. Much later (in 1996) one of the present authors (AC) encountered a very similar syndrome in a mother and her daughter both of whom were consuming enteroquinol (chemically somewhat similar to clioquinol) continuously for few years (without medical supervision). Very satisfactory symptomatic improvement occurred months after offending drug withdrawal (unpublished data). Infrequent occurrences of such isolated cases would certainly call for continued surveillance on habitual amoebicidal drug users (presumably for irritable bowel disease) in tropical countries like India, even when clioquinol is not now marketed anywhere in the world.

Tobacco and Alcohol-related Optic Neuropathy

Slowly progressive binocular optic neuropathy has been described in patients who consume heavy doses of tobacco or alcohol and who seem to have no other reasons for optic nerve disease.

Evidence for the independent toxicity of tobacco is weak. Many people smoke; few have optic neuropathy. The testimonials to the reversibility of visual loss with smoking cessation alone are unconvincing. Tobacco toxicity is said to result from an accumulation of cyanide moieties that impair oxidative phosphorylation and cause demyelination. A genetically low level of vitamin B12, which binds cyanide ions, and low dietary intake of amino acids (methionine, cysteine, and cystine) needed to detoxify cyanide may confer sensitivity to the toxic effects of tobacco. The cyanide hypothesis has been used to justify treatment with hydroxycobalamin, a form of vitamin B12 especially effective in binding cyanide. Cyanide toxicity from eating the staple cassava was blamed for an epidemic of bilateral optic neuropathy (tropical amblyopia), sensorineural deafness, myelopathy, and peripheral neuropathy in Nigeria.

Direct neurotoxicity of alcohol has been established experimentally. However, like tobacco, alcohol abuse is prevalent, yet few alcoholics get optic neuropathy. Alcohol neurotoxicity seems to require genetic predisposition and dietary or absorption deficiencies, particularly of B-complex vitamins (see nutritional deficiency optic neuropathy later). In classic studies on prisoners of war, conducted a half century ago, optic neuropathy remitted with dietary supplementation of thiamine or B-complex vitamins, even when the patients continued heavy drinking and smoking.

Nutritional Deficiency Optic Neuropathy

The principal dietary deficiencies implicated in optic neuropathy involve the B-complex vitamins. Thiamine (B1) is a cofactor in the energy-yielding breakdown of glucose to acetyl coenzyme A. Folate and B12 detoxify cyanide and formic acid, both of which interfere with mitochondrial oxidative phosphorylation (oxphos). Dysfunction of oxphos impairs axoplasmic transport in the longest axons (causing peripheral neuropathy) and conduction in the smallest, least myelinated axons such as those of the papillomacular bundle (causing central scotoma). Thus, the pathogenesis may be similar to that of LHON. Indeed, the LHON mutation has been found among abusers of alcohol and tobacco who develop optic neuropathy. Tobacco, alcohol, and ethambutol ingestion, and B12 and folate deficiency could be factors that cause optic neuropathy in persons predisposed by a mitochondrial mutation.

Vitamin B-complex Deficiency Optic Neuropathy

Several lines of evidence support B-complex vitamin deficiency as a contributor to optic neuropathy and other neurologic deficits. In most cases, no single vitamin deficiency alone has been implicated. Dietary supplementation with riboflavin, nicotinic acid, and other B-complex vitamins restored some vision in the World War II prisoners who had been malnourished. Thiamine B-complex vitamin treatment resulted in visual improvement in the Korean War prisoners.

Among case reports of the power of B-complex vitamins to restore sight, the 1991–1993 Cuban epidemic stands out. Poor nutrition set off an outbreak of optic neuropathy, myelopathy, sensorineural deafness, and peripheral neuropathy. A case-control study eventually implicated two familiar toxins—tobacco (especially cigars) and cassava (cyanide?), especially in undernourished persons. Reduced risk was associated with consumption of foods high in antioxidants. Vitamin B-complex and folate treatment improved sight. This modern case study epitomizes the complex inter-relationships between dietary deficiencies and toxins, suggests oxphos as a common pathogenic pathway, and justifies the use of antioxidants for prevention and treatment.

The role of B12 deficiency in optic neuropathy is strongly supported by experimental, pathologic, electrophysiologic, and clinical observations. Although optic neuropathy is subclinical in most cases of B12 deficiency, it may be a prominent manifestation in pernicious anemia, after gastrointestinal procedures that interfere with vitamin B-complex absorption and in fish tapeworm infestation.

Folate Deficiency Optic Neuropathy

The independent toxicity of folate on the optic nerves or spinal cord has never been firmly established. However, there are isolated reports of folate-deficient alcohol and tobacco abusers whose optic neuropathy improves with folate therapy alone.

OPTIC ATROPHY AND NEUROPATHIES: SOME INDIAN OBSERVATIONS

Menon et al. looked at the etiological profile of 484 cases of optic atrophies in India. Bilateral optic atrophy was more common than unilateral ones in hospital practice. Intracranial tumors especially pituitary chromophobe adenoma accounted for most cases of bilateral optic atrophy. However in younger individuals craniopharyngiomas were more common. Traumatic optic atrophy emerged as a major cause of unilateral optic atrophy in males while no definite factor could be elicited in unilateral optic atrophy in females. Surprisingly no clear mention of optic atrophies secondary to demyelinating optic neuropathies (including Devic's disease) has been mentioned in this study.

Menon et al. from All India Institute of Medical Sciences, New Delhi, reported on isolated cases of unusual optic neuritis related to ankylosing spondylosis, subacute sclerosing panencephalitis, cysticercosis, snake bite and herpes zoster ophthalmicus.

APPROACH TO PATIENTS WITH NON-COMPRESSIVE AND NONINFLAMMATORY BILATERAL OPTIC NERVE DISEASE

Patients who present with slowly progressive binocular visual loss, dyschromatopsia and maculopapillar bundle field loss should be suspected of having toxic, deficiency, or hereditary optic neuropathy. It is always advised to undertake appropriate imaging studies to exclude a chiasmal pathology as bilateral cecocentral scotomas may be difficult to distinguish from bitemporal hemianopias. If optic disks do not or doubtfully appear pale, evoked potential studies are justified to exclude psychogenic visual loss. If possible, an electroretinography is also indicated to exclude cone-rod dystrophy, which can manifest itself as optic disk pallor and central scotomas. An exhaustive laboratory workup is often needed and should usually include full blood count with RBC morphological indices, standard biochemical profile, protein electrophoresis, serum B12 and folate assay, serologic tests for sexually transmitted disease and Lyme's disease, plasma lead level, cerebrospinal fluid study to exclude occult inflammation and lastly molecular genetic study for LHON.

If all findings are negative, it may be advisable to treat patients with thiamine, multivitamins and possibly cyanocobalamin. It is not known if methylcobalamin may be superior. Patients must stop smoking and alcohol consumption.

TRAUMATIC OPTIC NEUROPATHY

The optic nerve may be damaged in injuries of the globe, orbit or brain. The cause of this injury may be blunt trauma, penetrating injury or a high-velocity injury caused by a gunshot. Regarding the optic nerve itself, it is important to recollect that this nerve is not a true nerve but an extension of the brain. Hence, the axons in the optic nerve cannot regenerate once damaged, a fact which imposes severe limitations to therapeutic options available in optic nerve injuries. It is also important to recall that for convenience the optic nerve is anatomically divided into four parts—intraocular, intraorbital, intracanalicular, and intracranial.

Trauma to different portions of the optic nerve may be considered separately:

- *Trauma to the intrabulbar portion:* This almost invariably occurs with a serious injury to the globe. These injuries are associated with intraocular hemorrhages which make fundoscopy unrewarding. Some investigators describe marginal hemorrhages extending to the disk, which disappear in a short time to be followed by a white scar. Visual field examination reveals a sector defect extending from the blind spot to the periphery.
- Trauma to the intraorbital portion: Isolated injury here is uncommon, except in penetrating gunshot wounds. Concomitant severe injuries to orbital contents exist, and there is usually proptosis, blindness, and multiple cranial nerve palsies.
- Trauma to the intracanalicular portion: This is the most vulnerable part in trauma. Although the cause may be penetrating injuries, in most cases the patient sustains closed head injury. Injury here results in monocular blindness, a dilated pupil with an absent direct pupillary and a brisk consensual pupillary response. The initial fundoscopic examination is unremarkable, but disk atrophy develops over weeks. In conscious patients, the diagnosis of optic nerve injury may be easy, but in unconscious patients with severe head injury, visual evoked responses may be useful. A good correlation exists between the initial visual evoked response and the ultimate visual acuity. In fact, Greenberg et al. showed that visual evoked responses are more accurate than clinical examination for assessing visual acuity in head trauma patients.
- *Trauma to the intracranial portion:* Isolated injuries here are extremely rare. Isolated bitemporal hemianopia has been documented in only 10% of patients identified to have clinical evidence of trauma to the intracranial

portion of the optic nerve or the chiasm. Most cases with injuries documented here have been associated with basifrontal fractures extending to the sellar region, resulting in stretch to the chiasm associated with interstitial hemorrhages and contusions. Vascular insufficiency may also play a role. In many patients with injuries here, neurological signs attributable to other structures in this region are discernible and include pituitary insufficiency, diabetes insipidus, carotid artery injury, caroticocavernous fistulae, cerebrospinal fluid fistulae, and other cranial nerve palsies.

Pathology

The pathogenesis of optic nerve injuries is mainly inferential. Most pathologial information has been obtained from postmortem studies of patients who died with severe head injuries. Gjerris has summarized the pathological abnormality as follows: The primary lesion is rarely a total section or laceration, but is usually a contusion, necrosis, ischemic necrosis or interstitial hemorrhage due to the blow or shearing at the time of impact. The pathogenesis of an immediate partial lesion is presumably the same, and in both cases tearing or injury to the pial vessels can lead to edema and infarction. The secondary edema occurs sporadically but is significant in those patients where visual deterioration occurs 2–6 days after the primary injury. A reaction to traumatic subarachnoid hemorrhage may lead to late-onset arachnoiditis and secondary loss of vision. Occasionally, after fracture, a callus may develop in the region of the optic foramen and this may cause progressive compression of the optic nerve.

Prognosis

The prognosis for visual recovery after a significant optic nerve injury is very poor. An extensive review of literature revealed that 50% of the patients remained blind, and as many as 75% showed no improvement in visual acuity or improvement of a visual field defect. If improvement is to occur, it begins within the first few days, and continues for 4–6 weeks, after which visual functions generally reach a plateau. It has been shown that the prognosis is slightly better for those patients whose visual acuity is diminished, but who retain a good pupillary response to light.

Medical Management

Once optic nerve injury is confirmed by neuro-ophthalmic examination, a high-resolution CT scan of the orbit should be supplemented with an MR scan of the orbit and brain. Treatment with steroids should be commenced as soon as possible. The recommended dose of methylprednisolone is 30 mg/kg intravenous stat followed by 15 mg/kg in the next 2 hours. Thereafter maintenance dose of methylprednisolone is used in a dose of 15 mg/kg every 6 hours, while evaluating response, as shown in the flowchart 1 below.

Surgical Management

Kline et al. have extensively reviewed the subject of surgical intervention for optic nerve injury. Their data shows that a significant number of patients with indirect injury to the optic nerve have spontaneous improvement, and the results of surgery largely are far from impressive. The only clear indication for operative intervention is when vision is initially good after trauma, and then progressive deterioration occurs thereafter. In such cases, especially if CT-scan shows bone fragments in the optic canal, surgical intervention should be prompt. No strict criteria exist for surgical intervention in patients with complete or partial loss immediately after killer trauma, patients with demonstrable fractures of the optic canal with or without visual loss, and patients with vision improving after trauma.

Traditionally the route of approach by neurosurgeons has been transcranial, but in a patient with brain swelling after trauma, the lateral orbital approach may be a better choice for reaching the optic nerve.

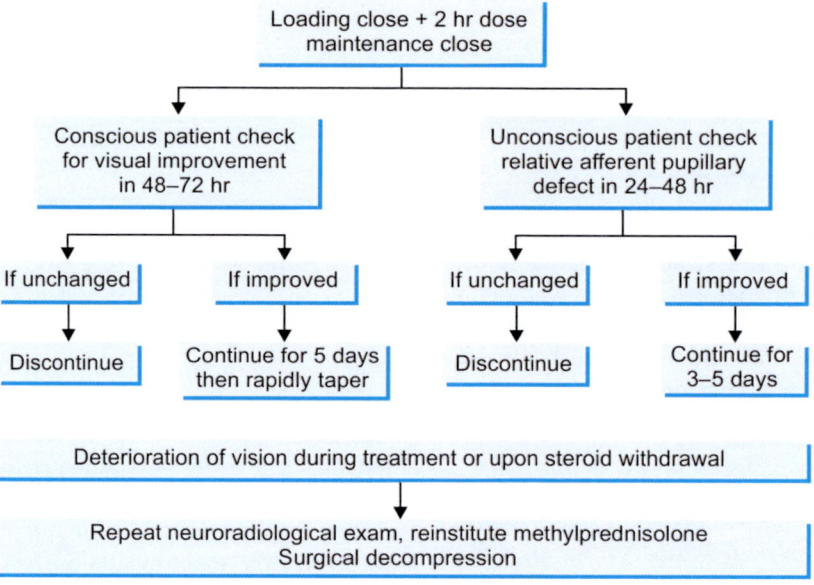

FLOWCHART 1: Approach To Traumatic Optic Neuropathy.

SUGGESTED READINGS

1. Adams RD, Kubik CS. Subacute combined degeneration of the brain in pernicious anemia. N Engl J Med. 1944;231:1-9.
2. Altrocchi PA, Reinhardt PH, Eckman PB. Blindness and meningeal carcinomatosis. Arch Ophthalmol. 1972;88:508-12.
3. Asayama T. Two cases of bitemporal hemianopsia due to ethambutol. Jpn J Clin Ophthalmol. 1969;23:1209.
4. Beck RW, Servais GE, Heyreh SS, et al. Anterior ischemic optic neuropathy. IX. Cup-to-disc ratio and its role in pathogenesis. Ophthalmology. 1987;94:1503-8.
5. Boghen DR, Glaser JS. Ischaemic optic neuropathy: The clinical profile and history. Brain. 1975;98: 689-708.
6. Carroll FD. Nutritional amblyopia. Arch Ophthalmol.1966;76:406-11.
7. Carroll FD. Optic nerve complications of cataract extraction. Trans Am Acad Ophthalmol Otolaryngol. 1973;77:623-9.
8. Clantz MJ, Burger PC, Friedman AH, et al. Treatment of radiation-induced nervous system injury with heparin and warfarin. Neurology. 1994;44:2020-7.
9. Cromptom MR, Layton DD. Delayed radionecrosis of the brain following therapeutic X-radiation of the pituitary. Brain. 1961;84:85-101.
10. Cullen JF, Coleiro JA. Ophthalmic complications of giant cell arteritis. Surv Ophthalmol. 1976;20:247-60.
11. Cullom ME, Heher KL, Miller NR. Leber's hereditary optic neuropathy masquerading as tobacco-alcohol amblyopia. Arch Ophthalmol. 1993;111:1482-5.
12. Devita EG, Miao M, Sadun AA. Optic neuropathy in ethambutol-treated renal tuberculosis. J Clin Neuro-ophthalmol. 1987;7:77-86.
13. Eiberg H, Kjer B, Kjer P, et al. Dominant optic atrophy (OPA1) mapped to chromosome 3q region, 1: Linkage analysis. Hum Molec Genet. 1994;3:977-80.
14. Ellis W, Little HL. Leukemic infiltration of the optic nerve head. Am J Ophthalmol. 1973;75:867-71.
15. Filley CM, Kelly JP. Alcochol and drug-related neurotoxicity. Curr Opin Neurol Neurosurg. 1993;6:443-7.
16. Fry CL, Carter JE, Kanter MC, et al. Anterior ischemic optic neuropathy is not associated with carotid artery atherosclerosis. Stroke. 1993;24:539-42.
17. Gjerris F. Traumatic lesions of the visual pathways. In: Vinken PJ, Bruyn GW, eds. Handbook of Neurology. New York; Elsevier,1976;24:27-57.
18. Golnik KC, Schaible ER. Folate-responsive optic neuropathy. J Neuro-ophthalmol. 1994;14:163-9.
19. Goodwin JA. Temporal arteritis. In Vinken PJ, Bruyn GW (eds): Handbook of Clinical Neurology, vol 39. Neurological Manifestations of Systemic Diseases, pt II. Amsterdam: Elsevier-North Holland, 1980.
12. Greenberg RP, Becker DP, Miller JD, et al. Evaluation of brain function in severe human head trauma with multimodality evoked potentials. Part 2: Location of brain dysfunction and correlation with post-traumatic neurological conditions. J Neurosurg. 1981;47:163-77.
13. Gudas PP Jr. Optic nerve myeloma. Am J Ophthalmol. 1971;71:1085-9.
14. Hamilton HE, Ellis PP, Sheets RE Visual impairment due to optic neuropathy in pernicious anemia: report of a case and review of the literature. Blood. 1959;14:378.

15. Harding AE, Sweeney MG, Govan GG. Pedigree analysis in Leber hereditary optic neuropathy families with a pathogenic mtDNA mutation. Am J Hum Genet. 1995;57:77-86.
16. Hayreh SS, Anterior ischemic optic neuropathy IV. Occurrence after cataract extraction. Arch Ophthalmol. 1980;98:1410-6.
17. Hayreh SS, Joos KM, Podhajsky PA, et al. Systemic diseases associated with nonarteritic anterior ischemic optic neuropadiy. Am J Ophthalmol. 1994;118:766-80.
18. Hayreh SS, Zimmerman MB, Podhajsky P, et al. Nocturnal arterial hypotension and its role in optic nerve head and ocular ischemic disorders. Am Ophthalmol. 1994;117:603-24.
19. Hunder GG, Michet C. Giant cell arteritis and polymyalgia rheumatica. Clin Rheum Dis. l985;11:471-83.
20. Huston KA, Hunder GG, Lie JT, et al. Temporal arteritis: A 25-year epidemiologic, clinical and pathologic study. Ann Intern Med. 1978;188:162-7.
21. Jefferson A. Ocular complications of head injuries. Tans Ophthalmol Soc UK. 1961;81:595-612.
22. Johns DR, Heher KL, Miller NR, et al. Leber's hereditary optic neuropathy. Clinical manifestations of the 14484 mutation. Arch Ophthalmol. 1993;111:495-8.
23. Johns DR, Newman NJ. Hereditary optic neuropathies. Semin Ophthalmol. 1995;10:203-13.
24. Johns DR. Mitochondrial DNA and disease. N Engl J Med. 1995;333:638-44.
25. Johnston PB, Gaster RN, Smith VC, et al. A clinicopathologic study of autosomal dominant optic atrophy. Am J Ophthalmol. 1979;88:868-75.
26. Jonasson F, Cullen JF, Elton RA. Temporal arteritis: A 14-year epidemiological, clinical and prognostic study. Scott Med J. 1979;11:111-9.
27. Kakisu Y, Adachi E, Mizota K. Pattern electroretinogram and visual evoked cortical potential in ethambutol optic neuropathy. Doc Ophthalmol. 1987;67:327-34.
28. Karnik PP, Maskati BT, Kirtane MV, et al.. Optic nerve decompression in head injuries. J Laryngol Otol. 1981;95:1135-40.
29. Katz DM, Trobe JD, Cornblath WT, et al. Ischemic optic neuropathy after lumbar spine surgery. Arch Ophthalmol. 1994;112:925-31.
30. Keltner JL. Giant-cell arteritis: Signs and symptoms. Ophthalmology 1982; 89;1101-10.
31. Kermode AG, Moseley IF, Kendall BE. Magnetic resonance imaging in Leber's optic neuropathy. J Neurol Neurosurg Psychiatry. 1989;52:671-74.
32. King JH, Passmore JW. Nutritional amblyopia: A study of American prisoners of war in Korea. Am J Ophthalmol. 1955;39:173-86.
33. Kjer P. Infantile optic atrophy with dominant mode of inheritance. A clinical and genetic study of 19 Danish families. Acta Ophthalmol Suppl. 1959;164(Supp 54):1-147.
34. Kline LB, Glaser JS. Dominant optic atrophy: The clinical profile. Arch Ophthalmol. 1979;97:1680-6.
35. Kline LB, Kim JY, Ceballos R. Radiation optic neuropathy. Ophthalmology. 1985;92:1118-26.
36. Kline LB, Morawetz RB, Swaid SU. Indirect injury of the optic nerve. Neurosurgery 1984;14:756-64.
37. Kraus AM, O'Rourke JO. Lymphomatous optic neuritis. Arch Ophthalmol. 1963;70:173-5.
38. Kumar A, Sandramouli S, Verma L, et al. Ocular ethambutol toxicity: Is it reversible? J Clin Neuro-ophthalmol. 1993;13:15-7.
39. Lancaster FE. Alcohol, nitric oxide, and neurotoxicity: Is there a connection? A review. Alcohol Clin Exp Res. 1992;16:539-41.
40. Leibold JE. Drugs having a toxic effect on the optic nerve. Int Ophthalmol Clin. 1971;11:137-57.
41. MacDonal DR, Rottenberg DA, Schultz JS, et al. Radiation-induced optic neuropathy [Abstract]. Neurology. 1981;31:43-4.
42 Manchester PT, Calhoun FP. Dominant hereditary optic atrophy with bitemporal field defects. Arch Ophthalmol. 1958;60:479-84.
43. Manryjarvi MI, Nerdrum K, Tuppurainen K. Color vision in dominant optic atrophy. Clin Neuro-Ophthalmol. 1992;12:89-93.
44. Manzo L, Locatelli C, Candura SM, Costa LG. Nutrition and alcohol neurotoxicity. Neurotoxicology. 1994;15: 555-65.
45. Martin SG, Weidle PJ, Rismondo V, et al. A case of isoniazid (INH)-induced optic neuropathy in an asymptomatic HIV-infected woman and review of the literature. Int Conf AIDS. 1996;11:88.
46. McDonnell PJ, Moore W, Miller NR. Temporal arteritis: A clinicopathologic study. Ophthalmology 1986;93:518-30.
47. McLean DR, Jacobs H, Mielke BW. Methanol poisoning: A clinical and pathological study. Ann Neurol. 1980;8:161-7.
48. Menon V, Arya AV, Sharma P, Chhabra KK. An etiological practice of optic atrophy. Acta Ophthalmol (Copenh). 1992;70:725-9.
49. Nakissa N, Rubin P, Strohl R, et al. Ocular and orbital complications following radiation therapy of paranasal sinus malignancies and review of the literature. Cancer. 1983;51:980-6.
50. Newman NJ, Wallace DC. Mitochondria and Leber's hereditary optic neuropathy. Am Ophthalmol. 1990;109:726-30.
51. Newman NJ. Leber's hereditary optic neuropathy: New genetic considerations. Arch Neurol. 1993;50:540-8.
52. Nikoskelainen E, Hoyt WF, Nummelin K. Ophthalmoscopic findings in Leber's hereditary optic neuropathy. II. The fundus findings in the affected family members. Arch Ophthalmol. 1983;101:1059-68.
53. No Authors Listed. Optic nerve decompression' surgery for nonarteritic anterior ischemic optic neuropathy (NAION) is not effective and maybe harmful. The Ischemic Optic Neuropathy Decompression Trial Research Group. JAMA. 1995;273:625-32.
54. Osuntokun BO, Osuntokun O. Tropical amblyopia in Nigerians. Am J Ophthalmol. 1971;72:708-16.

55. Repka MX, Savino PJ, Schatz NJ, et al. Clinical profile and long-term implications of anterior ischemic optic neuropathy. Am J Ophthalmol. 1983;96:478-83.
56. Ridley H. Ocular manifestations of malnutrition in released prisoners of war from Thailand. Br J Ophthalmol. 1945;29:861-5.
57. Rizzo JF III, Lessell S. Posterior ischemic optic neuropathy during general surgery. Am J Ophthalmol. 1987;103:808-11.
58. Rizzo JF, Lessell S. Tobacco amblyopia. Am Ophthalmol. 1993;116:84-7.
59. Rizzo JF. Adenosine triphosphate deficiency: A genre of optic neuropathy. Neurology. 1995;45:11-6.
60. Roden D, Bosley TM, Fowble B, et al. Delayed radiation injury to the optic nerves and chiasm. Clinical syndrome and treatment with hyperbaric oxygen and corticosteroids. Ophthalmology. 1990;97:346-51.
61. Rose FC. History of subacute myelo-optic neuropathy (SMON) and its clioquinol connection. In: Some Aspects of History of Neurosciences. Ed. Sinha KK, Jha DK. Association of Neuroscientists of Eastern India. Ranchi. 2003;P159-76.
62. Roth AM, Milsow L, Keltner JL. The ultimate diagnoses of patients undergoing temporal artery biopsies. Arch Ophthalmol. 1984;102:901-3.
63. Sadda SR, Nee M, Miller NR, et al. Clinical spectrum of posterior optic neuropathy. Am J Ophthalmol. 2001;132:743-50.
64. Sadun AA, Martone S, Mucimendoza R. Epidemic optic neuropathy in Cuba. Eye findings. Arch Ophthalmol. 1994;112:691-9.
65. Sadun AA, Rubin RM. Annual (almost) review in neuro-ophthalmology: The anterior visual pathways-II (Part One). J Neuro-ophthalmol. 1996;16:137-51.
66. Salomon O, Huna-Baron R, Kutz S, et al. Analysis of prothrombotic and vascular risk factor in patients with nonarteritic anterior ischemic optic neuropathy. Ophthalmology. 1999;196:739-42.
67. Sandvig K. Pseudoglaucoma of autosomal dominant inheritance. A report on three families. Acta Ophthalmol. 1961;39:33-43.
68. Schatz NJ, Lichtenstein S, Corbett JJ. Delayed radiation necrosis of the optic nerves and chiasm. In: Glaser JS, Smith JL (eds). Neuro-ophthalmology: Symposium of the University of Miami and the Bascom Palmer Eye Institute vol 8. St. Louis. Mosby-Year Book. 1975;131-9.
69. Sergott RC, Cohen MS, Bosley TM, et al. Optic nerve decompression may improve the progressive form of nonarteritic ischemic optic neuropathy. Arch Ophthalmol. 1989;107:1743-54.
70. Sharpe JA, Hostovsky M, Bilbao JM. Methanol optic neuropathy: A histopathologic study. Neurology. 1982;32:1093.
71. Shukovsky LJ, Fletcher GH. Retinal and optic nerve complications in a high-dose irradiation technique of ethmoid sinus and nasal cavity. Radiology. 1972;104:629-34.
72. Smith JI, Hoyt WF, Susac JO. Ocular fundus in acute Leber optic neuropathy. Arch Ophthalmol. 1973;90:349-54.
73. Smith KH, Johns DR, Heher KL, Miller NR. Heteroplasmy in Leber's hereditary optic neuropathy. Arch Ophthalmol. 1993;111:1486-90.
74. Stone EM, Newman NJ, Miller NR. Visual recovery in patients with Leber's hereditary optic neuropathy and the 11778 mutation. Clin Neuro-ophthalmol. 1992;12:10-4.
75. The Cuba Neuropathy Field Investigation Team. Epidemic optic neuropathy in Cuba: Clinical characterization and risk factors. N Engl J Med. 1995;333:1176-82.
76. Troncoso J, Mancall EL, Schatz NJ. Visual evoked responses in pernicious anemia. Arch Neurol. 1979;36:168.
77. Waardenburg PJ. Different types of hereditary optic atrophy. Acta Genet. 1957;7:287-90.
78. Wadia NH. An introduction to Neurology in India. Tropical Neurology. Ed. Spillaine JD. Oxford University Press. Oxford. 1972. P. 28-36.
79. Wakamura M, Yokoe J. Evidence for preserved direct papillary light response in Leber's hereditary optic neuropathy. Br J Ophthalmol. 1995;79:442-6.
80. Wilson J. Cyanide in human disease: A review of clinical and laboratory evidence. Food Appl Toxicol. 1983;3:397-9.
81. Woon C, Tang RA, Pardo G. Nutrition and optic nerve disease. Semin Ophthalmol. 1995;10:195-202.
82. Young WC, Thornton AF, Gebarski SS, et al. Radiation-induced neuropathy: correlation of MR imaging and radiation dosimetry. Radiology. 1992;185:904-7.
83. Zimmerman CF, Schatz NJ, Glaser JS. Magnetic resonance imaging of radiation optic neuropathy. Am J Ophthalmol. 1990;110:389-94.

CHAPTER 11

Chiasmal Disorders

Sandip Chatterjee

INTRODUCTION

The term chiasmal disorders encompasses all the pathology around the optic chiasm, and include a variety of special tumors and tumor-like conditions which are peculiar to the region. Roughly about 25% of all intracranial tumors arise in the chiasmal area; of the lesions causing chiasmal compression, 50% are pituitary adenomas, 25% are craniopharyngiomas, and 10% are meningiomas. Hence, this chapter will attempt to discuss briefly about general features of lesions in this region before going into details about these common tumors of the region. However, no discussion of chiasmal problems can begin without a reference, however, brief to the regional anatomy.

REGIONAL ANATOMY

The two optic nerves meet in the midline to form the optic chiasm. This is a flattened oblong structure having 12 mm in transverse diameter, 8 mm in anteroposterior diameter, and 4 mm in thickness. The chiasm forms the anteroinferior wall of the third ventricle, and at this point is tilted 45° from the horizontal plane. Its anatomic relations superiorly are the lamina terminalis, anterior commissure, and the third ventricle; posteriorly the pituitary stalk, tuber cinereum, mammillary bodies, and oculomotor nerves; and inferiorly the diaphragma sellae and the pituitary gland. It must be pointed out that the optic nerve and the carotid artery are medial to the anterior clinoid process. The optic nerve pursues a posterolateral course to meet its fellow of the opposite side in the chiasm, whereas the carotid artery travels posterolaterally to its bifurcation.

The normal chiasm overlies the diaphragma sellae and the pituitary gland, a relationship which is maintained in 70% of cases. Of the remaining 30%, half are prefixed and half are postfixed. A prefixed chiasm overlies the tuberculum sellae, whereas the postfixed chiasm overlies the dorsum sellae. Technical difficulties in the transcranial approach to the pituitary gland may be encountered in cases where the chiasm is prefixed in position, thus obscuring the surgeon's view of the sellae (Figs. 1 and 2).

The pituitary gland itself is a relatively small gland which measures roughly 1.5 cm by 1 cm by 0.5 cm and resides in the sella turcica, being attached to the hypothalamus by the stalk or infundibulum. The anterior lobe is larger than the posterior lobe, occupying about 75% of the gland, and appears darker than the posterior part on sectioning.

The position of the chiasm in reference to the pituitary gland and diaphragma sellae may also affect the pattern of visual field changes in patients with pituitary tumors. For instance, with a prefixed chiasm, an expanding tumor may cause a bitemporal scotomatous hemianopia rather than the classical superior bitemporal quadrantanopia as a result of posterior infrachiasmal compression. Further, pituitary tumors in patients with postfixed chiasms involve the junction of the chiasm with the optic nerve, and thus may present with anterior chiasmal syndrome, which consists of an ipsilateral visual field loss and a contralateral superior temporal quadrantanopia (junctional scotoma).

One of the other important structures in close proximity to the optic chiasm is the cavernous sinus on each side. It is particularly important to the neurosurgeon performing pituitary surgery because the medial border is often exposed during transsphenoidal surgery. Anatomically, the cavernous sinus is irregular in shape and fits

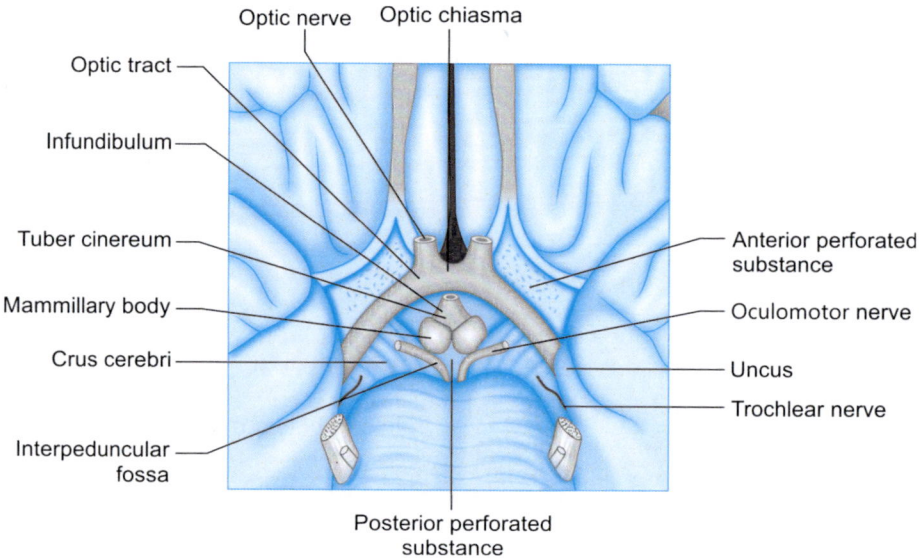

FIG 1: The Interpeduncular fossa.

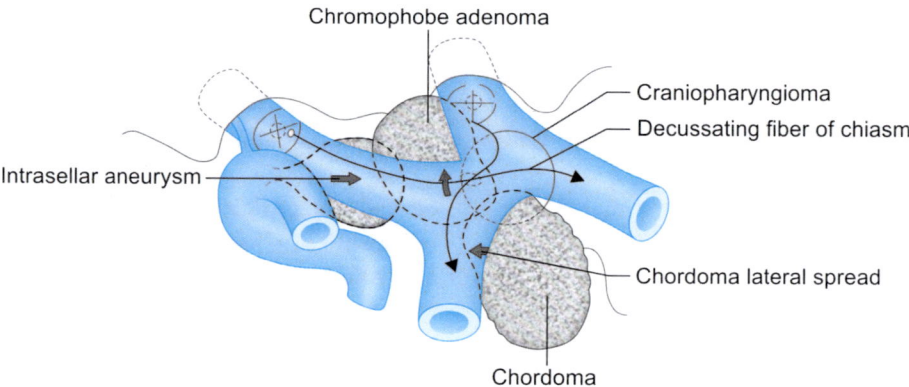

FIG. 2: Masses around the optic chiasm.

into the space between the body of the sphenoid bone and the dura forming the medial boundary of the middle cranial fossa. In an anteroposterior direction, it extends from the superior orbital fissure to the apex of the temporal bone. On its lateral wall, one can identify from top to bottom the following structures: oculomotor nerve, trochlear nerve, the ophthalmic and maxillary divisions of the trigeminal nerve; and suspended by fibrous trabeculae between the lateral wall of the sinus and the sphenoid bone are the abducens nerve and the internal carotid artery.

CLINICAL FEATURES

The clinical features of any space-occupying lesion in this region may be grouped into essentially one of two categories: (1) mass effects on surrounding structures, predominantly the optic pathway causing compromise of visual fields or impairment of visual acuity, and (2) endocrine effects caused by interference with any part of the hypothalamic-pituitary pathway. These may be hypersecretory states or insufficiency syndromes. Both these need to be discussed in some details.

Mass Effects

Mass effects are mainly observed with nonfunctional larger macroadenomas, often associated with panhypopituitarism. The most common manifestation of mass effect is headache—which may be retro-orbital, bifrontal, or even bitemporal in nature. The pain is probably caused by stretching of the dura or distortion of the diaphragma sellae, the latter being innervated by the first division of the trigeminal nerve. Headaches have been noted in about one-third of the patients with pituitary tumors, although it may be pointed out that in these patients headaches sometimes spontaneously disappear as the tumor progresses upward beyond the diaphragma sellae.

The characteristic visual field defect caused by a pituitary tumor is bitemporal hemianopia. In a typical case, the superior temporal quadrants are affected initially followed by the inferior temporal quadrants. In instances of progressive chiasmal compression, thereafter the inferior nasal followed by the superior nasal quadrants are affected, followed by blindness. Another type of visual abnormality that frequently occurs in association with lesions around the chiasm is a junctional scotoma.

Anatomically lesions producing these deficits are located at the optic nerve immediately adjacent to the chiasm. Involvement of the optic nerve itself produces unilateral central scotoma, whereas involvement of the crossing inferior nasal fibers from the opposite optic nerve that loop forward in the involved optic nerve (von Wilbrand's knee) accounts for the superior temporal quadrantanopia in the contralateral eye. It may be pertinent to point out that the pathophysiological mechanism responsible for the visual impairment may be mechanical compression or ischemia or both. In a study by Hollenhorst and Younge of 1,000 patients with pituitary tumors presenting to the Mayo Clinic, the most common types of visual field defects encountered were bitemporal hemianopia (30%), superior bitemporal defects (10.1%), blindness in one eye, and a superior temporal defect in the other eye (8.1%). It may be pointed out that in our experience of about 400 pituitary adenomas we have operated upon, a classical bitemporal field defect was encountered in only 58 patients (14.5%) (unpublished observation).

The presence of optic disk pallor on fundoscopy may represent ischemia of the optic nerve and may result in optic atrophy with associated visual impairment. Papilledema as such is rare in pituitary tumors but commonly encountered in suprasellar masses, such as meningiomas or craniopharyngiomas.

Another mass effect of tumors in this region is production of extraocular muscle paralysis. The oculomotor nerve is most commonly involved, followed next by the abducens nerve and then the trochlear nerve. With suprasellar tumors or suprasellar extensions of sellar tumors, there may develop obstruction of the third ventricle producing hydrocephalus, and this may produce headache of raised intracranial pressure.

Endocrine Effects

Suprasellar tumors may produce mass effect on the hypothalamic–pituitary neurovascular axis and interfere with both anterior and posterior pituitary function in one of several ways, but these are uncommon modes of presentations for them. On the other hand, pituitary tumors often present with endocrinopathies. Three commonly encountered clinical syndromes that result from a hormone-producing pituitary adenoma, are in order of frequency: (1) the amenorrhea–galactorrhea syndrome (hyperprolactinemia), (2) acromegaly (excess growth hormone), and (3) Cushing's disease (excess adrenocorticotrophic hormone with hypercortisolism).

Pituitary tumors producing excess of thyrotropin and gonadotropin have been described but are rare. Nelson's syndrome is a result of a pituitary adenoma that develops in a patient who has undergone bilateral adrenalectomy for Cushing's disease. The tumors associated with Nelson's syndrome are usually biologically aggressive tumors. Current opinion seems to hold that the pituitary tumor was present before the adrenalectomy and caused the Cushing's disease.

Patients harboring prolactinomas have distinct clinical features. Women give a history of amenorrhea ranging from months to several years, and may or may not have spontaneous galactorrhea. Impotence and hypogonadism in males have been attributed to the hyperprolactinemia.

The appearance of patients with well-established Cushing's disease and acromegaly is so characteristic that a clinician rarely has trouble in recognizing either of these two entities. The clinical features of Cushing's disease include the characteristic facies, centripetal obesity, hypertension, thin skin, purple striae, ecchymoses, osteoporosis, amenorrhea and hirsutism, glucose intolerance, and emotional disorders. The clinical features of acromegaly include overgrowth of the head, hands and feet, prognathism, arthritic manifestations, impairment of glucose tolerance, cardiomyopathy, and hyperhidrosis. These classical clinical manifestations will be described in some details later.

Compression of the normal pituitary gland by large tumors can be seen commonly in nonsecretory tumors, and result in hypopituitary states. It may be pointed out that the different components of the pituitary gland have different tolerances to chronic compression—the gonadotrophs are most sensitive, followed by the thyrotrophs, the somatotrophs, and the corticotrophs.

NEURORADIOLOGICAL EVALUATION

Over the past few decades, significant advances have been made in neuroradiological techniques that have influenced the diagnostic workup of patients with tumors in the region of the optic chiasm. This discussion will focus on various radiological techniques in chronological order of use.

Skull Films

A single lateral skull X-ray should be obtained in all patients who are undergoing evaluation for a sellar and parasellar mass. Although modern imaging modalities like magnetic resonance imaging (MRI) have almost made the skull X-ray redundant, it is pertinent to recall anatomical information obtainable from this film. A normal lateral sellar X-ray is shown in Fig. 3.

Computed Tomography and Magnetic Resonance Techniques

Magnetic resonance imaging is the preferred neurodiagnostic study in evaluating the sellar and parasellar areas. For pituitary tumors, most MR studies are done on a 1.5 tesla magnet, and the protocol consists of high-resolution T1-weighted sagittal and coronal images of the sellar region

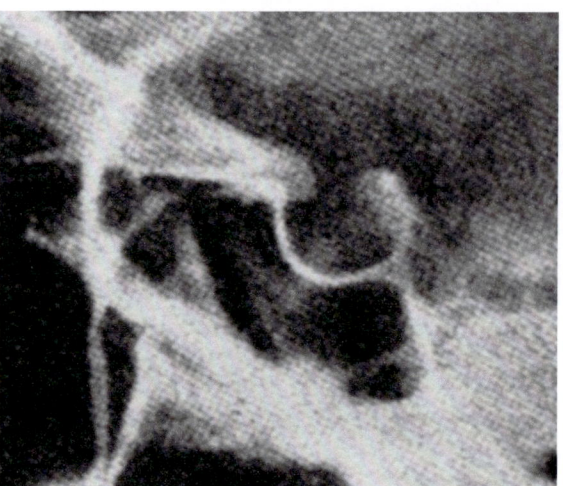

FIG. 3: Lateral skull film—normal sella turcica.

performed before and after administration of gadolinium-chelated compounds. A T2-weighted coronal image is also obtained. The T1 and T2-weighted images are done with thin sections (3 mm slice thickness) with a 10% gap, a small field of view (15–18 cm), a 256 × 160 matrix, and multiple averages. In cases in which a parasellar abnormality is suspected, a brain protocol is used. This usually consists of sagittal T1-weighted images, axial or coronal proton-density and T2-weighted images (fast spin-echo technique), and appropriate axial and coronal pregadolinium and postgadolinium studies.

In selected cases, computed tomography (CT) scan of the region is obtained. Precontrast and postcontrast examinations are performed with the patient in a prone position with the head tilted up in a head holder. Contrast dynamic studies of the pituitary gland improve visualization of the microadenomas by showing displacement of the vascular tuft seen on the superior aspect of the pituitary gland. Dynamic magnetic resonance (MR) studies have also been with techniques based on the modification of regular spin-echo, fast spin-echo, and gradient-echo sequences. In patients with Cushing's disease, Miller and Doppman described the technique of inferior petrosal sinus sampling as extremely valuable in lateralizing the functional microadenoma in the pituitary gland. One final word about pituitary imaging is that adenomas less than 1 cm in diameter are called "microadenomas," whereas those greater than 1 cm in diameter are called "macroadenomas."

Pituitary microadenoma is the most common sellar mass in adults. On unenhanced CT scan or MRI studies, microadenomas are relatively hypodense or hypointense relative to the normal pituitary gland. On T2-weighted sequences, they have variable signal intensity. Following contrast administration, the microadenomas are seen as hypodense or hypointense masses relative to the strongly-enhancing normal pituitary tissue and cavernous sinus. On the other hand, on imaging studies, the macroadenomas are usually isointense with the brain on T1-weighted images and enhance intensely on contrast studies (Fig. 4). On T2-weighted studies, variable signal intensity is noted. There may be erosion of the sellar floor and extension of the tumor into the sphenoid sinus (Fig. 5). Similar invasion into the cavernous sinus may be documented.

Empty sella syndrome refers to the herniation of the subarachnoid space into the sella through a widely opened diaphragma sellae, where the pituitary gland is compressed to one side. In most cases, empty sella is not associated with clinical manifestations, although a number of patients in our experience in Eastern India have presented with spontaneous cerebrospinal fluid (CSF) rhinorrhea. Intrasellar cysts in the pituitary gland are found in 20% of autopsy specimens. On CT or MRI studies, these lesions are usually hypodense or hypointense. In contrast, dermoid cysts in this region are hyperintense on both T1-weighted and T2-weighted images.

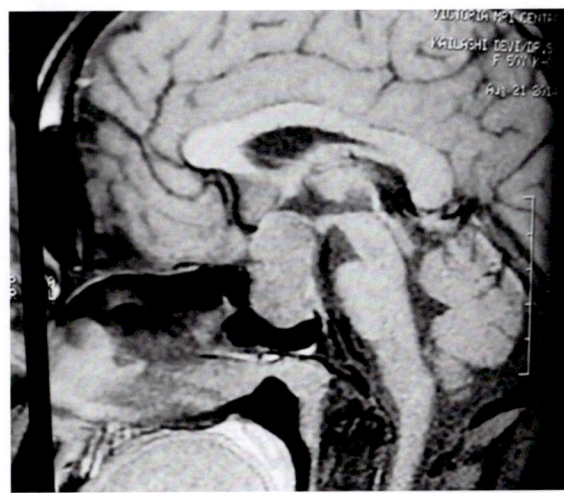

FIG. 5: T1 sagittal MR image showing invasion of sphenoid sinus.

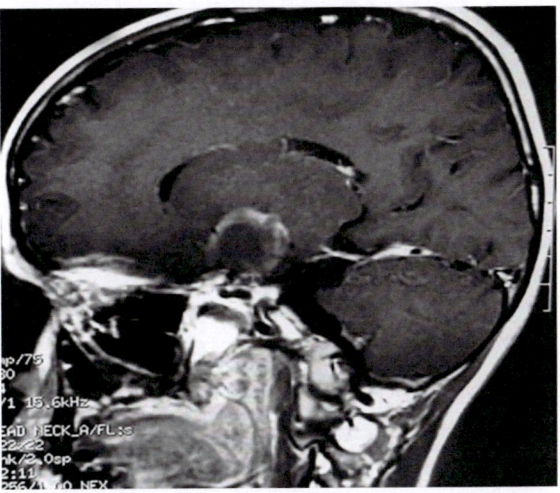

FIG. 6: T1-Gad enhanced MR scan showing craniopharyngioma with central fluid and peripheral enhancement.

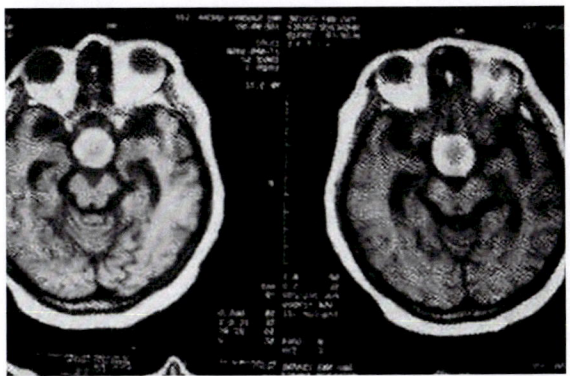

FIG. 4: Pituitary macroadenoma—magnetic resonance (MR) axial.

Craniopharyngiomas are epithelial tumors which arise primarily in this location. Sartoretti-Scefer et al. have described MRI correlation of craniopharyngiomas with the pathological classification of adamantinous and papillary types. The former are tumors of childhood and young adults and are characterized by the presence of large cysts. On MRI, the cysts are hyperintense on T1-weighted images and pathologically correlate with high protein content and free methemoglobin within the cysts. The squamous papillary subtype is found in adults, and these tumors are frequently solid and enhance intensely. Calcifications may be present but not as frequently as in adamantinous type.

Gliomas of the visual pathway constitute about 5% of primary brain tumors in childhood and 2% in adults. In children,12 20–50% are associated with neurofibromatosis type I. CT scans may show an enlarged optic canal with a focal isodense mass of the optic nerve that variably enhances after contrast administration. MRIs show the enlarged optic nerve or chiasm, which is hypointense to isointense on T1-weighted images, and hyperintense on T2-weighted images (Figs. 8 and 9). Hypothalamic gliomas have similar imaging characteristics.

Giant aneurysms of the cavernous or supraclinoid internal carotid artery may present as large masses in the sellar and suprasellar regions. CT scans may show erosion of the adjacent bony wall around the cavernous sinus, with circumferential or lamellated calcification within the wall of the aneurysm. On MR scans, the aneurysm shows a circumscribed area of flow void, with associated phase artifacts corresponding to the disturbed flow within the lumen. Meningiomas may also present in this situation.

PITUITARY ADENOMAS

Nonfunctional Pituitary Adenoma

The nonfunctional pituitary adenoma is defined as an adenoma that does not cause a clinically apparent endocrinopathy. These tumors thus come to medical attention because of mass effects, usually visual impairment, or because of discovery during the course of other clinical investigations. Since operative morbidity is very low particularly for the transsphenoidal approach, even small suprasellar and parasellar tumors should be operated upon. It is only the so-called "incidentalomas", small adenoma-like conditions found incidentally on MR scans that do not need to be operated

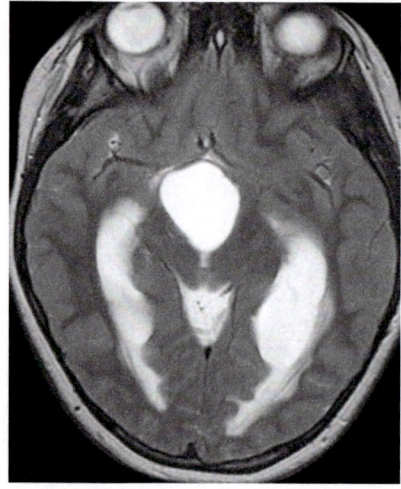

FIG 7: T2 weighted image of cystic craniopharyngioma.

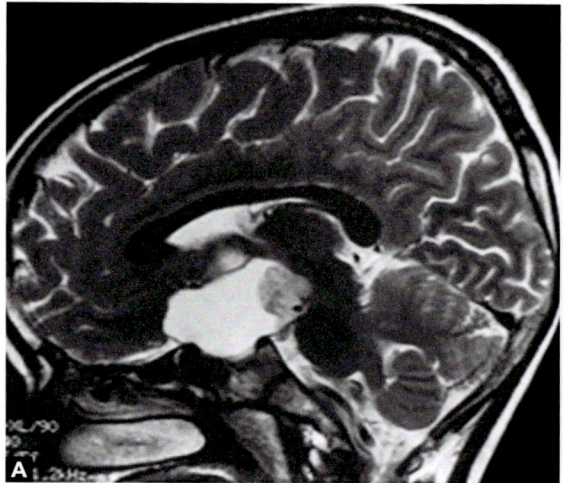
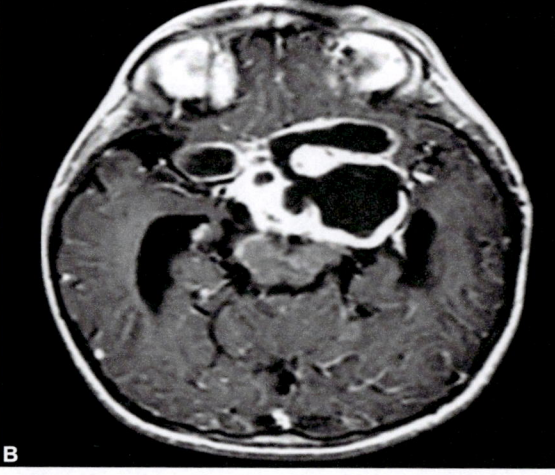

FIG 8: Optic Glioma - MR scan images showing mixed signal changes and brain invasion.

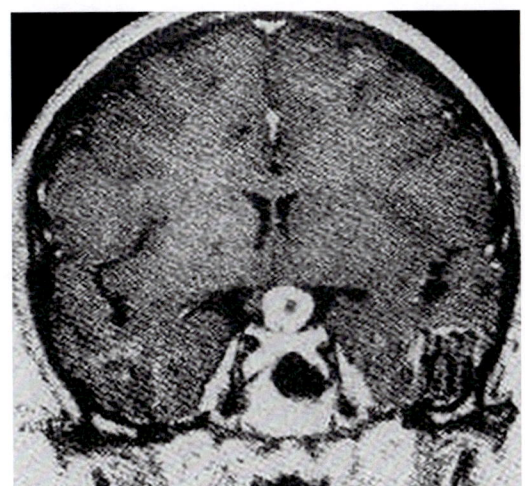

FIG. 9: Chiasmatic glioma (contrast enhanced).

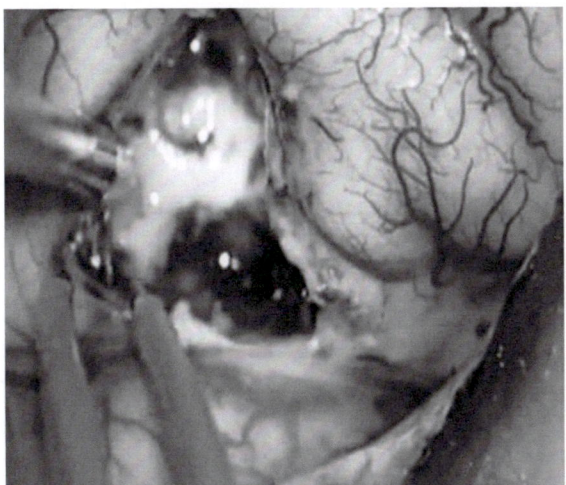

FIG. 10: Optic pathway glioma in a probable Neurofibromatosis 1 patient. *(For color version, see Plate 1)*

upon. Endoscopic transsphenoidal surgery is indicated in all sellar tumors with sphenoidal sinus extension, or symmetrical suprasellar extension, and is relatively contraindicated in tumors with asymmetrical suprasellar or parasellar extensions. The transsphenoidal microsurgical procedure has been replaced by an even less invasive endoscopic15 transsphenoidal procedure where the nasal mucosal dissection is not necessary and the natural sphenoidal ostium is used to gain entry into the sphenoidal air sinus.

Adjuvant therapy is indicated in patients with significant residual tumor or in those cases where the tumor showed radiological or operative features of invasiveness. The mean radiation dose used is 48 Gy.

Prolactinomas

Prolactinomas constitute the largest group of pituitary adenomas and make up 30% of these tumors. These tumors autonomously secrete prolactin, a polypeptide hormone, and they occur most commonly in women of reproductive age.

Prolactin is produced and secreted by acidophilic cells in the anterior pituitary gland, and it needs to be recalled that hypothalamic modulation of prolactin release is mainly through inhibitory factors. Pituitary stalk section or lesions that produce mass effect on the pituitary stalk can therefore, cause hypersecretion of prolactin, although unlike in the case of prolactinomas, the rise in serum prolactin levels in these instances is mild to moderate only.

Clinical manifestations of the hyperprolactinemia caused by these tumors vary in between the sexes. In women, the principal effects are amenorrhea, galactorrhea, and reproductive dysfunction. Men with prolactinomas may present with loss of libido, impotence, or oligospermia, and it has been found that prolactinomas in men tend to be much larger at diagnosis because women are perhaps more sensitive to the effects of hyperprolactinemia.

In patients with pituitary tumors who have a moderately elevated serum prolactin level (e.g. 60–150 µg/L), it is difficult to identify the cause of hyperprolactinemia. A fasting level of greater than 150 µg/L is highly suggestive of a pituitary adenoma being the cause of the hypersecretion. Very high levels of serum prolactin (> 1000 µg/L) suggest invasiveness, which usually means that the tumor has extended into the cavernous sinus.

In certain situations, no treatment may be required, e.g. in the case of a young woman with a small tumor with modest hyperprolactinemia and no mass effect who does not desire pregnancy. These patients can be followed with serial imaging studies. However, conservative approach is not indicated in any patient with a macroadenoma, unless the patient is unfit for surgical intervention due to some other cause. Medical treatment revolves around use of dopamine agonists. The most common one is the ergot derivative bromocriptine, which acts by inhibition of prolactin messenger ribonucleic acid (mRNA) transcription. As might be expected, there is a variable response to the drug. Bromocriptine binds to the D2 dopamine receptors found on the lactotrophs, and its effectiveness has been found to correlate with the number of receptors present. Therefore, it cannot always be recommended as the panacea for this condition. Moreover, treatment with bromocriptine is often lifelong, and given that it has a lot of side effects (nausea, vomiting, dizziness, postural hypotension, and headaches), patient compliance is often poor. However, patients with prolactinomas can be treated by bromocriptine in one of two ways. Bromocriptine may be used as the primary therapy, or it may be used as an adjunct to surgical intervention. Cabergoline is a long-acting dopamine agonist that is useful in the treatment of prolactin-secreting tumors even if these are bromocriptine resistant.

Surgical intervention is considered where there is no response to bromocriptine or where the patient does not desire lifelong medications. Prolactinomas with significant mass effect or cystic components, or those associated with pituitary insufficiency in spite of medical therapy, prolactinomas with pituitary apoplexy or CSF rhinorrhea, and prolactinomas in women who desire pregnancy are indications of surgical intervention.

Radiotherapy is used as an adjunct therapy only and may be in the nature of conventional or stereotactic radiotherapy. Clinical advantages of radiotherapy need to be balanced by the adverse effects of brain irradiation, including hypopituitarism, optic apparatus injury, and delayed brain radionecrosis.

Adrenocorticotropic Hormone Producing Adenomas

Cushing's syndrome is broadly defined as pathological hypercortisolemia. The causes are broadly divided into those that are adrenocorticotrophic hormone (ACTH)-dependent and those that are not ACTH-dependent.

Adrenocorticotrophic hormone-dependent Cushing's syndrome accounts for roughly 80% of cases and can be caused by a pituitary adenoma, pituitary hyperplasia, ectopic tumor secreting ACTH; whereas ACTH-dependent cases account for approximately 20% of cases and include adrenal adenomas, carcinomas, and adrenal hyperplasia. Most patients with endogenous Cushing's syndrome have Cushing's disease caused by oversecretion of ACTH by a corticotroph adenoma. Approximately 90% of these are microadenomas, and are often not identifiable on MR scans. The clinical features of this condition are well known and include redistribution of body fat causing centripetal obesity, muscle weakness, osteoporosis, hyperglycemia, hypertension, skin changes, hirsutism, as well as neuropsychiatric and immunological changes.

After the clinical suspicion of Cushing's syndrome has been raised, the first step is to biochemically demonstrate hypercortisolism. This can be done by: (a) measurement of basal 24-hour urine-free cortisol, or (b) by the 1 mg overnight dexamethasone suppression test. It may be pointed out that the normal 24-hour urine-free cortisol has a normal range up to 2,480 nmol/L. The normal response after overnight dexamethasone suppression is a cortisol level less than 140 nmol/L. The next step in the biochemical diagnostic algorithm is to check the serum ACTH level as a means of distinguishing ACTH-dependent causes from ACTH-independent Cushing's syndrome. Once ACTH-dependant Cushing's syndrome has been established, MR scan is performed to try and identify the adenoma. Unfortunately, this detects lesions in only 50–70% of cases. In cases where the MR scan is not found to be useful, the next step is to perform bilateral inferior petrosal sinus sampling using bovine corticotropin-releasing hormone (CRH) and to record a central to peripheral ACTH gradient in the samples.

After control of hypertension and hyperglycemia, surgical intervention is considered for Cushing's disease. The indications of surgery are mass effect on surrounding structures, establishment of a diagnosis, and control of endocrinopathy. However, even with surgery, a remission of hypercortisolism can be induced in only 70% of patients.

Growth Hormone-secreting Adenomas

The classical description of a patient with acromegaly is that of enlargement of hands, feet, and bones of the face resulting in large spade-like hands and feet, frontal bossing, dental malocclusion, and a large lower jaw. Sleep apnea, cardiovascular disease, hyperlipidemia, and increased colonic polyps are lesser known problems associated with this condition. An unfortunate fact about this disease is the delay in diagnosis and most series have reported symptoms of the disease for 10–20 years before it is diagnosed. Serum insulin-like growth factor-1 (IGF-1) measurement is a useful test to diagnose oversecretion of growth hormone. Oral administration of 75 grams of glucose with measurement of serum glucose and growth hormone levels is the definitive test for acromegaly. Most patients with growth hormone-secreting tumors have a nadir growth hormone level greater than 1.5 ng/L. It may be pointed out that a random serum growth hormone level is of little use unless it is extremely high at 60 ng/L or higher.

There are two classes of drugs that lower growth hormone levels: (1) the dopamine agonists like bromocriptine, and (2) the 8-amino acid somatostatin analog octreotide. However, for the overwhelming number of patients, surgical intervention is the treatment of choice. An interesting point regarding surgery is that most often prompt regression of symptoms occurs and this includes immediate alteration in facial appearances. However, durable endocrine remission is possible in only 60–70% of patients, and the remaining requires radiotherapy to achieve control of their growth hormone levels.

Pituitary Apoplexy

The progression of visual field defects with pituitary tumors is usually slow. A rather dramatic form of chiasmal syndrome called "pituitary apoplexy" is associated with sudden visual loss, which may be accompanied by headache, ocular motility disturbances, and loss of consciousness. This occurs because of rapid expansion of a pituitary tumor owing to infarction or hemorrhage. Rapid tumor growth outstripping its blood supply or compression of the tumor's vascular supply by the mass itself may cause ischemic necrosis of the tumor. With modern imaging technique, hemorrhage may be detected without a dramatic clinical event. Hence, evidence of intratumor hemorrhage is seen more frequently nowadays than the clinical syndrome of pituitary apoplexy.

The headache is usually of sudden onset, generalized, or retrobulbar and severe enough to be mistaken for a ruptured aneurysm.

Ophthalmoplegias are frequent. Associated visual acuity or visual field loss points to the diagnosis. CSF is usually bloody but may only show xanthochromia, pleocytosis, or may be normal. Patient may be blind in both eyes over a period of few hours or few days. Loss of consciousness may not be universal. A strong clinical suspicion is the clue to early diagnosis.

Magnetic resonance imaging is the diagnostic procedure of choice for suspected pituitary apoplexy since it best identifies areas of hemorrhage in the tumor except within the first 24 hours when CT may be better.

Factors implicated in precipitating apoplexy include—radiation therapy, trauma, pregnancy, and dynamic testing of anterior pituitary function.

Corticosteroid replacement therapy is the first therapeutic measure for pituitary apoplexy. Neurosurgical decompression of the anterior visual pathways should be performed urgently if vision is decreased.

Craniopharyngiomas

Craniopharyngiomas account for 2.5–4% of all brain tumors, but are about 20% of tumors in the region of the optic chiasm. They are considered benign tumors and are thought to arise from the squamous cell nests located along the pituitary stalk. This is why most of these tumors are adherent to the pituitary stalk and may present with posterior pituitary problems.

Craniopharyngiomas follow definite growth patterns. Those arising from the distal portion of the pituitary stalk tend to grow within the sella turcica and anatomically mimic pituitary adenomas. Those arising from the central portion of the pituitary stalk are typically midline, grow within the subarachnoid space, and are located in the suprasellar compartment frequently extending into the third ventricle. Those arising from the proximal portion of the stalk grow predominantly within the third ventricle, impinging on the foramen of Monro, and causing secondary hydrocephalus. The tumors can be cystic, or solid with calcifications in their walls. When the optic chiasm is prefixed in location, the tumor tends to fill the entire suprasellar region and the optic apparatus is pushed anteriorly and superiorly. In cases where the chiasm is postfixed, the tumors grow from the suprasellar region downward in between the two optic nerves which are thus pushed laterally.

Although craniopharyngiomas grow in an expansile fashion, they tend to become adherent to major arteries of the anterior circulation, which somewhat limits the safe total resection of these tumors. The blood supply of these tumors is from small vertebral feeders of the anterior part of the circle of Willis.

Growth failure occurs in 93% of children diagnosed with craniopharyngiomas. In adults, a decreased sexual drive in men and menstrual irregularities in females have been reported in about 80–85% of cases. As these tumors grow extra-axially, they often grow to a large size before they are diagnosed. Visual disturbance, headaches, psychiatric symptoms, and cognitive deficits especially related to memory loss are other common presentations of these tumors.

Depending on the location and size of the tumor, different approaches can be used to remove them. Intrasellar tumors can be removed with a standard transnasal-transsphenoidal approach. Larger tumors with suprasellar extension or smaller tumors in the suprasellar space are removed with a pterional-transsylvian approach. Tumors extending significantly into the third ventricle may be best tackled by a transcallosal approach as described by Yasargil et al.

Craniopharyngiomas are considered radiosensitive tumors. A number of studies have shown better results in craniopharyngiomas treated by surgery followed by radiation therapy compared to those treated by surgical excision alone, with significant improvement in recurrence-free survival interval. In cystic tumors, intracystic radiation therapy has been well described.

GLIOMAS OF THE VISUAL PATHWAY

Unilateral optic nerve tumors may be intraorbital, intracanalicular, intracranial, or a combination of the earlier. Although the first category is outside the purview of this present discussion, the second is often present with the intracranial tumor. All these tumors present with ipsilateral visual loss with poor perception of color and brightness. In instances particularly in this part of the world where the tumor grows slowly, the patient may be unaware of the visual impairment until the normal eye is covered.

In the presence of a tumor involving the optic nerve, the acuity in the affected eye will be reduced and there will usually be difficulty in reading the Ishihara charts. With extrinsic compression, e.g. by a meningioma, the visual field shows a central scotoma, with "breakthrough" as the defect increases. This finally leaves a peripheral crescent of preserved vision. The optic disk itself is normal in the early stages and then gradually becomes pale and atrophic. An afferent pupillary defect accompanies the earlier findings.

The two important optic nerve tumors which may present intracranially are (1) optic nerve gliomas and (2) meningiomas in the region. The optic nerve gliomas usually present in childhood, usually involve an intra-orbital or hypothalamic component as well, and may be part of manifestations of neurofibromatosis type I. In childhood, they often present with slow visual loss and proptosis. Primary gliomas of the chiasm present in childhood with unilateral or bilateral loss of vision, "amblyopia", strabismus, optic atrophy, or nystagmus. Chakravarty et al. have described a single patient with optic pathway glioma, Chiari type 1 anomaly, syringomyelia, and kyphoscoliosis but no cutaneous lesions (Figs. 8A and 8B). They argued in favor of considering this entity a variant form of neurofibromatosis type 1 (NF1).

Meningiomas arising in this region arise from the posterior optic foramen, the tuberculum sellae, or the anterior clinoid process, and usually present with features of an unilateral progressive optic nerve lesion (Fig. 11). Rarely, they may show features of chiasmal involvement.

Children with optic pathway gliomas with or without NF1 are managed according to symptoms

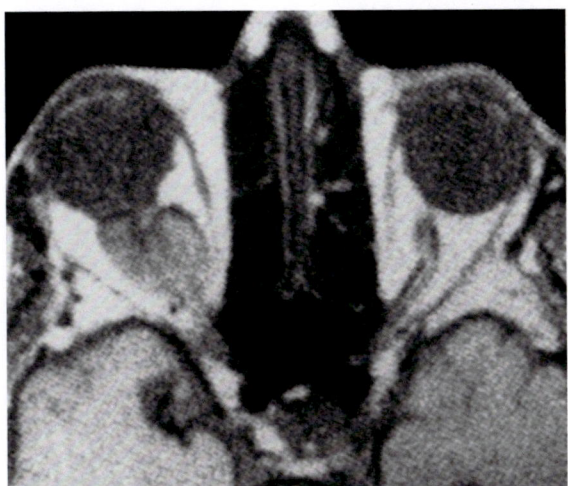

FIG 11: Right optic nerve sheath meningioma.

If the symptoms are minimal, the patient may be kept under surveillance with serial MR scans. If there is progression of proptosis and visual loss, some treatment is required. Patients with no useful vision in the affected eye and proptosis are treated with radical resection of the mass. Radiotherapy or chemotherapy has not been established to have any value. Chiasmal or hypothalamic astrocytomas particularly in the setting of NF1 require no surgical intervention nor biopsy, and only require serial clinical and radiological surveillance.

INDIAN DATA ON CHIASMAL LESIONS

Pituitary tumors constitute by far one of the most common tumors in this region. From the data on 1,250 intracranial space-occupying lesions collected by Dastur et al. in 1991, 145, i.e. 11.6% were pituitary adenomas. Out of these 24 were exclusively intrasellar (quite in contrast to Western statistics), and the remaining were all extrasellar, i.e. parasellar or suprasellar in extension. Craniopharyngiomas in the same series constituted 2.6% of all intracranial neoplasms, and 16.8% of all intrasellar tumors. Suprasellar meningiomas constituted 38 out of the total of 473 meningiomas reported from SCTIMST over a 10-year period from 1983 to 1993. It may be pointed out that meningiomas reported from India tend to occur mainly at an age less than reported in Western literature. In the suprasellar area, craniopharyngiomas constitute 6–9% of all tumors in the pediatric age group.

SUGGESTED READINGS

1. Alford FP, Arnott R. Medical management of pituitary tumors. Med J Aust. 1992;157:57-60.
2. Bailey P. Hypophyseal adenomas. In: Thomas CC (Ed). Intracranial Tumors. United States: Springfield; 1983.
3. Barrow DL, Mizuno J, Tindall GT. Management of prolactinomas associated with very high serum prolactin levels. J Neurosurg. 1988;68:554-8.
4. Bergland RM, Ray BS, Torack RM. Anatomical variations in the pituitary gland and adjacent structures in 225 human autopsy cases. J Neurosurg. 1968;28:98-9.
5. Chakravarty A, Bhargava A, Nandy S. A patient with optic pathway glioma, scoliosis, Chiari type 1 malformation and syringomyelia—is it neurofibromatosis type I? Neurology India. 2002;50:520-1.
6. Choux M, Lena G, Genitori L. Craniopharyngiomas in children. Neurochirurgie. 1991;37:1-174.
7. Cunnah D, Besser M. Management of prolactinomas. Clin Endocrinol (Oxford). 1991;34:231-5.
8. Cushing H, Walker CB. Distortions of the visual fields in cases of brain tumour: Chiasmal lesions, with special reference to bitemporal hemianopsia. Brain. 1915;37:41-400.
9. Dastur DK, Manghani DK, Gaitonde PS, et al. Craniopharyngiomas (A) against a perspective of brain tumor and (B) Some histological features. Neurology India. 1991;39:5.
10. Davis DH, Laws ER, Ilstrup DM, et al. Results of surgical treatment for growth hormone-secreting pituitary adenomas. J Neurosurg. 1993;79:70-5.
11. Deopujari CE, Kumar A, Karmakar VS, et al. Pediatric suprasellar lesions. J Pediatr Neurosci. 2011;6:S46-55.
12. Escourolle H, Abecassis JP, Bertagna X, et al. Comparison of computerized tomography and magnetic resonance imaging for the examination of the pituitary gland in patients with Cushing's disease. Clin Endocrinol. 1993;39:307-13.
13. Farmer J, Hoyt C. Monocular nystagmus in infancy and early childhood. Am J Ophthalmol. 1984;98:504-9.
14. Hollenhorst RW, Younge BR. Ocular manifestations produced by adenomas of the pituitary gland: analysis of 1,000 cases. In: Kohler PO, Ross GT (Eds). Diagnosis and Treatment of Pituitary Disorders. Amsterdam: Excerpta Medica; 1973. pp. 53-68.
15. Jho HD, Carrau RL, Ko Y, et al. Endoscopic pituitary surgery: an early experience. Surg Neurol. 1997;47:213-23.
16. Kachara R, Misra BK, Nair S, et al. Suprasellar meningiomas: surgical outcome. Abstracts of papers. Ann Neurol Soc India; 1992.

17. Kobayashi T, Kageyama N, Ohara K. Internal irradiation for cystic craniopharyngiomas. J Neurosurg. 1981;55:896-903.
18. Kulkarni MV, Lee KF, McArdle CB, et al. 1.5-T MR imaging of pituitary microadenomas: technical considerations and CT correlation. AJNR Am J Neuroradiol. 1988;9:5-11.
19. Laws ER. Conservative surgery and radiation for childhood craniopharyngiomas. J Neurosurg. 1991;74:1025-6.
20. Listernick R, Charrow J, Greenwald M, et al. Optic gliomas in children with neurofibromatosis type 1. J Pediatr. 1989;114:788-92.
21. Lyle TK, Clover P. Ocular symptoms and signs in pituitary tumors. Proc R Soc Med. 1961;54:611-9.
22. MacLeod RM, Lehmeyer JE. Suppression of pituitary tumor growth and function by ergot alkaloids. Cancer Res. 1973;33:849-55.
23. Miki Y, Matsuo M, Nishizawa S, et al. Pituitary adenomas and normal pituitary tissue: enhancement patterns on gadopentetate-enhanced MR imaging. Radiology. 1990;177:35-8.
24. Miller D, Doppmann J. Petrosal sinus sampling techniques and rationale. Radiology. 1992;185:143-7.
25. Miller N, Iliff W, Green W. Evaluation and management of gliomas of the anterior visual pathways. Brain. 1974;97:743-54.
26. Ontjes DA, Nay RL. Pituitary tumors. Cancer Clin. 1976;26:330-50.
27. Oxenhandler D, Sayers M. The dilemma of childhood optic gliomas. J Neurosurg. 1978;48:34-41.
28. Rhoton AL, Hardy DG, Chambers SM. Microsurgical anatomy and dissection of the sphenoid bone, cavernous sinus and sellar region. Surg Neurol. 1979;12:63-104.
29. Rodriguez L, Edwards M, Levin V. Management of hypothalamic gliomas in children: an analysis of 33 cases. Neurosurgery. 1990;26:242-7.
30. Samii M, Bini W. Surgical treatment of craniopharyngioma. Zmtralbl Neurochir. 1991;52:17-23.
31. Sartoretti-Scefer S, Wichmann W, Aguzzi A, et al. MR differentiation of adamantinous and squamous-papillary craniopharyngiomas. AJNR Am J Neuroradiol. 1997;18:77-88.
32. Stoffel-Wagner B, Springer W, Bidlingmaier D, et al. A comparison of the different methods for diagnosing acromegaly. Clin Endocrinol. 1997;46:531-37.7
33. Trainer PJ, Lawrie HS, Veerheist J, et al. Trans-sphenoidal resection in Cushing's disease: undetectable serum cortisol as the definition of successful treatment. Clin Endocrinol. 1993;38:73-8.
34. Yasargil MG, Curcic M, Kiss M, et al. Total removal of craniopharyngiomas: approaches and long-term results in 144 patients. J Neurosurg. 1990;73:3-11.
35. Zervas NT. Surgical results in pituitary adenomas: results of international survey. In: Black PC, Zervas NT, Ridway EC (Eds). Secretory Tumors of the Pituitary Gland. New York: Raven Press; 1984. pp. 377-85.

12 Retrochiasmal Visual Impairments

K K Sinha

INTRODUCTION

In a vast majority of cases of visual loss, the cause of impairment is located within the eyeball, the retina, the optic nerves, and the optic chiasm, but often many such problems may have their origin in the retrochiasmal part of the visual pathway from the optic tract to the occipital cortex and its connections with other parts of cerebral cortex. This chapter predominantly focuses on retrochiasmal disorders that lead to complex visual problems.

CHARACTERISTICS OF THE VISUAL LOSS CAUSED BY RETROCHIASMAL LESIONS

The hallmark of the visual field defects caused by retrochiasmal lesion is homonymous hemianopia and as a general rule, the pattern of the defect in each eye becomes increasingly congruous as the lesion approaches the occipital lobe. In such cases, the visual acuity is unaffected by the hemianopia but infrequently, patients are not aware that the field defect is in both eyes. They report that the vision is reduced in the eye on the side of the temporal hemianopia.

BILATERAL RETROCHIASMAL PATHWAY DAMAGE

If the retrochiasmal pathways are damaged bilaterally, cerebral blindness might occur. The pupils and fundi in such conditions are usually normal except in optic tract lesions. Neuroimaging, especially a high-resolution magnetic resonance imaging (MRI) is essential to make a correct diagnosis in any patient with suspected retrochiasmal visual loss.

A homonymous hemianopia results from lesions in the contralateral optic tract, lateral geniculate body, optic radiation, or occipital cortex, but visual acuity in the intact homonymous field in each eye should be normal under such conditions.

Complete homonymous hemianopia in an individual patient essentially does not have any anatomically localizing value since it may originate from a lesion at any point in the retrochiasmal pathway; however, as told earlier, as a general rule, the more congruous a partial homonymous defect is more likely is the lesion to be found in the posterior retrochiasmal region in the visual system. In these cases, the associated clinical deficits usually have a greater localizing value. Examples of some of these accompanying deficits include hemisensory and hypothalamic dysfunction in optic tract lesions, hemiparesis, hemisensory loss, and aphasia in lesions involving optic radiation, etc.

The frequency of different etiologic lesions and their anatomical locations have been found to be variable in different studies. But in one such study of 100 patients with homonymous hemianopia, Smith reported that 42% had a vascular origin, while 38% were caused by tumors; also 40% had lesions located in the occipital lobe, 33% in the parietal lobe, and 24% in the temporal lobe. Lesions in the optic tract and lateral geniculate body were rare.

Another study reported that in those patients, who presented with isolated homonymous hemianopia, 89% were of vascular origin and 86% of these patients had occipital lobe infarction, caused by posterior cerebral artery occlusion. In contrast, all cases under the age of 30 years had nonvascular causes.

CLINICAL CHARACTERISTICS OF OPTIC TRACT LESIONS

Optic tract lesion usually cause grossly incongruous homonymous hemianopia often associated with unilateral or bilateral impairment of central visual acuity and sometimes a classical ipsilateral temporal optic disk pallor and contralateral wedge or butterfly band pattern. Ultimately, it might cause bilateral optic atrophy, since the tract fibers are really the ganglion cells axons derived from both eyes.

Involvement of neighboring neural structures may cause contralateral hemiparesis, hypothalamic dysfunction, or ipsilateral optic atrophy. Compressive lesion that leads to chiasmal syndrome may also be responsible for optic tract defects if they extend laterally and posteriorly.

CHARACTERISTICS OF LATERAL GENICULATE NUCLEUS LESIONS

These are a rare cause of homonymous hemianopia but usually have a distinctive and surprisingly a congruous wedge-shaped homonymous hemianopia that straddles the horizontal meridian in a pattern that reflects either lateral or anterior choroidal artery occlusion. Infarction in the distribution of the anterior choroidal artery may also result in optic tract dysfunction.

CLINICAL CHARACTERISTICS OF LESIONS OF OPTIC RADIATION

The presence of noncongruous superior homonymous wedge defects localizes the lesion to the contralateral temporal lobe with involvement of the portion of the optic radiation known as Meyer's loop. Other associated features might include complex partial seizures or disorders of language. Deep parietal lobe lesions, such as tumors or hematomas involve the upper fibers of optic radiation and tend to produce more inferior homonymous field defects.

CLINICAL FEATURES OF OCCIPITAL LOBE LESIONS

Lesions affecting the occipital lobe usually produce either a complete homonymous hemianopia with or without "macular sparing" or congruous homonymous scotomata, which are usually caused by lesions located in the calcarine sulcus. When a meticulous perimetry is performed, one may notice a slight lateral shift of the field defect from the midline, which is usually less than 15°. This is called "macular sparing" and which is very common in patients with complete homonymous hemianopia caused by lesions of the occipital lobe (Fig. 1).

Gordon Holmes prepared a classical map of the visual cortex, which is well recognized, where he showed topographic representation of the contralateral visual hemifield in the striate cortex. The central 15° of the visual field in this classic map was shown to represent approximately 25% of the total surface area of the striate cortex. Recently, in studies using high-resolution MRI, this clinico-anatomical correlation has been revised. In this revised scheme, the area of striate cortex that serves the striate cortex has been considerably enlarged and that devoted to peripheral vision has been reduced. The phenomenon of macular sparing with homonymous hemianopia of occipital lobe origin is more easily seen with this new enlarged central visual field mapping.

Macular sparing is attributed to the double vascular supply of the occipital pole by the posterior as the well as middle cerebral arteries that occur in majority of people. Because the representation of the central visual field is so magnified in the posterior half of the striate cortex, perfusion by the middle cerebral artery preserves the function of a significant portion of the region following posterior cerebral artery occlusion particularly the area of the cortex devoted exclusively to macular vision. This sparing of macular vision occurs to a variable degree in different cases. This is the reason why macular sparing in homonymous hemianopia suggests occipital cortex as the site of the lesion (Fig. 2).

Some Important Clinical Syndromes Produced by Occipital Lobe Lesions

A number of clinical syndromes are found to occur in people with different kinds of lesions of the occipital cortex. Some of these are outlined here.
- *The syndrome of ipsilateral eye pain with contralateral homonymous hemianopia:* This

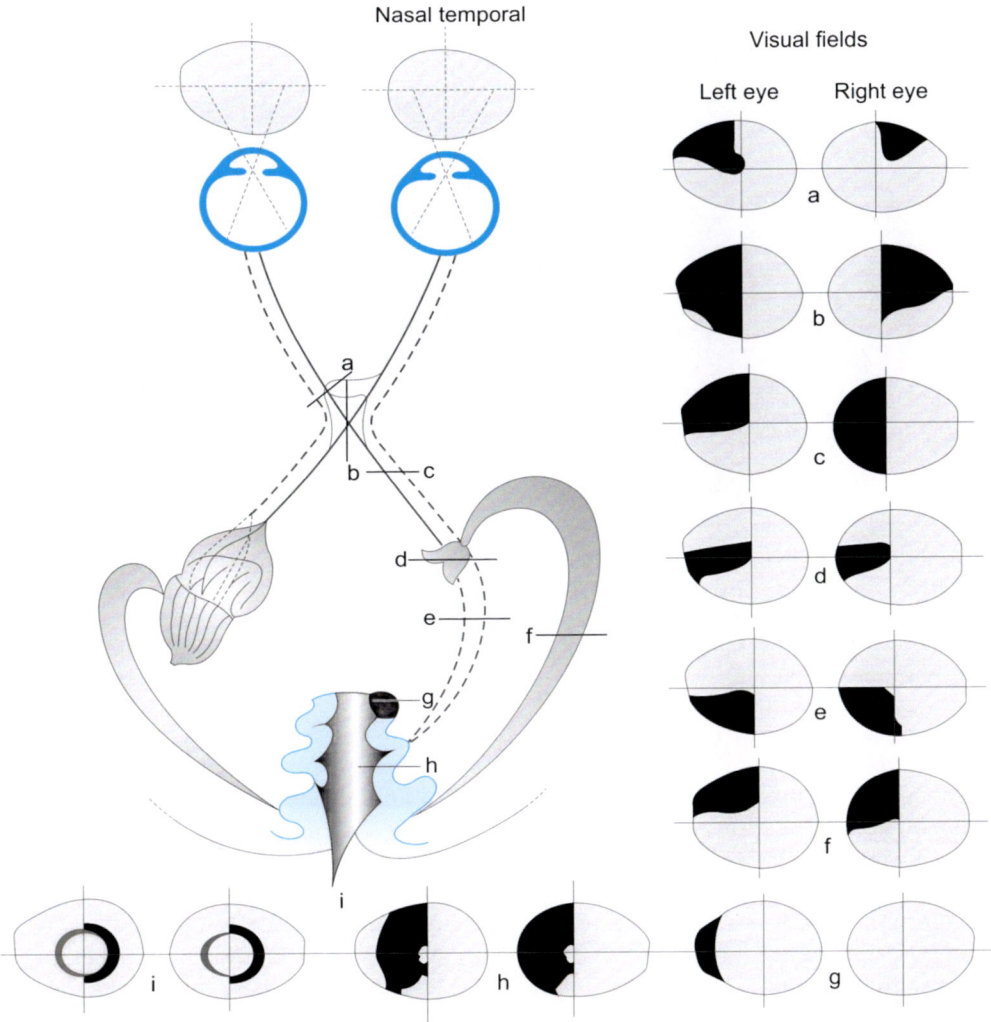

FIG. 1: Diagram to show the effects on the fields of vision produced by lesions at different points along the optic pathways.

syndrome is usually caused by an embolic posterior cerebral artery occlusion, resulting in occipital lobe infarction. Such patients need cardiac evaluation, and carotid studies are usually not indicated, because the infarct is in the area of supply of the posterior cerebral artery.

- *The syndrome of alexia (word blindness) without dysgraphia and right homonymous hemianopia:* This specific syndrome strongly indicates infarction of the left occipital lobe extending to the splenium of the corpus callosum. Because alexia can sometimes be associated with right homonymous hemianopia, all such patients must have their reading ability tested as a part of their neurological examination.
- *The syndrome of monocular peripheral visual field loss (absence of temporal crescent in one-half of visual field):* This syndrome sometimes occurs with lesions of posterior optic radiation or that of anterior occipital lobe which may damage the projection of the unpaired peripheral nasal retinal fibers. Also in those cases of homonymous hemianopia that do not involve the anterior visual cortex,

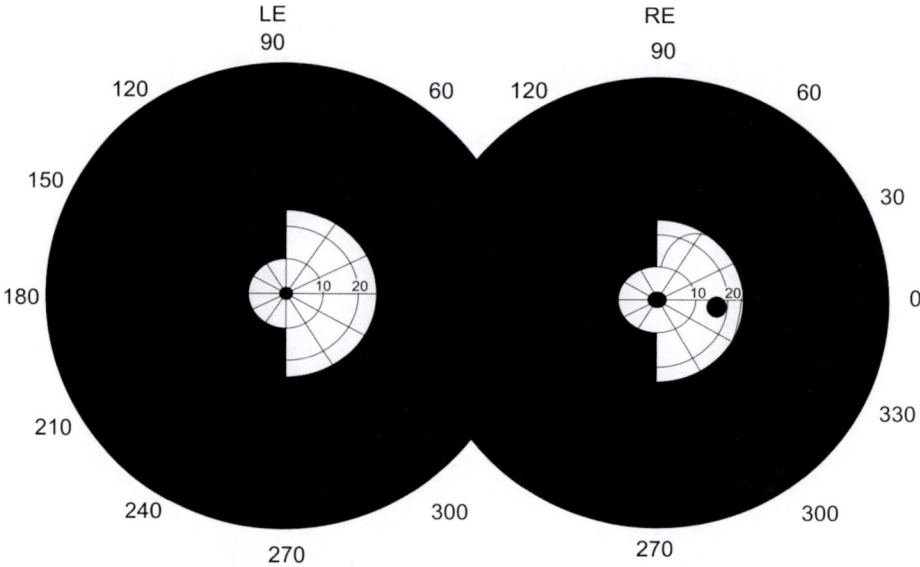

FIG. 2: Bilateral homonymous hemianopia as plotted on a visual field chart. The smaller area of preserved vision in the left hemifield of each eye indicates retrochiasmatic damage on both sides with macular sparing.

the monocular temporal crescent may be absent. However, occipital lobe lesions that result in visual field defects, confined entirely to monocular temporal crescent, are rare. But, however, it must be stressed that monocular peripheral temporal visual field defects are more commonly produced by retinal lesions and not by occipital lesions. Therefore, in all such cases, the nasal part of retina should be carefully examined before an occipital lobe lesion is suspected or diagnosed.

- *Syndrome of isolated homonymous congruous quadrantic visual deficit with well-defined horizontal border:* This is a syndrome, which has higher degree of specificity for lesions of the occipital lobe rather than lesions of temporal or parietal lobes. In these cases, when the field defect respects the horizontal meridian in a meticulously performed perimetric examination, it suggests specific involvement of the extrastriate cortex as well as the upper or lower calcarine striate cortex. These lesions are often small and arise from occlusion of smaller branches of vertebrobasilar vascular tree. These often escape detection by the CT scan, if they present acutely. On the other hand, the visual field defects caused by lesions of the optic radiation in either the parietal or temporal lobe are often incongruous and often have sloping borders that fail to respect the horizontal meridian precisely. Also, patients with lesions of optic tract such as those that occur occasionally following surgical lesions of globus pallidus interna (GPi) for Parkinson's disease, usually have incomplete homonymous quadrantic defect that do not respect the horizontal meridian and are often accompanied by homonymous paracentral scotomas.

- *Syndrome of bilateral homonymous paracentral scotoma:* Very rarely occipital lobe lesions may also cause bilateral homonymous paracentral scotomas that are mistaken for bilateral optic nerve lesions with cecocentral scotomas. However, with occipital lobe lesions producing bilateral homonymous paracentral scotomas, the pupillary reflexes are normal, in contrast to a similar syndrome caused by optic nerve lesions where it may be reduced or absent.

Statistically, the occipital lobe is the most common location for lesions causing an isolated homonymous hemianopia. These lesions are usually vascular, such as embolic occlusion of the posterior cerebral artery. In such cases, abrupt onset of homonymous hemianopia is often associated with pain in the ipsilateral eye or eyebrow on the side ipsilateral to the stroke and contralateral to the field defect. MRI of the brain in such cases shows a discrete lesion without mass effect in the involved occipital cortex, consistent with infarction. Embolic occlusion of the posterior cerebral artery is a common lesion and the echocardiogram may demonstrate clot in the left atrium or the left ventricle. Such patients need urgent anticoagulation to prevent further showers of embolism. Such patients also have several associated risk factors for cerebral infarction, such as valvular heart disease, atherosclerotic heart disease, smoking, diabetes, and previous attacks of myocardial or cerebral infarction. Uncommonly, prolonged hypotension may result in watershed infarction at the parieto-occipital junction with resulting homonymous hemianopia or cortical blindness.

Infrequent causes of retrochiasmal visual loss include arteriovenous malformations trauma, demyelinating diseases, progressive multifocal leukoencephalopathy, Alzheimer's disease, Creutzfeldt–Jakob disease, chemotherapeutic agents, poisons, and viral encephalitis.

SPECIAL FEATURES OF VISUAL LOSS OF CEREBRAL ORIGIN

It is now clear that visual impairment caused by lesions of that part of visual system which is located in the cerebrum, including the lateral geniculate nucleus, optic radiation, and calcarine occipital cortex, has some special features. As stated earlier, unilateral damage to the lateral geniculate nucleus, optic radiation, and calcarine occipital cortex typically results in contralateral hemianopia. The severity and magnitude of hemianopia in such cases are determined by the precise anatomy of the lesion and the degree of resulting neural dysfunction. On the one hand, hemianopia can be so severe that a patient cannot perceive any stimulus whatsoever within the affected hemifield; on the other hand, it can be so mild that it can only be detected by careful perimetric testing. Visual acuity is usually preserved even in severe "macular splitting" hemianopia, because these patients very effectively use the intact half of field to visualize the images. If acuity is impaired, it points to bilateral involvement of the central visual pathways and if the cause is located in the brain, the visual loss will be equal in both eyes.

Bilateral hemianopia impairs visual acuity, if the most posterior portion of the central visual field area is damaged. However, only rarely bilateral hemianopia is perfectly symmetrical; therefore, it is important that the differences between the right and left hemifield be defined with a perimetric examination. The papillary and fundoscopic examinations are normal. MRI shows a high T2 signal throughout the white and gray matter of posterior cerebral hemispheres. Such visual impairments are seen as common complications of eclampsia and hypertensive encephalopathy. Complete visual loss from cerebral lesions in these situations is rare and even if it appears as an acute episode, it does not usually persist.

Almost all patients with chronic lesions of occipital lobe show sparing of vision in some region of their visual fields.

Blindsight is a term that is used to indicate subtle evidence of visual preservation in patients with severe or complete destruction of occipital cortex. This phenomenon was originally described by Riddoch in 1917, who reported the loss of object discrimination with sparing of motion perception in soldiers of World War I with occipital lesions as a result of war wounds. Blindsight has been reported most commonly after damage to primary visual cortex but has also been reported after optic nerve lesion. This is thought to be due to sparing of small islands of neurons in calcarine cortex, which remain undetected on initial testing.

Some patients with severe visual loss caused by extensive bilateral damage to occipital cortices fail to recognize their deficits. This is a kind of visual anosognosia and has been termed "Anton syndrome". Patients with Anton syndrome are virtually blind, but they do not realize that they are blind and would often remark, "Why are the lights off?"

Such patients deny their visual loss and will often confabulate. This syndrome is not always specific of extensive bilateral occipital lobe damage because it has also rarely been seen in blindness caused by severe ocular and optic nerve diseases.

In all cases of cerebral visual loss, fundoscopy and papillary function are normal and may help to locate the site of lesion in the visual cortex, however, these examinations are not always reliable. For example, in visual loss caused by macular disease, visual changes may be so subtle that they are not easy for a neurologist to detect. Also, patients with bilaterally symmetrical retrobulbar optic neuropathy may show normal pupillary functions and the fundi may appear normal if they are examined before optic atrophy has set in. A meticulously carried out perimetric examination, therefore, remains the only essential tool for localization of such visual disturbances. Perimetry distinguishes bilateral hemianopia from nonspecific visual field constriction and can also distinguish functional visual loss caused by hysteria or malingering.

INVESTIGATING CAUSES OF CEREBRAL VISUAL LOSS

Once the clinical and perimetric evaluation suggests a cerebral cause for visual loss, the next step is to establish the anatomicopathologic diagnosis. Here, neuroimaging with MRI or CT scan (preferably with MRI) is critical, as vast majority of etiologies would show evidence of structural image. Sometimes, where imaging is not helpful, electrophysiological tests can be helpful. These include mainly electroencephalogram (EEG) and visual evoked potentials (VEPs), and it is the EEG, which is more helpful of the two. The alpha rhythm is often lost and the EEG is usually unresponsive to eye opening in the leads placed over the damaged area.

Causes of Cerebral Visual Loss

The causes of cerebral visual impairment can be classified on the basis of whether they are acute, chronic, or transient.

- *Acute onset visual loss:* Acute visual loss, which persists, indicates in the vast majority of cases, a vascular cause, such as infarction in the territory of posterior cerebral artery. This is usually thromboembolic in origin with the source of embolus located either in the heart or in the vertebrobasilar arterial system. Occlusion at the distal end of the basilar artery causes acute ischemia in the distribution of both cerebral arteries. In addition to the visual loss, such patients often have confusion, marked memory deficits, vertical gaze palsy, and quadriparesis, including bilateral paralysis of lower cranial nerves. This condition has been described in the neurologic literature as "top of the basilar" syndrome. Transtentorial herniation may occasionally result in ischemia in the distribution of either one or both posterior cerebral arteries, which results in unilateral or bilateral hemianopia. Other causes of acute onset visual loss of cerebral origin include sagittal sinus thrombosis or bacterial meningitis and head trauma.
- *Chronic visual loss*: Chronic onset cerebral visual loss may be caused by a number of conditions including tumors, abscesses, adrenoleukodystrophy, subacute sclerosing panencecphelitis, Creutzfeldt–Jakob disease, demyelinating disorders, and chronic mercury poisoning as in Minamata disease.
- *Brief visual impairment:* Brief visual impairment of cerebral origin occurs typically in migraine with aura. Several kinds of visual perceptions have been described by migraineurs during attacks. Most of them describe it as aura before the onset of headache. These visual phenomena generally last 15–30 minutes, but evolve to a peak in a few minutes after onset. Most often, these visual phenomena begin at the center of the visual field, which then gradually expands outward and finally disappears.

Short spells of bilateral visual dimming lasting few seconds may occur as a presyncopal feature in cases of postural hypotension, vasovagal attacks, or in cardiac arrhythmia. In the background of hypoperfusion of the brain, as in postural hypotension, they are associated with a feeling of giddiness, lightheadedness, paresthesiae of various kinds, tinnitus, and excessive sweating. Loss of consciousness in such situations has been termed "gray out" and "black out", in common man's vocabulary. Focal transient ischemic attacks in the vertebrobasilar territory have been well publicized as the cause of transient visual loss, but are much less common than global hypoperfusion. Such attacks usually result in transient hemianopia and last for seconds, minutes, or hour and are often associated with other symptoms of transient brainstem dysfunction. Transient visual loss may also occur postictally following simple partial or secondarily generalized seizures. Visual hallucinations and brief visual loss may occur as aura in partial onset seizures with an epileptogenic focus in the occipital cortex. They are typically accompanied by other epileptic features, such as visual hallucinations and gaze deviation. Rarely, postictal visual loss usually manifesting as unilateral hemianopia, and very rarely, bilateral hemianopia may last for several hours and has been referred to as visual equivalent of Todd's motor paralysis.

Brief visual loss may also occur after head trauma particularly in children, even if the injury is mild. It often starts within hours of injury but does not last for more than a day.

Visual Inattention

Vision does not only mean perceiving visual stimuli. High-level vision involves many other processes, such as object and event recognition, selective attention, and vasomotor action. Selective attention is a set of processes that directs selection of some stimuli over others which then leads to performance of several tasks in a coordinated and sensible stepwise or chain-like maner. The term attention commonly appears in layman's language but this intuitive psychologic use of the word does not provide solid definition of what exactly it means. Attention is directed to localization by all sensory modalities and thoughts but specially visual and auditory ones. It can be disturbed in many pathological processes involving the occipital and other sensory cortices, and it is then called inattention and if it involves the higher visual process, it is called "visual inattention". Inattentional blindness indicates the importance of attention in conscious awareness.

Inattentive patients neglect stimuli presented contralateral to the lesion. This is more often seen in the setting of acute unilateral cerebral infarction. Hemineglect of vision usually accompanies defects in attention in other sensory modalities as well. However, it differs in severity from severe neglect with practically no awareness of objects or movements in contralateral space to subtle neglect, which can only be detected by very careful testing.

Severe visual hemineglect can be difficult to distinguish from hemianopia resulting from geniculocalcarine damage. With hemineglect alone, responses to stimuli in the affected visual field tend to be inconsistent and depend on the intensity of distracting stimuli in the normally attended area of visual field. Patients with visual inattention are usually unaware of their problem and do not make eye and head movements to explore contralateral space. But patients with an isolated hemianopia usually do show awareness of their deficit and more adaptive head movement to compensate for the defect.

Perceptual Rivalry and Double Simultaneous Stimulation Test to Recognize Unilateral Visual Inattention

Perceptual rivalry is the perceptual rearrangement that occurs when the brain is confronted with at least two mutually exclusive images simultaneously. It has a complex underlying mechanism but is primarily mediated by interocular, interstimulus, and interhemispheric competition. It correlates with neural activity in all higher cortical areas including temporal, parietal, and occipital.

The phenomenon of perceptual rivalry has been used in diagnosing unilateral visual inattention. Mild forms of unilateral visual inattention can be demonstrated by the well-known clinical test called "double simultaneous stimulation" which is commonly used by neurologists all over the world at the bedside. In this test, small stimuli are presented in the right and left hemifields simultaneously. Patients with hemineglect fail to identify the stimulus appearing in their impaired hemifield. Simultaneous wiggling of index finger in the temporal fields bilaterally by the examiner is a very common method that is used to test for visual hemineglect and hemianopia. Contralateral visual inattention is most closely correlated with right parietal lobe lesion. This has been seen in human experiments using functional MRI. These functional neuroimaging studies have demonstrated that the right parietal lobe subserves attention in both visual hemifields, while the left parietal lobe serves only the right hemifield. Bilateral damage in the area of intraparietal fissure results in severe visual attentional deficit (Fig. 4). It is called Balint

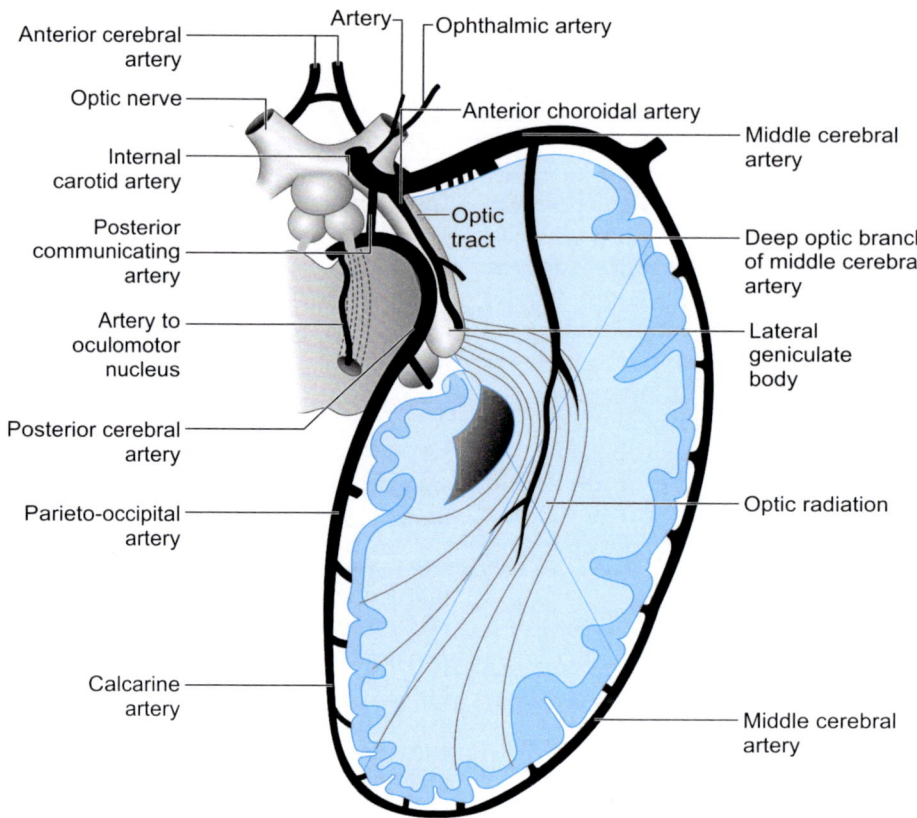

FIG. 3: Blood supply to the visual pathways.

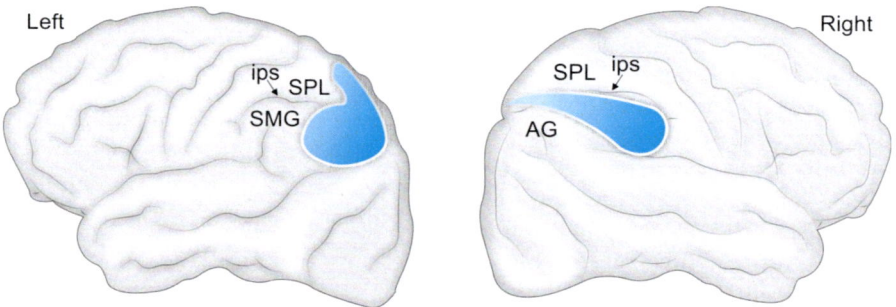

AG, angular gyrus; IPS, intraparietal sulcus; SMG, supramarginal gyrus; SPL, superior parietal lobule.
FIG. 4: Projected locations of bilateral lesions on the superolateral surface of the hemisphere in a subject with Balint syndrome.

syndrome in which patients are inattentive to stimuli outside the central fixation area. Because these patients lose interest in the peripheral visual field, they have a paucity of exploring eye movements, often stare straight, and look as if they are blind.

Simultagnosia

Simultagnosia refers to a condition in which patients can identify only one portion of the visual scene at a time and, therefore, fail to include all components of a complex illustration into a whole meaningful picture. Alzheimer's disease may sometimes lead to visual deficiency, which resembles Balint syndrome and simultagnosia as a result of early posterior parietal lobe dysfunction.

SOME SPECIAL VISUAL LOSS SYNDROMES CAUSED BY CEREBRAL DYSFUNCTION

There are some patients with a focal cerebral lesion who show descrete features of visual perception and recognition as a result of isolated dysfunction of cortical processing at a higher level particularly that which involves transfer of information from one cortical region to another. Almost any aspect of higher cortical visual process can be impaired discretely, including color vision, perception of form, facial recognition, spatial orientation, visual motion perception, and reading. And this can be explained by the current views on integration of the retinal information into higher cortical processing. The brain is an enormously intricate organ and even within a circumscribed domain, such as visual image creation or imagery, it seems to process information received from the retina in complex and subtle ways. The current understanding proposes that visual signals are segregated in the retina according to their information contents, and this segregation is supposed to continue throughout the subsequent steps of visual sensory processing. There is also a kind of division of labor in the visual system of humans and other primates. For example, in monkeys, two distinct types of retinal ganglion cells project to different layers of lateral geniculate nucleus, where one type of neuron, called the P cells, is thought to transfer motion and spatial information, whereas another class, called M cells, transmits information for color and discrimination of fine form. From the lateral geniculate ganglion, information is transferred to calcarine cortex and from calcarine cortex to different cortical regions, which have different functions. The processing stream that is meant to detect color and fine form projects to the ventromedial part of occipitotemporal lobe.

Motion and spatial information is extracted in a dorsolateral area extending from the junction of the temporal and occipital lobes to the posterior parietal region.

The complete expression of a selective visual disorder usually requires presence of bilateral lesions affecting homologous areas of each cerebral hemisphere. But unilateral lesions can also cause perceptual defects limited to the contralateral visual hemifield or less severe defects affecting both hemifields. In unilateral lesions affecting either the left or right hemispheres, there are different types of visual disturbances. These differences are based on hemispheric specialization for higher visual functions.

Some of these selective visual loss syndromes include color achromatopsia, color anomia, pure alexia, alexia without agraphia, visual inattention, visual agnosia including prosopagnosia, and defective spatial orientation.

Cerebral Achromatopsia

This is a term used to indicate deficient color perception. Patients with cerebral achromatopsia are unable to name colors. It is caused by bilateral damage affecting the fusiform and lingual gyri, which are parts of temporal and occipital lobes. It is likely that achromatopsia constitutes a family of disorders, where the variable nature of color impairment is a consequence of the pattern of damage to the extent of color center or to a cluster of visual cortical regions.

Color Anomia

It is a term used to indicate color vision deficiency where color matching is normal but the patients have difficulty in naming colors. Patients with simple achromatopsia do not have problems with naming of colors. Color anomia is often associated with alexia and both these symptoms are usually caused by left hemispheric lesions that do not allow inputs for the ventromesial visual processing circuits from reaching the angular gyrus.

Agnosia and Visual Agnosia

The term agnosia means "not knowing", and it indicates a group of neuropsychological disorders in which patients fail to recognize familiar objects, even in the presence of adequate perception, memory, language, and adequate intellectual ability. Of all the agnosias, it is the visual agnosia, which seems to be the most common, with a number of subtypes and the probable reason is that in the human brain, more tissue is devoted to vision than for any other sense. The concept of visual agnosia was originally introduced by Lissauer, who demonstrated great insight into the nature of the disorder based on the observations of a single case. He proposed that in early stages of visual processing, the processing of color, form, and motion might be affected separately as a result of brain damage. Based on the theory that visual recognition required processing through two distinct stages, he suggested that visual agnosia could be basically of two types: (1) apperceptive and (2) associative. Patients with apperceptive visual agnosia, have a complex visual perceptual process. They are not blind and can describe their visual experience, yet they do not have sufficient higher-level visual perception to recognize the object in question. In contrast, patients with associative visual agnosia show impaired recognition of visually presented objects, but they perform well on tests of perception.

Akinetopsia

The term akinetopsia refers to a selective motion perception deficit and was coined by Zeki. Bilateral lesions in lateral occipitotemporal cortex, result in a deficit of conscious motion discrimination.

Prosopagnosia

It is a term, which refers to a specific form of agnosia where patients cannot recognize familiar people by their faces alone and must rely on other cues for recognition, such as the voice, or distinctive clothing or hairstyle. In the past, it was attributed to a combination of generalized cognitive and visual disturbance and indeed, impaired face recognition does occur in disorders with more generalized problems of cognitive perception and memory, such as in Alzheimer's disease and Huntington's disease. But the term, prosopagnosia, is best reserved for patients in whom the facial recognition deficit is an isolated defect or at least more severe than any other recognition deficit that may be present. Patients with prosopagnosia are usually aware of their social difficulty, except in some cases with childhood onset disorder. Prosopagnosia is caused by lesions in the lingual and fusiform gyrus of the medial occipitotemporal cortex and sometimes in more anterior temporal lobe. There is increasing pathologic and imaging evidence in the majority of cases, that the responsible lesion is located in the right hemisphere.

Topographic Agnosia

Refers to a severe form of spatial dysperception in which patients have difficulty in recognizing previously familiar environmental landmarks, which they used as a guide when they were normal but they fail to use them as a guide in the diseased state. It may be associated with prosopagnosia and in that case, it may arise from bilateral damage either in the parietal lobes or in the fusiform and lingual gyri.

Alexia with and without Agraphia

Selective impairment of reading which is not associated with other language deficits is called pure alexia or alexia without agraphia. Reading is a relatively recent cultural acquisition in the evolution of mankind and is usually acquired only by special instruction with considerable effort. It differs from spoken language and many of the mechanisms for processes in which the written language diverges from those that determine the ability to produce and comprehend vocal speech. The purpose of the written word is to convey sound and meaning to the reader. Brain damage can affect reading in a previously literate individual without any associated impairment of spoken language or of spelling or writing. But in many cases, it is associated with agraphia, which means failure to write a word or sentence, which the patient knows well. Alexia without agraphia or pure alexia is caused by lesions that disconnect the left angular gyrus from visual inputs from both hemispheres without damaging the gyrus itself.

Vision is vital to our survival. It provides us with more information than any other sensory system to meet the essential requirements in identifying objects, manipulating our activities, and navigating in this world. However, our understanding of its basic mechanisms is very recent. The often-cited similarity between the eye and a camera is too simplistic and is correct up to a certain limit. The eyeball is an absolutely essential component of the visual system and because it is located anteriorly it catches our attention, but there are many other components outside the eyeball which are equally important and without them, one would never have the useful vision that one has. In reality, our visual system is a computerized camera, where the visual and other cortices act as the computer and they are just as important as the cornea, the lens, the aperture, or the retina. It is the cerebral substrates of the vision that really help us give the sharpness and the meaning to vision that we all possess. Our understanding on the cerebral mechanisms is only decades old and it is still rapidly evolving and in future, many new theories, concepts, and hypotheses of cerebral organization of vision will be developed to give us a better understanding of what we know now.

SUGGESTED READINGS

1. Adams AJ, Verdon WA, Sprivey BE. Colour vision. In: Tasman W, Jaeger EA (Eds). Duane's Foundations of Clinical Ophthalmology. Philadelphia: Lippincott-Raven; 1997.
2. Allport A. Attention and control. Have we been asking the wrong questions? A critical review of twenty-five years. In: Meyer DE, Kornblum S (Eds). Attention and Performance. Cambridge: MIT Press; 1993.
3. Benton A. Facial recognition. Cortex. 1990;26:491-9.
4. Biousse V, Newman NJ, Carroll C, et al. Visual fields in patients with posterior GPi pallidotomy. Neurology. 1998;50:258-65.
5. Damasio AR, Damasio H. The anatomic basis of pure alexia. Neurology. 1983;33:1873-83.
6. Fendrich R, Wessinger CM, Gazzaniga MS. Speculations on the neural basis of islands of blindsight. Prog Brain Res. 2001;134:353-66.
7. Foster DH. Inherited and Acquired Colour Vision Deficiencies: Fundamental Aspects and Clinical Studies. Boca Raton: CRC Press; 1991.
8. Gegenfurtner KR, Reiger J. Sensory and cognitive contributions to the recognition of natural scenes. Curr Biol. 2000;10:805-8.
9. Grochowicki M, Vighetto A, Berquet S, et al. Pituitary adenomas: automatic static perimetry and Goldmann perimetry. A comparative study of 345 visual field charts. Br J Ophthalmol. 1991;75:219-21.
10. Hillis AE, Cramazza A. Cognitive and neural mechanisms underlying visual and semantic processing applications from optic aphasia. J Cog Neurosci. 1995;7:457-78.
11. Holmes GM. The organization of the visual cortex in man. Proc R Soc Lond (Biol). 1945;132:348-61.
12. Horton JC, Hoyt WF. Quadrantic visual field defects. A hallmark of lesions in extrastriate (V2/V3) cortex. Brain. 1991;114:1703-18.
13. Horton JC, Hoyt WF. The representation of the visual field in human striate cortex. A revision of the classic Holmes map. Arch Ophthalmol. 1991;109:816-24.
14. Jacobson DM. The localizing value of quadrantopia. Arch Neurol. 1997;54:401-4.
15. Landis T, Regard M, Blieste A, et al. Prosopagnosia and agnosia for noncanonical views. Brain. 1988;111:1287-97.
16. Lee SH, Blake R. Rival ideas about binocular rivalry. Vision Res. 1997;37:175-83.
17. Lissauer H. Ein fall von seelenblindheit nebst einem beitrage zur theorie derselben. Arch Psychiatr Nervenkr. 1890;21:222-70.
18. Logothetis NK, Leopold DA, Scheinberg DL. What is rivaling binocular rivalry? Nature. 1996;380:621-4.
19. Luck SJ, Vecera SP. Attention from tasks to mechanisms. In: Yantis S (Ed). Steven's Handbook of Experimental Psychology. New York: Wiley; 2002. pp. 235-86.
20. Luco C, Hoppe A, Schweitzer M, et al. Visual field defects in vascular lesions of the lateral geniculate body. J Neurol Neurosurg Psychiatry. 1992;55:12-5.
21. Lumer ED, Friston KJ, Rees G. Neural correlates of perceptual rivalry in the human brain. Science. 1998;280:1930-4.
22. Mack A, Rock I. Inattentional blindness: perception without attention. In: Write RD (Ed). Visual Attention. Oxford: Oxford University Press; 1988. pp. 55-76.
23. McFadzean R, Brosnahan D, Hadley D, et al. Representation of the visual field in the occipital striate cortex. Br J Ophthalmol. 1994;78:185-90.
24. McFadzean RM, Hadley DM. Homonymous quadrantopia respecting the horizontal meridian. A feature of striate and extrastriate cortical disease. Neurology. 1997;49:1741-6.
25. Meadows JC. Disturbed perception of colours associated with localized cerebral lesions. Brain. 1974;97:615-32.
26. Mendez MF, Martin RJ, Smyth KA, et al. Disturbances of person identification in Alzheimer's disease. A retrospective study. J Nerv Ment Dis. 1992;180:94-6.
27. Miller SM, Liu GB, Ngo TT, et al. Interhemispheric switching mediates perceptual rivalry. Curr Biol. 2000;10:383-93.
28. Mishkin M, Ungerleider LG, Macko KA. Object vision and spatial vision: two cortical pathways. Trends Neurosci. 1984;6:414-7.
29. Pomeranz HD, Lessel S. Palinopsia and polyopia in the absence of drugs or cerebral disease. Neurology. 2000;54:855-9.
30. Poppel E, Held R, Frost D. Leter: Residual visual function after brain wounds involving the central visual pathways in man. Nature. 1973;243:295-6.
31. Riddoch G. Dissociation of visual perceptions due to occipital injuries with special reference to appreciation of movement. Brain. 1917;40:15-57.
32. Rizzo M, Smith V, Pokorny J, et al. Color perception profiles in central achromatopsia. Neurology. 1993;43:995-1001.
33. Smith JL. Homonymous hemianopsia: a review of one hundred cases. Am J Ophthalmol. 1962;54:616-22.

34. Takahashi N, Kawamura M, Hirayama K, et al. Prosopagnosia: a clinical and anatomical study of four patients. Cortex. 1995;31:317-29.
35. Tanaka J, Weiskopf D, Williams P. The role of colour in high level vision. Trends Cog Sci. 2001;5:211-5.
36. Trobe JD, Lorber ML, Schelzinger NS. Isolated homonymous hemianoposia. Arch Ophthalmol. 1973;89:377-81.
37. Weiskrantz L, Warrington EK, Sanders MD, et al. Visual capacity in the hemianopic field following a restricted occipital ablation. Brain. 1974;97:709-28.
38. Wüst S, Kasten E, Sabel BA. Blindsight after optic nerve injury indicates functionality of spared fibers. J Cogn Neurosci. 2002;14:243-53.
39. Zeki S, Flytche DM. The Riddoch syndrome: insights into the neurobiology of conscious vision. Brain. 1998;121:25-45.
40. Zeki S. A century of cerebral achromatopsia. Brain. 1990;113:1721-77.
41. Zeki S. Cerebral akinetopsia (visual motion blindness): a review. Brain. 1991;114:811-24.
42. Zihl J, von Cramon D, Mai N. Selective disturbance of movement vision after bilateral brain damage. Brain. 1983;106:313-40.

CHAPTER 13

Visual Illusions and Hallucinations

Ambar Chakravarty

INTRODUCTION

Most disturbances of the visual pathway give rise to "negative" symptoms, such as reduced acuity or visual field defects. Some disturbances produce "positive" symptoms, such as alterations in the shape, size, position, or motion of viewed objects or flashing or flickering lights, geometric shapes, and animated objects or scenes. A single disturbance may produce a combination of negative and positive symptoms.

Positive visual phenomena are divided into two types: (1) illusions, or misperceptions of viewed object; and (2) hallucinations, or visual experiences that are based on endogenous neural activity rather than on exogenous, viewed objects. A simple way to distinguish between illusions and hallucinations is to ask the patient whether they disappear when the eyes are closed. Those that do are illusions; the rest are hallucinations.

Why bother separating illusions from hallucinations? Because their origins may be different. Both types of positive visual phenomena emanate from disturbances of the neural visual pathway, but illusions may also be caused by optical abnormalities, whereas hallucinations are always neural events.

The optical disorders that generate illusions include improper refractive corrections (causing altered shape) and cataractous or dislocated lenses (causing multiple images and altered color). The neural disorders that generate illusions include photoreceptor dysfunction (causing micropsia, metamorphopsia, and xanthopsia), visual association cortex dysfunction (causing altered size, shape, position, distance, motion, and multiple images), and oculomotor or vestibular system dysfunction (causing altered position and motion). By contrast, visual hallucinations originate from disorders of the retina, optic nerve, or the vision-related areas of the occipital, parietal, or temporal cortex.

Positive visual phenomena may arise from a focal or a diffuse disturbance. Focal processes are always responsible for the following four phenomena:

1. Illusions confined to a hemifield are caused by dysfunction of the contralateral occipital, parietal, or temporal vision-related cortex
2. Very brief flashes of white or colored light exacerbated by eye movement are caused by physical deformation of retinal receptors by vitreous-tug or retinal tear or detachment
3. Sparkling lights confined to one eye generally indicates dysfunction of the outer retina or optic nerve
4. Sparkling lights with zigzag shape are indicative of dysfunction of the contralateral visual cortex. The differential diagnosis includes migraine, occipital ischemia, and occipital seizures. Progression of the scintillation across the hemifield over a period of 20–30 minutes identifies migraine as the cause.

Most positive visual phenomena are not caused by focal disturbances, but rather by diffuse cerebral disorders that interfere with normal sensory inputs to the visual system. This interference, or "deafferentation", allows emergence of endogenous visual activity that is ordinarily suppressed by normal cognitive activity (release phenomena). These visual release phenomena are associated with exposure to psychoactive, recreational or medicinal agents, toxic or inflammatory meningoencephalitis, dementia, psychosis, sleep deprivation, or impaired vision.

Illusions and hallucinations must be distinguished from delusions, thought disorders marked by defective reality testing. Patients who are having altered sensory experiences, whether illusory or hallucinatory, are suffering from delusions if they believe that the images they see are real. Enduring delusions usually betoken psychosis. However, temporary delusions are common and do not always indicate an ongoing psychiatric disorder. For example, believable hallucinations are often experienced by children and suggestible adults, especially during trance-like or sleep-like states.

A concise stepwise approach to a patient complaining of visual illusions or hallucination is presented here. It is important to establish whether the positive visual phenomenon is experienced by one eye, one hemifield in both eyes, or the entire visual field in both eyes. Great care need to be exercised to establish these distinctions as causative pathologic lesions would vary and misinterpretation by patients is common.

MONOCULAR ILLUSIONS

Multiple Images

When one eye sees two images (actually one clear image and a ghost image around it), the explanation is nearly always an ocular media aberration. The diagnosis is made by the finding that the pinhole eliminates the accessory image. Corneal surface irregularities, myopic astigmatism, and early cataract are common causes. If refractive correction is not helpful, a topical miotic may attenuate the diplopia. If the pinhole dies not eliminate the secondary images, the problem is likely to be psychogenic.

Altered Size or Shape

The illusion is often caused by a refractive correction problem—a new corrective lens prescription that contains a power, axis, or base curve change for one eye only. The patient reports that edges of objects appear tilted or bowed and that viewing them induces a deep-seated ache about the eyes. Although patients often adapt in time, prescribing a refraction that creates a substantial image size difference between the two eyes (aniseikonia) is unwise.

If the patient complains of seeing images of different sizes in the two eyes, the cause may be a refractive correction problem or a maculopathy. As the cones become separated by edema, inflammation, or blood, fewer of them are stimulated by the viewed object, and the object is perceived as smaller than normal (micropsia). As the edema is not evenly distributed, the object may also appear distorted (retinal metamorphopsia). The receptors may be drawn abnormally close together in the healing phase to produce an illusion of macropsia. If maculopathy is not evident, the problem is likely to be psychogenic.

Altered Color

Monocular alterations in color are of three types: (1) brunescence, (2) cyanopsia, and (3) erythropsia. Brunescence refers to the yellowish-brown tint that discolors images seen by an eye with cataract. Cyanopsia is the blue discoloration seen by patients who have recently undergone cataract extraction and have become pseudophakic or aphakic. Erythropsia refers to the reddish cast to the vision of aphakic or pseudophakic patients when they are exposed to bright sun or snow. Its mechanism is unknown. Fortunately, it lasts no more than 48 hours. Erythropsia may also be experienced by patients who suffer from anterior chamber or vitreous hemorrhage. When the appropriate ocular abnormalities are not found, the symptom is likely to be psychogenic.

Decreased Brightness

Many patients who have suffered from optic neuropathy report that the image appears dimmer when viewed with the affected eye. The objective correlate of their complaint is the afferent pupillary defect. The same complaint can be generated by a dense anterior chamber or vitreous hemorrhage but not by a dense corneal scar or cataract, both of which scatter light rather than absorbing it.

Prolonged Afterimage

Patients who report that their vision is impaired after viewing a bright light usually do not have an organic correlate for their complaint. On occasion, however, they may be describing a pathologically prolonged afterimage, the result of delayed photopigment regeneration in outer retinal ischemia or maculopathy.

MONOCULAR HALLUCINATIONS

Hallucinations seen by only one eye always originate from dysfunctional photoreceptors or optic nerve. The nature of the hallucinations is a clue to their origin.

Spontaneous, Concussive, or Eye Movement-induced Flashes

These momentary hallucinations derived from photoreceptor deformation. When the flashes (phosphenes, Moore's lightning flashes) are spontaneous or induced by eye movement, a contracting vitreous or a vitreous detachment should be suspected. An indirect ophthalmoscopic examination is advisable to rule out a retinal tear, detachment, or tumor. It can be an early symptom of optic as well especially when eye movements are painful.

Sound-induced Flashes

If a sudden sound triggers a flash of light (phosphene) in one eye, the patient has an optic neuropathy, usually demyelinating. These sound-induced phosphenes, or auditory-visual synesthetic phenomena, usually arise when the patient is in a state of repose or near sleep.

Flickering Lights

Monocular silvery scintillations likened to "snow" on a television set may be a symptoms of inner or outer retinal ischemia (reduced arterial flow or impaired venous drainage), inflammation [multiple evanescent white dot syndrome (MEWDS), paraneoplastic retinopathy], or degeneration (retinitis pigmentosa). The same symptom is occasionally reported by persons with acute optic neuropathy (demyelinating, ischemic) and by young patients who have no evidence of retinal disease and who may have a history of migraine. In these cases, the attacks are called "retinal migraine" or "cilioretinal migraine". The mechanism may be ischemia from vasospasm, but that remains indeterminate.

BINOCULAR HEMIFIELD ILLUSIONS OR HALLUCINATIONS

Binocular hemifield illusions or hallucinations have three possible causes: (1) migraine, (2) occipito-parieto-temporal lesions, or (3) vertebrobasilar transient ischemic attack (TIA).

Binocular illusions confined to a hemifield are usually caused by unilateral lesions of the occipito-parieto-temporal region. The lesions are tumors, infarcts, dysplasias, or inflammations. In most cases, they also cause a hemianopic visual field defect. Vertebrobasilar TIA must be considered as another cause. Finally, migraine may cause transient illusions of this sort (the Alice in Wonderland syndrome), especially in children.

Illusions

Illusions caused by occipito-parieto-temporal lesions consist of alterations in shape, position, motion, and duration of a perceived object, often in combination. These striking illusions suggest a fresh, large, or expanding lesion or one that is causing seizures.

Altered Shape

Patients typically describe elongations of forms along one plane with overlapping of one object onto another (cerebral metamorphopsia or illusory spread; coneheads may grow out of shoulders and gigantic fingers from elbows, rather like a cubist image). Such illusions may be episodic or persistent, but they usually disappear spontaneously within days to weeks of onset. They often coexist with palinopsia (see later) or visual hallucinations.

Altered Position

Patients see the image of a previously viewed object as displaced into the opposite hemifield (visual allesthesia). For example, a figure standing to the right of fixation, will a moment later, appear to be standing to the left of fixation. When the inciting visual stimulus for allesthesia is still within view, patients report double vision (cerebral diplopia) or multiple vision (cerebral polyopia for stationary objects). The allesthetic image is almost always displaced into a partial homonymous hemianopic field.

This altered visual experience may be an epileptic phenomenon. During the episode, patients often have either an altered sensorium, focal tonic-clonic movements, or a focal discharge on electroencephalogram (EEG). Antiepileptic medications may be effective.

Preservation

Patients with this visual illusion report seeing a previously viewed scene, such as a household setting or a highway signpost, suddenly "played back" before their eyes. This is a form of visual preservation in time, or "palinopsia" (palinopia, paliopia). The preservative illusion may occur immediately after the object has been viewed or hours later. The longer the interval, the more likely it is to be considered a hallucination rather than an illusion.

In some patients, the palinopsic experience appears to be part of a focal seizure. Right posterior hemisphere lesions have outnumbered left hemisphere lesions. Whereas the episodes generally subside within weeks, they sometimes persist. In such cases, anticonvulsant therapy is worth a try.

Altered Motion

Patients who have occipital lesion may see objects that move smoothly across their path of vision like a sequence of snapshots or as trailed by a comet-like tail. Called "cerebral polyopia for moving objects", it differs from "cerebral polyopia for stationary objects", an illusion that results from visual allesthesia (see Altered Position, earlier). A lesion in the same region may also give rise to the sensation of continuous or episodic motion of stationary viewed objects.

Hallucinations

Like illusions, hemifield hallucinations are produced by migraine, vertebrobasilar TIA, or an occipito-parieto-temporal lobe lesion. Transient hemifield hallucinations are usually produced by migraine, and less commonly by vertebrobasilar TIA. On the other hand, persistent hemifield hallucinations always reflect an occipito-parieto-temporal lobe structural lesion.

Migraine

Migraine is a common paroxysmal neurologic condition usually represented by headache. In classic migraine (migraine with aura), the headache is preceded by a transient neurologic disturbance called an "aura". In order of frequency, auras include positive or negative visual phenomena, paresthesias, aphasia, and hemiparesis.

Among the auras that affect migraineurs, the most common is an unformed visual hallucination. In fact, migraine accounts for most episodes of binocular unformed visual hallucinations, not just in youth but among elderly persons. Nearly every conceivable visual pattern has been described, but the scintillating scotoma, a twinkling zigzag shape, accounts for about 30%. Likened to the outline of a medieval Roman fortress, the scintillating scotoma has also been called a "fortification" or a "teichopsia", from the Greek word teichos, meaning city wall. Its evanescent quality has given rise to the term "fortification spectrum" (as in spectral, or ghostly). An estimated 25% of migraineurs with visual aura report a 20–40 minutes march (migration, expansion, spread, and buildup) of the scotoma across the hemifield. The speed of spread is 3–5 mm/minute which is the same as the speed of march of the cortical spreading depression which causes hallucination by possibly producing cortical hypoperfusion. If scotoma is produced by cortical hypoperfusion, what may be the explanation of the shining fortification? The bars in the fortification arc show that they consist of two parallel bright lines with a dark gap between. These shimmering and oscillating in brightness, with all the inside lines "on" when all outside lines are "off", and vice versa producing a boiling or rolling motion. This suggested that there is a network of reciprocal inhibition, with depression of activity enhancing the spontaneous neural activity in adjacent regions.

The marching scintillating scotoma is reported very rarely in vertebrobasilar TIA and is uncommon during posterior hemispheric surface electrode stimulation or electrographically documented spontaneous seizures. However, it has been documented in single case reports of patients who have occipito-parieto-temporal lesions, particularly arteriovenous malformations (AVMs).

Among 70 patients with occipital lobe AVMs, "migraine-like visual phenomena" occurred in 15 patients (21%). In two occipital AVM cases, the migraine-like episodes disappeared after the AVM was excised. Therefore, we regard the marching scintillating scotoma merely as a reaction pattern that occurs mostly in an idiopathic disorder called migraine and rarely with focal injury to primary visual cortex.

Although the marching scintillating scotoma is common in migraine, many patients with classic migraine report other visual phenomena, such as stationary sparkling lights or pinwheels. In many cases, these scintillations are not confined to a hemifield. In a large proportion of migraineurs, especially those older than 50 years, headache does not follow the visual hallucination (acephalgic, dissociated migraine).

An important feature that helps to distinguish migraine from vertebrobasilar TIA and occipito-parieto-temporal lesions is an additional aura such as the "marching paresthesia". With a time course similar to that of the marching scintillating scotoma, the marching paresthesia begins 5–30 minutes after the onset of the visual aura. Aphasia may follow. By contrast, the latency of the sensory auras of a seizure generally is much briefer, and in vertebrobasilar TIA, multiple neurologic manifestations typically occur simultaneously. Migraine rarely causes formed hallucinations. When a focal disorder is responsible, the manifestation will be partial seizures emanating from injured or deafferented parietal or temporal cortex.

Migraine with visual aura is relatively uncommon in Indian population occurring in only 2–3% of cases. Distinction from epileptic visual aura (with or without headache) is often needed. A commonly quoted distinguishing feature is that migraine visual aura is usually monochromatic (black and white) while epileptic aura in general is colored. This rule of the thumb generally works well in routine clinical practice.

Vertebrobasilar Transient Ischemic Attacks

Vertebrobasilar TIA may cause transient negative or positive visual phenomena. The visual manifestations may be the only abnormality; in one series, they were the first or only symptoms in 10% of cases. The hallucinations take many forms: tadpoles, soap flakes, snowflakes, sparklers, pinwheels, or glowing light. As in migraine, they may occupy the whole visual field or be restricted to a hemifield, depending upon whether the hypoperfusion affects one or both posterior cerebral arteries.

Vertebrobasilar TIAs rarely produce the zigzag shape or the 20–30 minute march across the hemifield that is typical of migraine. The visual disturbance usually lasts only seconds. If it lingers beyond a few hours, expect to find a persistent homonymous visual field defect and imaging evidence of occipital infarction. After occipital infarction, the hallucinations usually regress within weeks, although some field loss usually persists.

Distinguishing vertebrobasilar TIA from migraine depends in part on the presence of features of brainstem ischemia, such as vertigo, disequilibrium, drop attack, diplopia, altered consciousness, nausea, extremity weakness, and numbness. These symptoms, one or more of which are present in 90% of patients suffering from a vertebrobasilar TIA, are infrequent in migraine. There is, however, an adolescent form of migraine (basilar migraine, Bickerstaff migraine) that can also produce many of these symptoms.

Occipito-parieto-temporal Lesion

Lesions in this posterior region of the cerebrum often give rise to episodic or persistent binocular visual hallucinations, sometimes as isolated manifestations. Three mechanisms have been proposed to explain these events: (1) classic migraine auras triggered by the lesion; (2) partial seizures triggered by the lesion; and (3) release phenomena in visual association cortex disinhibited by lack of input from primary visual cortex.

Partial seizures with unformed visual hallucinations originate in primary visual cortex. Typically, the hallucination begins in one hemifield, but sometimes it spreads quickly over the entire field. Anatomic abnormalities are usually evident on brain imaging, the exception being benign childhood epilepsy with occipital paroxysms (CEOPs), a self-limited condition that mostly affects preadolescent girls.

Our knowledge of the visual experiences produced by partial seizures comes from patients' description during surface electrode stimulation and during EEG recordings of spontaneous seizures. The visual hallucinations consist of stationary lines, squares, stars, circles, disks, sparkling dots, and zigzags. They last longer than those caused by vertebrobasilar TIA, and in contrast to migraine, marching zigzags are rare. In a series of 20 patients with occipital seizures, no one described zigzags.

Identifying partial seizures (or complex partial seizures) as cause of visual hallucinations depends on finding nystagmus, frequent blinking or eyelid fluttering, staring or other automatisms, tonic-clonic movements, or loss of consciousness. In one series of 25 patients with occipital lobe partial seizures, eye deviation was present in 16 patients (64%) and repeated blinking in 14 patients (56%).

In the Indian context, partial seizures with visual aura (with or without generalization), especially in children and young adults, are often caused by cysticercal lesions in the occipital region. However, the visual aura is often binocular probably due to rapid spread of epileptic discharge to the other side. In children, presentation is often with only visual aura (generally colored) associated with a vascular type of headache, mimicking classical migraine. Response to antiepileptics is generally very satisfactory.

Visual hallucinations associated with occipito-parieto-temporal lesions are not always manifestations of focal seizures. Such lesions can block input to vision-related cortex and allow the emergence of endogenous visual activity as release phenomena. In one large series of patients with visual hallucinations following occipital infarctions, EEG failed to document any seizures. Visual hallucinations developed only in those patients whose posterior hemispheric lesions spared much of visual association cortex and nearby white matter. The inference is that, for visual hallucinations to occur, association visual cortex must be intact and cut off from normal visual inputs by a lesion in the primary visual cortex region.

Among patients who are not exposed to psychoactive agents and who have intact mentation and adequate vision, formed hallucinations (images of animate objects or scenes) always originate in parietal or temporal vision-related cortex. They may be manifestations of a partial seizure or release phenomena.

Surface electrode stimulation of the cerebral cortex shows that partial seizures originating in temporal cortex often cause a dream-like state. The hallucinations evoke feelings of fear, pleasure, strangeness, or familiarity. By comparison, partial seizures of parietal origin create formed hallucinations whose details are so vivid and realistic that patients temporarily believe that they are actually seeing them.

Even though they are generated in a damaged hemisphere, formed hallucinations generally do not remain confined to the contralateral hemifield. In general, right posterior hemisphere lesions are more likely than left ones to produce formed hallucinations.

BINOCULAR FULL-FIELD ILLUSIONS OR HALLUCINATIONS

Illusions or hallucinations involving both eyes and not confined to hemifield may be initiated by the same focal processes identified earlier as causes of hemifield illusions or hallucinations. They can also result from nonlocalizing processes such as exposure to a psychoactive agent or an impaired mental or visual state. These nonlocalizing conditions should be ruled out first.

Exposure to Psychoactive Agent

When the patient has been exposed to a psychoactive agent, visual illusions and hallucinations must initially be considered pharmacologically induced. Virtually, every psychoactive medication or drug has been associated with the production of visual illusions and hallucinations. The medications most often implicated are those with anticholinergic, dopaminergic, or serotoninergic properties. Among hallucinogenic, street drugs, mescal, psilocybin, lysergic acid, and amphetamines are most cited. Withdrawal from habitual use of some of these agents, as well as from alcohol, may cause prominent illusions and hallucinations, often of animals (zoopsia). Although drug-induced or withdrawal-associated visual hallucinations may be accompanied by auditory hallucinations, psychotic thought disorder, or delirium, it is critical to recognize that the visual aberrations may be the most prominent, or the only manifestation.

Abnormal Mental State or Impaired Vision Present

Inflammatory or Metabolic Encephalopathy

Visual illusions and hallucinations are frequent manifestations of delirium, an altered behavioral and autonomic state brought on by infection, fever, metabolic imbalance, or hypoxia.

Dementia

Visual hallucinations are widely reported in the advancing stages of all dementing processes. Usually formed, and often reminiscent of earlier life experiences, they may arise spontaneously and are exacerbated when the patient is left alone in a darkened room or treated with psychoactive medications (sundowning). Any type of dementia can produce visual hallucinations, but they are especially common in diffuse Lewy body disease.

Psychosis

The visual hallucinations of psychosis are distinctive in being complex, delusional, and paranoid, and they are often integrated with auditory hallucinations.

Sleep-like States

Visual hallucinations usually occur just before sleep (hypnagogic hallucinations) or upon awakening (hypnopompic hallucinations). They are also a prominent feature of narcolepsy.

Vivid animate hallucinations associated with a sleep-like state may arise from lesions of the midbrain (peduncular hallucinosis). Because sleep-wake cycle disturbances are always present, these hallucinations probably represent dream intrusions generated by a damaged reticular activating system.

Trance-like States

Visual illusions and hallucinations are often reported during hypnosis, intense emotional stress, and religious rituals. The fertile imaginations of children quite normally conjure up imaginary playmates they regard as real.

Impaired Vision

When sight is poor, external visual stimuli can no longer shield the brain from its internal visual memories. Elderly patients who have 20/200 visual acuity or worse in the better eye often report seeing detailed floral or wallpaper patterns and unfamiliar faces (Charles Bonnet syndrome). Although these figments are usually pleasant, they sometimes have a paranoid component that frightens the patients. This phenomenon is more likely to occur against a background of dementia, but it can also occur in persons in a normal cognitive state. Social isolation is a prominent feature. Low-dose haloperidol, 0.5–1.0 mg/day, or another antipsychotic medication often relieves the symptoms.

Abnormal Mental State or Impaired Vision Not Present

When full-field binocular illusions or hallucinations cannot be attributed to the effects of a psychoactive agent, abnormal mental state or blindness, clues to precise localization come from the nature of the visual experience and the neuro-ophthalmologic findings.

Altered Color

Patients suffering from digitalis toxicity may report a yellowish-green tinge or frosting to their vision (xanthopsia), a manifestation of retinal photoreceptor damage.

Achromatopsia, the inability to sort or match colors, may result from inferior occipital lobe lesions involving the lingual and fusiform gyri. Patients also have superior altitudinal visual field defects to achromatic stimuli. Bilateral posterior cerebral infarctions are the most common cause.

Altered Spatial Relationships

Patients who have medullary ischemia from vertebrobasilar vascular insufficiency may see their environment as tilted or even upside down. Infarction of the dorsolateral medulla (Wallenberg's syndrome) may cause this illusion to persist for days to weeks. The diagnosis is based on eliciting other manifestations of brainstem damage.

Bilateral parieto-occipital lobe lesions may lead to great difficulty in judging the relative distances of objects in space and manifest as misreaching under visual guidance, bumping into furniture, or getting lost. Although patients may complain that objects appear displaced, their problem is not that they are experiencing illusions but rather that they cannot function within space (topographic agnosia). Their deficit is believed to result from disconnection between visual cortex and parietal cortex, where multiple sensory inputs are integrated.

Altered Motion

Illusions of motion may be caused by unilateral (or markedly asymmetric) optic neuropathy. When affected patients view a pendulum swinging in a place, they perceive its path as describing an ellipse (counterclockwise rotation if the right optic nerve is affected; clockwise rotation if the left optic nerve is affected). Called a "Pulfrich stereo-illusions", this misperception is believed to result from unequal conduction rates in the two optic nerves. Some patients who demonstrate the Pulfrich stereo-illusion also complain that they can no longer tell how fast the ball is moving or judge its distance from them. A ball thrown at them appears to curve as it approaches. Whether these complaints and the Pulfrich stereo-illusion are related is not known.

The most frequent illusions of motion do not arise from visual pathway lesions but from the oculomotor pathway. Oscillopsia is the name given to the illusion of movement of stationary objects. Oscillopsia is most clearly described by patients who have large-amplitude nystagmus. If the nystagmus is pendular (both phases are slow eye movements), patients perceive to-and-from movement. If the nystagmus is jerk (one phase is fast), they perceive the objects as moving only in the direction of the fast phase. Sometimes, patients cannot clearly distinguish movement and report a "shimmery" sensation that may be misinterpreted as a scintillation.

Oscillopsia may also be described by patients who do not have nystagmus but instead have a defective vestibulo-ocular reflex (VOR). When the VOR is functioning normally, head and body movements are synchronized perfectly with eye movements in the opposite direction, but when the VOR is defective, this synchrony is disturbed and the eyes cannot be held immobile in space during slight head or body movements. The result is that the patient sees stationary objects as blurred or "jiggling". The offending lesion lies in the vestibular pathways, in either the end organs, nerves, or brainstem connections.

Patients who have chronic lesions adapt quite well to VOR defects. Oscillopsia occurs more frequently in acute processes such as aminoglycoside ototoxicity and brainstem infarct, demyelination, or tumor. A simple way to verify that the VOR is the cause of the symptom is to have the patient read a Snellen near card while moving the head rapidly from side to side. Under normal circumstances, the VOR compensation ensures continued clear vision; if the VOR is defective, acuity is degraded by at least two Snellen lines.

Oscillopsia is never a complaint of patients with congenital nystagmus, even when the ocular oscillations are very large. Those persons report blurred vision but are not aware of movement.

SUGGESTED READINGS

1. Alvarez WC. The migrainous scotoma as studied in 618 persons. Am J Ophthalmol. 1960;49:489-504.
2. Anderson SW, Rizzo M. Hallucinations following occipital lobe damage: The pathological activation of visual representations. J Clin Exp Neuropsychol. 1994;16:651-63.
3. Asaad G, Shapiro B. Hallucinations: theoretical and clinical overview. Am J Psychiatry. 1986;143:1088-97.
4. Bender MB. Oscillopsia. Arch Neurol. 1965;49:489-504.
5. Bender MB. Polyopia and monocular diplopia of cerebral origin. Arch Neurol Psychiatry. 1945;54: 323-38.
6. Bickerstaff ER. The basilar artery and the migraine-epilepsy syndrome. Proc R Soc Med. 1962;55:167-9.
7. Brickner R. Oscillopsia: A new symptom commonly occurring in multiple sclerosis. Arch Neurol Psychiatry. 1936;36:586-9.
8. Brindley GS, Lewin WS. The sensations produced by electrical stimulation of the visual cortex. J Physiol. 1968;196:479-93.
9. Charles N, Froment C, Rode G, et al. Vertigo and upside down vision due to an infarct in the territory of the medial branch of the posterior inferior cerebellar artery caused by dissection of a vertebral artery. J Neurol Neurosurg Psychiatry. 1992;55:188-9.
10. Cogan DG. Visual hallucinations as release phenomena. Von Graefes Archklin Ophthalmol. 1973;188:139-51.
11. Crawford J. Living without a balancing mechanism. N Engl J Med. 1952;246:458-60.

12. Critchley M. Neurological aspects of visual and auditory hallucinations. Br Med J. 1939;2:634-9.
13. Critchley M. Types of visual preservation: "Palinopsia" and "illusory visual spread". Brain. 1951;74:267-99.
14. Cummings JL, Syndulko K, Goldberg Z, et al. Palinopsia reconsidered. Neurology. 1982;32:444-7.
15. Cummings JL. Clinical Neuropsychiatry. Orlando: Grune & Stratton; 1985. pp. 221-33.
16. Damasio AR. Disorders of complex visual processing: Agnosias, achromatopsia, Balint's syndrome, and related difficulties of orientation and construction. In: Mesulam MM (Ed). Principles of Behavioral Neurology. Philadelphia: F.A. Davis; 1985. pp. 259-88.
17. Damos J, Skelton M, Jenner FA. The Charles Bonnet syndrome in perspective. Psychol Med. 1982;12:251-7.
18. Davidoff RA. Migraine: Manifestations, Pathogenesis, and Management. Philadelphia: F.A. Davis; 1995.
19. Dobelle WH, Mladejorsky MG, Garvin JP. Artificial vision for the blind: Electrical stimulation of visual cortex offers hope for functional prosthesis. Science. 1974;183:440-4.
20. Drugs that cause psychiatric symptoms. Med Lett Drugs Ther. 1989;29:808.
21. Dunn DW, Weisberg LA, Nadell J. Peduncular hallucinations caused by brainstem compression. Neurology. 1983;33:1360-1.
22. Egdell HG, Kolven I. Childhood hallucinations. J Child Psychol Psychiatry. 1972;13:279-87.
23. Engel JL. Seizures and Epilepsy. Philadelphia: F.A. Davis; 1989. p. 146.
24. Fisher CM. Late-life migraine accompaniments as a cause of unexplained transient ischemic attacks. Can J Neurol Sci. 1980;7:8-17.
25. Fisher CM. The posterior cerebral artery syndrome. Can J Neurol Sci. 1986;13:232-9.
26. Fulan AJ, Whisnant JP, Kearns TP. Unilateral visual loss in bright light: an unusual symptom of carotid artery occlusive disease. Arch Neurol. 1979;36:675-6.
27. Gastaut H, Zifkin BG. Benign epilepsy of childhood with occipital spike and wave complexes. In: Andermann F, Lugaresi E (Eds). Migraine and Epilepsy: An Overview. Boston: Butterworths; 1987.
28. Hacaen H, Albert ML. Human Neuropsychology. New York: John Wiley & Sons; 1978. pp. 215-27.
29. Hachinski VC, Porchawka J, Steele JC. Visual symptoms in the migraine syndrome. Neurology. 1973;23:570-9.
30. Heron G, Dutton GN. The Pulfrich phenomenon and its alleviation with a neutral density filter. Br J Ophthalmol. 1989;73:1004-8.
31. Holmes G. Disturbances of visual orientation. Br J Ophthalmol. 1918;2:449-68.
32. Hornsten G. Wallenberg's syndrome. I. General symptomatology, with special reference to visual disturbances and imbalance. Acta Neurol Scand. 1974;50:434-46.
33. Hoyt WF. Transient bilateral blurring of vision. Considerations of an episodic ischemic symptom of vertebrobasilar insufficiency. Arch Ophthalmol. 1963;70:746-51.
34. Hupp SL, Kline LB, Corbett JJ. Visual disturbances of migraine. Surv Ophthalmol. 1989;33:221-36.
35. Jacobs I. Visual allesthesia. Neurology. 1980;30:1059-63.
36. Jacobs L, Karpik A, Bozian D, et al. Auditory-visual synesthesia: Sound-induced photisms. Arch Neurol. 1981;38:211-6.
37. Jacobson DM, Thirkill CE, Tipping SJ. A clinical triad to diagnose paraneoplastic retinopathy. Ann Neurol. 1990;28:162-5.
38. Jampol LM, Sieving PA, Pugh D, et al. Multiple evanescent white dot syndrome. I. Clinical findings. Arch Ophthalmol. 1984;102:671-4.
39. Kattah JC, Luessenhop AJ. Resolution of classic migraine after removal of an occipital lobe AVM. Ann Neurol. 1980;7:93.
40. Kolmel HW. Coloured patterns in hemianopic fields. Brain. 1984;107:155-67.
41. Kolmel HW. Complex visual hallucinations in the hemianopic field. J Neurol Neurosurg Psychiatry. 1985;48:29-38.
42. Kolmel HW. Complex visual hallucinations in the hemianopic field. J Neurol Neurosurg Psychiatry. 1985;48:29-38.
43. Kupersmith MJ, Vargas ME, Yashar A, et al. Occipital arteriovenous malformations: Visual disturbances and presentation. Neurology. 1996;46:953-7.
44. Lance JW, Smee RI. Partial seizures with visual disturbance treated by radiotherapy of cavernous hemangioma. Ann Neurol. 1989;26:782-5.
45. Lance JW. Simple formed hallucinations confined to the area of a specific visual field defect. Brain. 1976;99:719-34.
46. Leigh RJ. Management of oscillopsia. In: Barber HO, Sharpe JA (Eds). Vestibular Disorders. St. Louis: Mosby Year Book; 1988. pp. 201-11.
47. Lepore FE. Spontaneous visual phenomena with visual loss: 104 patients with lesions of retinal and neural afferent pathways. Neurology. 1990;40:444-7.
48. Lepore FE. Visual obscurations: Evanescent and elementary. Semin Neurol. 1986;6:167-75.
49. Lerner AI, Koss E, Patternson MB, et al. Concomitants of visual hallucinations in Alzheimer's disease. Neurology. 1994;44:523-7.
50. Lessel S, Cohen MM. Phosphenes induced by sound. Neurology. 1979;29:1524-6.
51. Lippman C. Certain hallucinations peculiar to migraine. J Nerv Mental Dis. 1952;116:346-51.
52. Ludwig BI, Ajmone C. Clinical ictal patterns in epileptic patients with occipital electroencephalographic foci. Neurology. 1975;25:463-71.
53. Mckee AC, Levine DN, Kowall NW, et al. Peduncular hallucinosis associated with isolated infarction of the substantia nigra pars reticulata. Ann Neurol. 1990;27:500-4.
54. McShane R, Gedling K, Reading M, et al. Prospective study of relations between cortical Lewy bodies, poor eyesight, and hallucinations in Alzheimer's disease. J Neurol Neurosurg Psychiatry. 1995;59:185-8.

55. Meadows JC. Disturbed perception of colors associated with localized cerebral lesions. Brain. 1974;97:615-32.
56. Michel EM, Troost BT. Palinopsia: Cerebral localization with computed tomography. Neurology. 1980;30:887-9.
57. Milder B, Rubin ML. The Fine Art of Prescribing Glasses Without Making a Spectacle of Yourself. Florida: Triad Publishing Company; 1984. pp. 404-8.
58. Minor RH, Kearns TP, Millikan CH, et al. Ocular manifestations of occlusive disease of the vertebrobasilar arterial system. Arch Ophthalmol. 1959;62:112-24.
59. Monteiro LR, Hoyt WF, Imes RK. Puerperal cerebral blindness. Arch Neurol. 1984;41:1300-1.
60. Newman DS, Levine SR, Curtis VL, et al. Migraine-like visual phenomena associated with cerebral venous thrombosis. Headache. 1989;29:82-5.
61. Page NC, Bolger JP, Sanders MD. Auditory evoked phosphenes in optic nerve disease. J Neurol Neurosurg Psychiatry. 1982;45:7-12.
62. Panayiotopoulos CP. Benign childhood epilepsy with occipital paroxysms: A 15-year prospective study. Ann Neurol. 1989;26:51-6.
63. Panayiotopoulos CP. Elementary visual hallucinations in migraine and epilepsy. J Neurol Neurosurg Psychiatry. 1994;57:1371-4.
64. Pearlman AL, Birch J, Meadows JC. Cerebral color blindness: An acquired defect in hue discrimination. Ann Neurol. 1979;5:253-61.
65. Penfield W, Jaspor H. Epilepsy and the Functional Anatomy of the Human Brain. Boston: Little Brown; 1954.
66. Penfield W, Perot P. The brain's record of auditory and visual experience. Brain. 1963;86:595-696.
67. Penfield W, Rasmussen J. The Cerebral Cortex of Man: A Clinical Study of Localization of Function. New York: Macmillan Publishers; 1950.
68. Piltz JR, Wertenbaker C, Lance SE, et al. Digoxin toxicity: Recognizing the varied visual presentations. J Clin Neuroophthalmol. 1993;13:275-80.
69. Plant GT. The fortification spectra of migraine. Br Med J. 1986;293:1613-7.
70. Riaz G, Hennessey JJ. Meningeal lesions mimicking migraine. Neuroophthalmology. 1991;11:41-8.
71. Robertson DM, Hollenhorst RW, Callahan JA. Ocular manifestations of digitalis toxicity: Discussion and report of three cases of central scotomas. Arch Ophthalmol. 1966;76:640-5.
72. Russel WR, Whitty WM. Studies in traumatic epilepsy. 3. Visual fits. J Neurol Neurosurg Psychiatry. 1955;18:79-96.
73. Sarbin TR, Juhasz JB. The social context of hallucinations. In: Seigel RK, West LJ (Eds). Hallucinations: Behavior, Experience, and Theory. New York: John & Sons; 1975. p. 256.
74. Schneider T, Dahlheim P, Zrenner E. Experimental investations of the ocular toxicity of cardiac glycosides in animals. Fortschr Ophthalmol. 1989;86:751-5.
75. Schultz G, Melzack R. Visual hallucinations and mental state: A study of 14 Charles Bonnet syndrome hallucinators. J Nerv Ment Dis. 1993;181:539-643.
76. Sokol S. The Pulfrich stereo-illusion as an index of optic nerve dysfunction. Surv Ophthalmol. 1976;20:432-4.
77. Steiner I, Shahin R, Melamed E. Acute "upside down" reversal of vision in transient vertebrobasilar ischemia. Neurology. 1987;37:1685-6.
78. Sternberg P, Fagadau WR, Massof RW, et al. Blizzard of '83 erythropsia. N Engl J Med. 1983;308:1482-3.
79. Teunisse RJ, Zitman FG, Raes DC. Clinical evaluation of 14 patients with the Charles Bonnet syndrome (isolated visual hallucinations). Compr Psychiatry. 1994;35:70-5.
80. Todd J. The syndrome of Alice in Wonderland. Can Med Assoc J. 1955;73:701-4.
81. Troost BT, Mark LE, Maroon JC. Resolution of classic migraine after removal of an occipital lobe AVM. Ann Neurol. 1979;5:199-201.
82. Vaphiades MS, Celesia GG, Brigell MG. Positive spontaneous visual phenomena limited to the hemianopic field in lesions of central visual pathways. Neurology. 1996;47:408-17.
83. Weinberger LM, Grant FC. Visual hallucinations and their neuro-optical correlates. Arch Ophthalmol. 1940;23:166-99.
84. Weiskrantz L, Warrington EK, Sanders MD, et al. Visual capacity in the hemianopic field following a restricted occipital ablation. Brain. 1974;97:709-28.
85. Weleber RG, Shults WT. Digoxin retinal toxicity: clinical and electrophysiologic evaluation of a cone dysfunction syndrome. Arch Ophthalmol. 1981;99:1568-72.
86. Williams D, Wilson TG. The diagnosis of the major and minor syndromes of basilar insufficiency. Brain. 1962;85:741-74.
87. Williamson PD, Thadani VM, Darcey TM, et al. Occipital lobe epilepsy: Clinical characteristics, seizures spread patterns, and results of surgery. Ann Neurol. 1992;31:3-13.

CHAPTER 14

Nuclear and Infranuclear Ophthalmoplegias

Ambar Chakravarty

INTRODUCTION

Ocular motility disorders result from supranuclear, nuclear, and infranuclear pathologies. Supranuclear lesions do not produce strabismus or diplopia. Nuclear and infranuclear lesions often lead to strabismus and diplopia. Such lesions produce oculomotor palsies with the resultant lesions lying at oculomotor nuclear levels in the brainstem, trunk of the oculomotor nerves, the myoneural junctions, or the bellies of the external ocular muscles. Diplopia is too exhaustive a topic to cover in one single chapter. Clinical approach to the problem of diplopia and strabismus would be discussed separately in the following chapter. The present chapter would cover pattern recognizing features and pathological lesions affecting the nuclear and infranuclear components of the oculomotor pathways from the brainstem to the ocular muscles.

SOME FUNDAMENTALS (FIG. 1)

The evolution of ocular motor nerve palsies is one of the most common neuro-ophthalmologic problems encountered by neurologists. The third cranial nerve passes through the rostral midbrain, subarachnoid space, and cavernous sinus on its way to innervate the extraocular (i.e., superior, inferior, and medial recti; inferior oblique; levator palpebrae) and intraocular (i.e., iris sphincter and ciliary) muscles. This course places it in harm's way by injury from a variety of brainstem lesions, leptomeningeal infiltrations or infections, extra-axial tumors, and aneurysms.

The trochlear nerve is unique because of two anatomical properties. It exits the dorsal brainstem (at the level of the caudal midbrain) and innervates a contralateral target (the superior oblique muscle). Ocular ductions appear full in many patients with fourth cranial nerve palsy, making it the most difficult of the ocular motor nerve palsies to diagnose. Moreover, the differential diagnosis of fourth cranial nerve palsy includes important neurologic and orbital disorders that must be sorted out when evaluating a patient with vertical double vision.

The sixth cranial nerve passes through the pons, climbs up the clivus, and courses through the cavernous sinus on its way to innervate the lateral rectus muscle. This cranial nerve is often injured by a variety of intra-axial and extra-axial lesions. In addition, sixth cranial nerve palsy may also represent a nonlocalizing sign of increased intracranial pressure from a brain tumor or other structural lesions.

A correct and timely diagnosis of the underlying cause of ocular motor nerve palsy is critical because of the realistic threat of serious neurological conditions. Even with the ready availability of computed tomography (CT) and magnetic resonance imaging (MRI), ominous lesions may be missed unless certain pitfalls are avoided.

EVALUATION OF THIRD CRANIAL NERVE PALSY

Nonisolated Third Cranial Nerve Palsy

If other neurologic symptoms or signs are present, they will, in most cases, direct one to the site along the oculomotor nerve pathway where the responsible lesion is likely to be residing (Box 1). For example, a patient with contralateral hemiparesis has a lesion in the midbrain ipsilateral to the third nerve palsy, while a patient with additional involvement of the sixth cranial nerve probably has a lesion in the ipsilateral cavernous sinus. In some cases, the presence of other neurologic or systemic features will suggest the specific disorder responsible for

Box 1: Causes of third nerve palsy by location of the responsible lesion

Brainstem:
- Congenital hypoplasia
- Infarction
- Hemorrhage
- Tumors
- Encephalitis
- Trauma (nonsurgical)
- Demyelination

Subarachnoid:
- Aneurysm—posterior communicating-internal carotid junction most common, basilar tip less common
- Leptomeningeal carcinomatosis
- Meningitis—e.g., tuberculosis, Lyme disease, opportunistic agents, fungi, syphilis
- Inflammation—e.g., Guillain–Barré syndrome, Miller Fisher variant
- Compression—uncal herniation at the tentorial edge
- Trauma—nonsurgical or surgical
- Tumors of the third nerve

Cavernous sinus/superior orbital fissure (Fig. 2 and 3):
- Tumors—e.g., pituitary adenoma, meningioma, craniopharyngioma, third nerve tumors
- Aneurysm—e.g., giant intracavernous carotid artery
- Carotid—cavernous fistula
- Cavernous sinus thrombosis
- Inflammation—e.g., Tolosa-Hunt syndrome
- Infection—e.g., herpes zoster

Uncertain or variable location:
- Peripheral nerve infarction
- Ophthalmoplegic migraine
- Congenital
- Infections
- Trauma

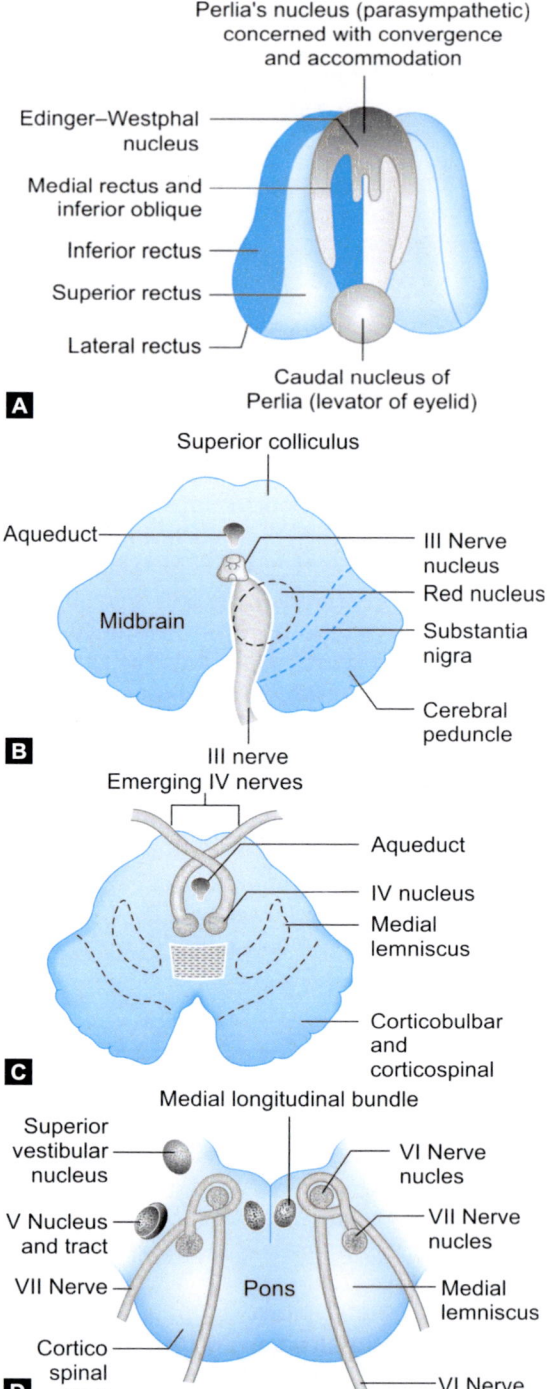

FIG. 1: A, The oculomotor (NIII) nuclear complex. B, Origin of the oculomotor nerve from midbrain at superior collicular level; C, Origin of the trochlear nerve from midbrain at inferior collicular level. Note its dorsal exit and decussation; D, Origin of the abducens nerve from pons. Note its close relation to the origin of the facial nerve.

the ophthalmoplegia, as in an elderly patient with headaches, weight loss, transient visual loss, and tenderness of the superficial temporal arteries who is most likely harboring giant cell arteritis.

Isolated Third Cranial Nerve Palsy

Many times, however, a patient develops third cranial nerve palsy without other neurologic or systemic symptoms or signs. In these patients, consideration of specific characteristics of the ophthalmoplegia (e.g., status of the pupil) and historical details (e.g., static versus progressive) will

Nuclear and Infranuclear Ophthalmoplegias | 129

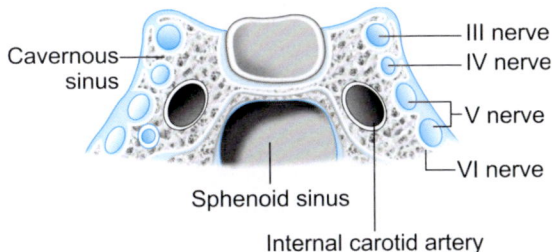

FIG. 2: Relationship of cranial nerves within the cavernous sinus.

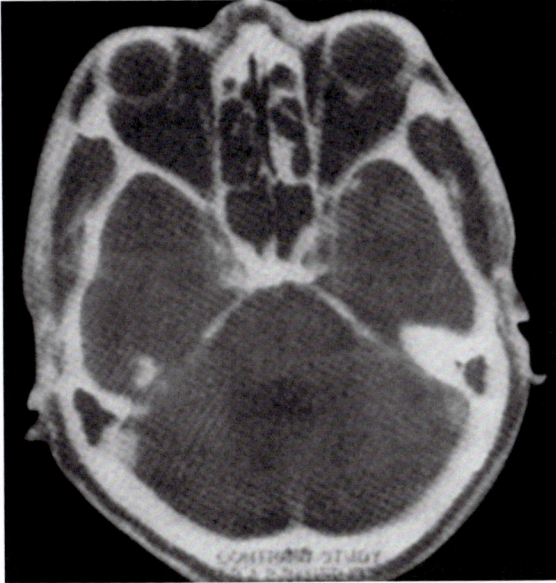

FIG. 3: Contrast-enhanced computed tomography of bilateral cavernous sinus thrombosis—showing enhancement of cavernous sinuses.

help guide one to the likely disorder responsible for the presentation.

The five important causes of acute third nerve palsy seen in routine clinical practice are:
1. Infarction of the peripheral cranial nerve
2. Compression by tumor
3. Compression by aneurysm
4. Trauma
5. Brainstem stroke.

This list should probably also include Tolosa–Hunt syndrome (THS) or painful ophthalmoplegia syndrome when considering clinical practice in the Indian context. However, the overall impression on the frequency of occurrence of this condition in India is probably somewhat overestimated and certainly the condition would not appear to be as prevalent if strict diagnostic criteria (neuroradiological) are employed (vide infra).

Most of the less frequent disorders causing oculomotor nerve palsy as well as trauma and brainstem stroke listed above, occur in patients with historical information or physical signs that implicate the underlying cause of ophthalmoplegia (i.e., nonisolated).

Therefore, the usual dilemmas facing a neurologist evaluating a patient with acute and neurologically-isolated third cranial nerve palsy include:
- Is it due to infarction or compression (by aneurysm)?
- Can one wait and watch, or do one need to image emergently?
- If one proceeds with imaging to exclude aneurysm, should one go directly to catheter angiography, or screen using a noninvasive test?

Ischemic third cranial nerve palsy is the most common pupil-sparing oculomotor palsy in middle-aged or older adults. It is usually the result of infarction of the extra-axial segment of the oculomotor nerve, although patients with similar clinical characteristics have been described who have documented midbrain strokes. This condition has traditionally been referred to as "diabetic third nerve palsy" or "diabetic ophthalmoplegia", since it frequency occurs in patients with established diabetes. However, the same condition may occur in patients who are not diabetic but who have other overt or unrecognized vascular risk factors, most notably left ventricular hypertrophy (LVH) associated with hypertension and polycythemia.

Patients with ischemic third nerve palsy have the following clinical profile:
- Age usually greater than 45 years. Occasionally, younger patients, those with long-standing diabetes in particular, may be affected
- Abrupt onset
- Often times associated with a dull, continuous pain around the ipsilateral brow, eye, or temple lasting a week or two, at most
- Pupil usually normal. About one-third of patients demonstrate small anisocoria (one millimeter or less), but the pupil characteristically remains

reactive to light. Anisocoria >1 mm, or a "blown" pupil, is not consistent with ischemic injury, and usually indicates that a mass lesion is compressing the oculomotor nerve
- Neurologically isolated. In particular, bilateral third nerve, or ipsilateral fourth or sixth nerve, involvement is not consistent with ischemic third nerve palsy
- Progression of external ophthalmoplegia during the subsequent 1–2 weeks occurs in about two-thirds of acutely-evaluated patients who have incomplete deficits at their first visit. Progression of deficits beyond this period indicates that the initial diagnosis was in error and that a mass lesion is compressing the third nerve. Of note, similar progression of ophthalmoplegia is often observed if a patient with sixth nerve palsy is seen acutely and their deficit is incomplete. The implication of ophthalmoplegia progressing beyond this period in such patients is similar to those with third nerve palsy
- Excellent prognosis. Spontaneous recovery (without signs of aberrant regeneration) is expected within 3 months in 90% of patients. Recurrent events involving the same or other ocular motor nerves occur in at least 15% of patients.

What is the work-up for a patient with pupil-sparing complete third nerve palsy?
- Fasting and 2-hour postprandial glucose tolerance test and, if known diabetes, hemoglobin A1c assay. It is not uncommon to identify unsuspected diabetes in a patient presenting with ischemic ocular motor nerve palsy. In those with established diabetes, poor glycemic control may be a predisposing factor
- Serial blood pressure measurements and electrocardiogram (looking for LVH). As with diabetes, it is not uncommon to identify previously unsuspected hypertension in this population
- Hemoglobin and hematocrit (seeking polycythemia)
- Other evaluations for vascular risk factors, as appropriate
- Erythrocyte sedimentation rate and/or C-reactive protein if older than 55 years to screen for giant cell arteritis

- Neuroimaging is generally not necessary unless:
  o Age less than 45 years
  o Vascular risk factors not present
  o No recovery within 3 months
  o Signs of aberrant regeneration develop
  o Pupil becomes involved with anisocoria >1 mm
  o Other neurologic signs develop.

Tumors that compress the third cranial nerve in ambulatory outpatients are usually located in the parasellar/cavernous sinus/orbital apex region. Common offenders include pituitary adenomas, meningiomas, craniopharyngiomas, and chodomas. They often injure additional neighboring structures, resulting in a combination of fourth or sixth cranial nerve palsy, trigeminal neuropathy, postganglionic Horner's syndrome, or produce visual loss due to compression of the optic nerve or chiasm. The pupil is usually dilated and poorly reactive when the third cranial nerve is compressed by tumor. If signs of aberrant regeneration are present, a chronic mass lesion within the cavernous sinus (e.g., meningioma or aneurysm) should be suspected. When a patient develops oculomotor palsy following seemingly minor head trauma, neuroimaging is indicated to exclude the presence of a previously unsuspected mass lesion at the base of the skull.

Aneurysms compressing the third cranial nerve classically produce acute, painful ophthalmoplegia with pupil involvement. Beware that chronic-progressive, painless, and pupil-sparing/relative pupil-sparing presentations are not inconsistent with aneurysm.

Three aneurysmal sites are most often encountered (Fig. 4):
1. Posterior communicating-internal carotid junction: This is the most common site of aneurysm that causes third cranial nerve injury. Unruptured aneurysms in this location usually do not produce other neurologic symptoms apart from ipsilateral headache. The pupil is "blown" (i.e., dilated and unresponsive to light) in one-half to two-thirds of patients, but may be normal in 14%, especially if external ophthalmoplegia is incomplete
2. Basilar tip: The posterior circulation is an often forgotten source of aneurysms that can

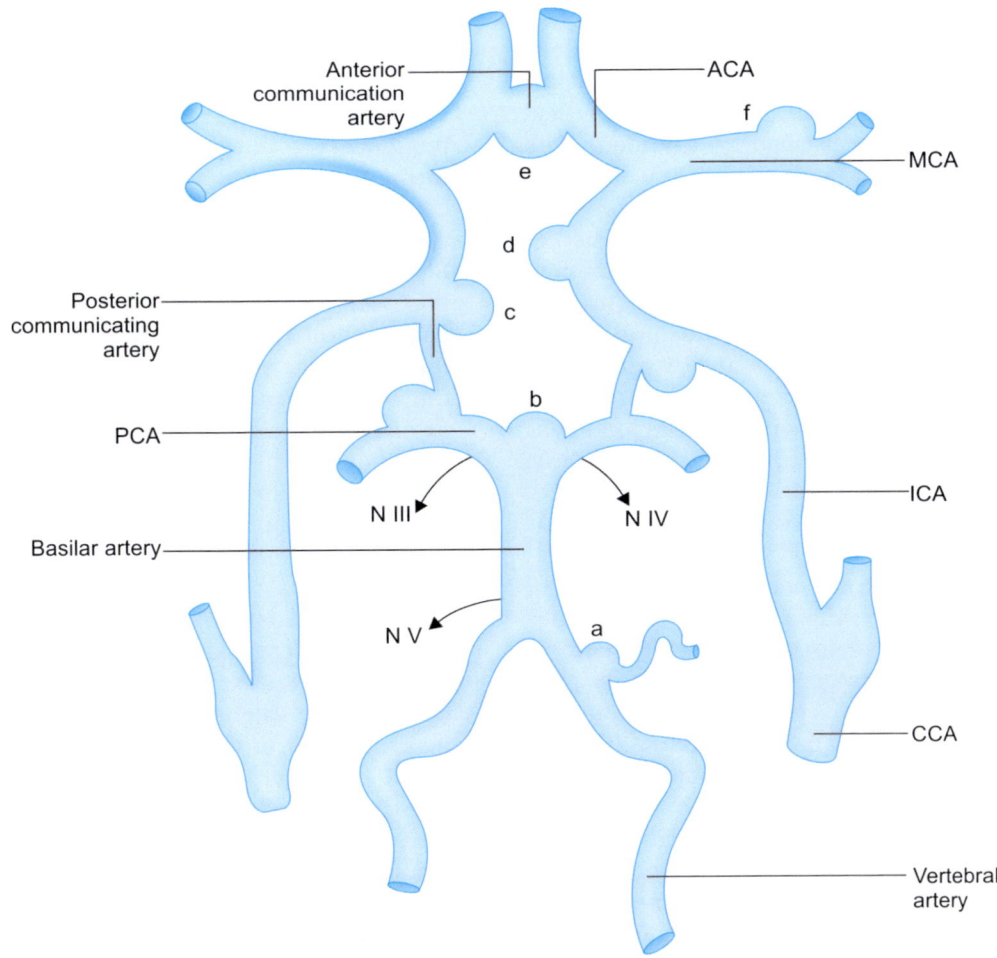

ACA, anterior cerebral arteries; CCA, common carotid artery; ICA, internal carotid arteries; MCA, middle cerebral arteries; PCA, posterior cerebral arteries.

FIG. 4: Common sites of intracranial aneurysms and the related oculomotor nerves; **a,** Posterior inferior cerebellar; **b,** basilar tip; **c,** posterior communicating; **d,** internal carotid; and **e,** anterior communicating.

compress the third nerve. They are often giant or fusiform in appearance. These aneurysms may compress the oculomotor nerve from below, sparing the pupillomotor fibers that are concentrated along the superior segment of the nerve, producing pupil-sparing or relative pupil-sparing ophthalmoplegia

3. Intracavernous carotid: These are often giant or dolichoectatic, and often produce other signs of the cavernous sinus syndrome, such as fourth or sixth nerve palsy, trigeminal neuropathy, or Horner's syndrome. If the pupillomotor fibers have been injured, the pupil may still appear normal in room light due to aberrant regeneration or superimposed oculosympathetic paresis. Evaluating the size of the pupils in bright light, however, will usually reveal that the affected pupil is larger than the fellow pupil because of iris sphincter paresis. In addition, evaluating the size of the pupils in darkness will reveal that the affected pupil is smaller than the fellow pupil if affected by either aberrant regeneration or Horner's syndrome. These aneurysms have a relatively

lower risk of rupture and, when they do, often cause signs of high-flow carotid-cavernous fistula rather than subarachnoid hemorrhage.

What elements of the history and physical examination can be used to try to differentiate ischemic from aneurysmal injury of the oculomotor nerve? The usual details—including age, presence of vascular risk factors, pain, and progression of ophthalmoplegia in the acute setting—are common enough in both disorders that none provide sufficient clinical power. The status of the pupil, on the other hand, is variable. The discriminating power of the pupil to differentiate third nerve infarction from compression by a mass lesion has become formalized into a clinical dictum, the "rule of the pupil". While this "rule" will work most of the time, there are important pitfalls that must be recognized in order to avoid missing aneurysms.

Simply put, the "rule" states that a normal pupil implies infarction while a dilated pupil implies compression (by aneurysm) of the oculomotor nerve. What is the anatomic basis of this "rule"? The pupillomotor fibers are concentrated peripherally along the superior to medial longitudinal segment of the third nerve as it courses from the interpeduncular fossa to the cavernous sinus. Aneurysms arising from the junction of the posterior communicating and internal carotid arteries typically expand downward and laterally, preferentially compressing the pupillomotor fibers as the third nerve becomes injured (producing pupil-involving third nerve palsy). In contrast, the core of the third nerve receives its blood supply via the vasa vasorum. Accordingly, the peripherally located pupillomotor fibers tend to be spared when the core of the third nerve is injured by ischemia (producing pupil-sparing third nerve palsy).

How reliable is the "rule" in clinical practice? In regards to aneurysms, Kissel et al. reviewed the course of 51 patients with third nerve palsy caused by angiographically-proven aneurysm at the junction of the posterior-communicating and the internal carotid arteries. A similar study was reported in a series of patients evaluated by a single investigator.

The main clinically relevant caveats to be derived from these series include:
- None of the patients in either series has pupil-sparing complete third nerve palsy. Pupil-sparing complete third nerve palsy is generally not a sign of aneurysm. Be aware, however, that exceptional reports exist
- Fourteen percent (14%) of Kissel's patients had pupil-sparing, but the ophthalmoplegia was incomplete in all. Beware that pupil-sparing can be a sign of aneurysmal compression in patients with incomplete ophthalmoplegia
- Five of seven patients in Kissel's series with pupil-sparing developed complete third nerve palsy (within 5 days in 4 patients). Re-evaluate those patients with pupil-sparing incomplete third nerve palsy within a week to identify pupil involvement, a sign signifying aneurysm.

There are four important settings where a patient with aneurysm and third cranial nerve palsy may have a normal appearing pupil. If one does not consider these traps, one may be at risk of missing an aneurysm:

1. When external ophthalmoplegia is incomplete: This usually refers to a patient with all third nerve innervated extraocular muscles affected, but not fully. Incomplete ophthalmoplegia may also refer to the situation where not all of the extraocular muscles are affected, as in point 2, an equally perilous trap
2. When the inferior division is spared: The oculomotor nerve travels within the dural lateral wall of the cavernous sinus where it bifurcates into a superior and inferior division near the superior orbital fissure. The superior division carries fibers that innervate the superior rectus and levator palpebrae, while the inferior division carries fibers that innervate the inferior rectus, medial rectus, inferior oblique, and iris sphincter muscles. Intracavernous carotid or basilar tip aneurysms are not uncommonly preferentially injure the superior division of the third cranial nerve, producing ptosis, and paresis of ocular elevation, but no anisocoria
3. When third nerve palsy is combined with Horner's syndrome: Giant intracavernous carotid artery aneurysms commonly injure the oculomotor nerve and, less often, the oculosympathetic pathway. If third nerve palsy and Horner's syndrome occur in the same patient, the size of the resulting pupil looks fairly similar to the other pupil in room light.

However, observing the pupils with added light will usually expose the paretic iris sphincter if the affected pupil looks slightly larger than the fellow pupil. In addition, the affected pupil usually dilates so poorly that it appears smaller than its fellow pupil if observed in darkness

4. When the injured third nerve has undergone aberrant regeneration: In some cases of chronic compression of the oculomotor nerve by a giant aneurysm of the cavernous sinus, regenerating fibers may become misswired, a process called aberrant regeneration. Fibers originally destined to innervate certain extraocular muscles become rerouted into pupillomotor fibers that innervate the iris sphincter. The enhanced tone of the iris sphincter that results from this process produces a pupil that is smaller than normal, reacts poorly to light but better to near, and dilates poorly in darkness.

The evaluation of a patient with third cranial nerve palsy must proceed urgently because of the threat of cerebral aneurysm, which may be as frequent as 30% in some series of isolated cases (Table 1). As discussed, the relationship between the degree of internal and external ophthalmoplegia is the best clinical predictor of whether neurologically isolated and acute third cranial nerve injury is due to compression or infarction. Except in those patients with pupil-sparing complete third nerve palsy, neuroimaging, preferably using MRI, is indicated to identify a mass lesion compressing the oculomotor nerve (e.g., pituitary apoplexy) or some other explanation for the presentation (e.g., midbrain stroke). If the study is unrevealing, one must then proceed emergently to exclude aneurysm.

While catheter angiography remains the "gold standard" for identifying aneurysm, it is not without risk. The complication rate is higher in certain patients in particular, including those greater than 70 years of age, as well as those with symptomatic atherosclerotic cerebrovascular disease, significant cardiovascular or renal disease, or Ehlers–Danlos syndrome. Improvements in three-dimensional time-of-flight magnetic resonance angiography (MRA) have made this tool a tempting alternative to catheter angiography. However, how sensitive is this screening test for detecting aneurysms causing third cranial nerve palsy? The answer depends, in part, on considering the ability of MRA to detect aneurysms of various sizes and the proportion of aneurysms in each size class associated with third nerve palsy. A recent meta-analysis disclosed estimates regarding aneurysms at the junction of the posterior communicating and internal carotid arteries. With aneurysm size ≥5 mm, the miss rate was 3%, whereas with sizes <5 mm, the miss rate exceeded 45%.

TABLE 1: Suggested neuroimaging evaluation of third cranial nerve palsy

Clinical characteristics	Study
Pupil-sparing complete third nerve palsy (iris sphincter normal, EOM totally impaired)	None
Pupil-blown third nerve palsy (iris sphincter totally impaired, EOM impaired)	MRI, then CA if negative
Relative pupil-sparing complete third nerve palsy (iris sphincter partially impaired, EOM totally impaired)	MRI, then MRA if negative*
Plus	
Age ≥40 years and vascular risk factors present Pupil-sparing incomplete third nerve palsy (iris sphincter normal, EOM partially impaired)	MRI, then MRA if negative*

*Catheter angiography recommended if: (i) Worsening of extraocular muscle or iris sphincter function continues beyond 14 days; (ii) iris sphincter impairment progresses to anisocoria >1 mm; (iii) no recovery of function occurs within 3 months; or (iv) signs of aberrant regeneration develop.
EOM, extraocular muscles; MRI, magnetic resonance imaging; CA, catheter angiography; MRA, magnetic resonance angiography.
Adopted from: Jacobson DM, Trobe JD. The emerging role of magnetic resonance angiography in the management of patients with third cranial nerve palsy. Am J Ophthalmol. 1999;128:94-6.

Due to the sensitivity of aneurysmal detection, using MRA has become sufficiently high, one may now substitute it for catheter angiography in the diagnostic evaluation of some, but not all, patients with third cranial nerve palsy. However, it should be considered a screening test to exclude aneurysm under certain clinical circumstances, namely, when the likelihood of aneurysm is relatively low (Table 1) and the risk of complication of catheter angiography is relatively high. Importantly, the use of MRA to detect aneurysm is subject to the following two crucial caveats:
1. Most importantly, the skill of the interpreting neuroradiologist must be first rate
2. Furthermore, the detection rate is dependent upon review of all imaging data, including source images, maximum intensity projections (the "angiogram"), multiplanar reformatted images, and spin echo images. If any short cuts are taken, the failure rate will increase.

Before using MRA to evaluate one's patients with third nerve palsy, one must first discuss its potential role with his/her radiologist. If there is any doubt about the quality of the study or its interpretation, stick with catheter angiography as the definitive study to rule out aneurysm for now.

Currently, many centers prefer CT angiography than time of flight MRA for aneurismal screening. Although CT angiography would need contrast use and at least a 64-slice scanner. A software is now available which can produce a bone subtraction effect producing very high quality images comparable to digital subtraction angiography (DSA) images. Most surgeons of course prefer a DSA if they need to operate or even go for coiling.

Lumbar puncture is generally not necessary when evaluating patients with acute and neurologically-isolated third cranial nerve palsy.

In India, isolated third nerve palsy may be an uncommon manifestation of central nervous system (CNS) tuberculosis. Cerebrospinal fluid (CSF) study is often warranted if third nerve palsy is preceded by systemic symptoms (fever, headache, vomiting, etc.), associated with other cranial nerve palsies (where imaging had been negative or noncontributory) and in immunocompromised subjects.

Two syndromes are discussed in this section as third cranial nerve palsy is often a prominent feature in these illnesses.

TOLOSA–HUNT SYNDROME AND PAINFUL OPHTHALMOPLEGIA

Almost any process causing ophthalmoplegia can be painful, with the possible exceptions of myasthenia gravis and chronic progressive external ophthalmoplegia. The physician should always be concerned about infections and tumors. However, there are a group of patients who present with painful, combined ophthalmoplegia due to a granulomatous inflammatory process that affects the cavernous sinus, extending forward to the superior orbital fissure, and orbital apex. Called the THS, it is usually a disease of middle or later life that may spontaneously remit and relapse.

Tolosa–Hunt Syndrome

In 1954 Tolosa followed a few years in 1961 Hunt and his colleagues described a small group of patients with unilateral orbital pain, visual loss in some, external ophthalmoplegia in all and reduced sensation in the first division of the trigeminal nerve. Cerebral angiography revealed narrowing of the intracavernous segment of the internal carotid artery. Surgical exploration of some such patients revealed essentially no definite pathological findings except some granulomatous inflammation in the carotid region. Hunt believed that the condition had been the result of some obscure etiology.

However, on the basis of clinical observations, they proposed the following diagnostic criteria for the condition:
- Pain preceding the ophthalmoplegia by several days, or may not appear until sometime later. Pain not a throbbing hemicranias occurring in paroxysms, but a steady pain behind the eye that is often described as "gnawing" or "boring"
- Neurological involvement not confined to the third cranial nerve alone, but may include the fourth, sixth, and first division of the fifth cranial nerves. Carotid sympathetic fibers and the optic nerve may be involved

- Symptoms lasting for days to weeks
- Spontaneous remissions occurring, sometimes with residual neurological deficit
- Attacks often recurring at intervals of months or years
- Exhaustive studies, including angiography and surgical exploration, producing no evidence of involvement of structures outside of the cavernous sinus. There is no systemic reaction.

Later, Hunt and coworkers reported the benefit of corticosteroids in relieving the symptoms in some patients. Smith and Taxdal introduced the eponym "THS" to this entity. They added five additional cases, "because there has been no previous report of this syndrome in the ophthalmology literature and to emphasize the use of steroids as a diagnostic test". The authors stated that "the administration of large doses of systemic steroids for 48 hours produces a dramatic response in painful ophthalmoplegia, which allows prompt differentiation of these cases".

Since these reports, several similar cases were reported from almost every corner of the world and therapy with corticosteroids became a standard procedure. Unfortunately, no real progress so as to understand the basic cause of inflammation had been made. However, advancement in neuroradiology have helped in defining the syndrome more accurately. Earlier, orbital venographic abnormalities had been described but later found to be nonspecific. On the other hand, using modern techniques of CT and MRI direct visualization of the cavernous sinus is possible and cavernous sinus abnormalities have now been described in THS.

Diagnostic Evaluation

In most cases, diagnosis can be made clinically with history of unilateral orbital pain associated with involvement of multiple ocular motor traversing the cavernous sinus/superior orbital fissure and involvement of the ophthalmic division of the trigeminal nerve. Neuroimaging is needed to exclude other pathologies and to demonstrate evidence of the granulomatous pathology in the parasellar/orbital apical region. The latter is possible in many but not all cases of THS. Ideally, contrast enhanced MRI to be performed with both axial and coronal sections through the area of interest.

Typical abnormality is an intermediate signal intensity on T1 and intermediate weighted images, consistent with an inflammatory process, which enhances with gadolinium. With steroid treatment along with improvement in clinical condition, this abnormality also improves. High-resolution CT can also demonstrate soft tissue changes in the region of the cavernous sinus/superior orbital fissure, but is less sensitive than MRI. Hence, even if CT is normal, MRI must still be performed to appropriately evaluate the region of the cavernous sinus or superior orbital fissure. The major limitation of MRI findings in THS is their lack of specificity. Similar signal abnormalities can be found in meningiomas, lymphoma, and sarcoidosis. Because of this fundamental limitation of initial imaging studies, resolution of imaging abnormalities after a course of systemic corticosteroids should be considered "diagnostic" of THS. Again such "remissions" can be found both with malignant conditions like lymphoma and benign conditions like vasculitis.

The International Headache Society published the following diagnostic criteria in 2018:
- Unilateral orbital or periorbital headache fulfilling criterion C
- Both of the following:
    - Granulomatous inflammation of the cavernous sinus, superior orbital fissure, or orbit, demonstrated by MRI or biopsy
    - Paresis of one or more of the ipsilateral third, fourth, and/or sixth cranial nerves.
- Evidence of causation demonstrated by both of the following:
    - Headache is ipsilateral to the granulomatous inflammation
    - Headache has preceded paresis of the third, fourth, and/or sixth nerves by ≤2 weeks, or developed with it.
- Not better accounted for by another ICHD-3 diagnosis.

Comments

Some reported cases of 13.8 THS had additional involvement of the fifth nerve (commonly, the first division) or optic, seventh or eighth nerves. Sympathetic innervation of the pupil is occasionally affected.

Careful follow-up is required to exclude other causes of painful ophthalmoplegia such as tumors, vasculitis, basal meningitis, sarcoid, or diabetes mellitus.

Pain and paresis of 13.8 THS resolve when it is treated adequately with corticosteroids. Non-specific abnormalities like raised erythrocyte sedimentation rate, C-reactive protein lupus erythematosus cell phenomenon have been including minor abnormalities in CSF study. These need not call for further investigations in most cases. However, if therapeutic response is not adequate further CSF study may be done and the question of biopsy raised. Biopsy from the region concerned would certainly be a hazardous procedure and the risk benefit ratio to be carefully assessed.

Treatment

Since the first documentation of the beneficial effect of corticosteroid therapy in THS, there is little new information as to optimal dosage, duration of treatment, or alternative forms of therapy. It is clear that spontaneous remissions may occur, but there is no doubt that corticosteroids markedly reduce the periorbital pain. No data are available as to whether treatment hastens recovery of the associated cranial nerve palsies. Although steroids are generally tapered over weeks to months, in some cases, prolonged therapy may be necessary. As cautioned previously, positive response to steroids has been reported in various parasellar neoplasms, including chordoma, giant cell tumor, lymphoma, and epidermoid.

Etiology

The etiology of THS is unknown. What triggers the granulomatous inflammatory process is not clear. It is possible that THS may represent a localized form of idiopathic form of inflammatory orbitopathy, commonly known as pseudotumor of the orbit. The present author feels that at least a proportion of THS cases could be a localized form of cranial pachymeningitis syndrome which may present with multiple cranial nerve palsies. In this connection, the relationship of such cases to the relatively recently described entity of immunoglobulin G4 (IgG4) syndrome need to be explored.

The author feels that at least a proportion of THS cases could be a localized form of cranial pachymeningitis syndrome which may present with multiple cranial nerve palsies. In this connection, the relationship of such cases to the relatively recently described entity of IgG4 syndrome need to be explored.

Differential Diagnosis

As the diagnosis of THS is essentially one of exclusion, the clinician needs to be familiar with the differential diagnosis of painful ophthalmoplegia (Box 2). In fact, during the initial patient evaluation,

Box 2: Diagnostic evaluation of Tolosa–Hunt syndrome

Hematological tests:
- Complete blood count
- Serum chemistry (glucose, electrolytes, liver and renal function
- Erythrocyte sedimentation rate
- C-reactive protein
- Glycosylated hemoglobin
- Fluorescent treponemal antibody test
- Antinuclear antibody
- Anti-dsDNA antibody
- Anti-sm antibody
- Serum protein electrophoresis
- Antinuclear cytoplasmic antibody
- Angiotensin converting enzyme

Cerebrospinal fluid:
- Opening pressure
- Cell count and differential
- Protein
- Glucose
- Culture: Bacterial, fungal, mycobacterial
- Serology
- Angiotensin converting enzyme
- Cytology

Neuroradiological studies:
- Magnetic resonance imaging
- Computed tomography
- Cerebral angiography

Biopsy:
- Nasopharynx
- Cavernous sinus

dsDNA, double stranded deoxyribonucleic acid.

there are often no clues in the history or physical examination to distinguish THS from other causes of painful ophthalmoplegia. Therefore, the clinician should be aware of: (i) causes of parasellar syndrome and (ii) other entities producing painful ophthalmoplegia.

CAUSES OF PARASELLAR SYNDROME

Craniocerebral trauma may produce painful ophthalmoplegia in various ways: basilar skull fracture with ocular motor nerve damage, intracavernous carotid artery injury with subsequent aneurysm formation, or carotid-cavernous fistula.

Various vascular causes may produce painful ophthalmoplegia, the most frequent being an intracavernous carotid artery aneurysm. Rarely, giant aneurysms of the posterior circulation, especially of the posterior cerebral artery may mimic THS. Carotid cavernous fistula and cavernous sinus thrombosis also have acute onset of symptoms and signs, and must be included in the differential diagnosis. Patients with carotid-cavernous fistulae rarely complain of severe pain and typically have dramatic ophthalmological signs including proptosis, "arterialised" conjunctival vessels, chemosis, increased intraocular pressure and retinal vascular abnormalities. A bruit is often present, cerebral angiography is the diagnostic procedure of choice, and interventional angiographic techniques are usually curative. Cavernous sinus thrombosis may be septic or aseptic in origin. In the septic type, there may be associated signs of sinusitis, otitis, gingivitis, or orbital cellulitis. Patients are febrile, have a leukocytosis, and if the infectious process spreads intracranially, seizures and altered mental states may occur. In the second type, cavernous sinus thrombosis may be associated with various hypercoagulable conditions including polycythemia, sickle cell disease, vasculitis, pregnancy, dehydration, trauma, and intracranial surgery. In both types, cavernous sinus thrombosis is characterized by orbital congestion, proptosis, eyelid swelling, chemosis, lacrimation, and ophthalmoparesis. Pain around or behind the eye is common. Treatment of cavernous sinus thrombosis usually involves anticoagulant drugs, at times thrombolytic agents, and in septic cases, appropriate antibiotic therapy. As outlined in box 3,

Box 3: Causes of parasellar syndrome producing painful ophthalmoplegia

1. **Trauma**
2. **Vascular**
- Intracavernous carotid artery aneurysm
- Posterior cerebral artery aneurysm
- Carotid-cavernous fistula
- Carotid-cavernous thrombosis
3. **Neoplasm**
- Primary intracranial tumor
   - Pituitary adenoma
   - Meningioma
   - Craniopharyngioma
   - Sarcoma
   - Neurofibroma
   - Gasserian ganglion neuroma
   - Epidermoid
- Primary cranial tumor
   - Chordoma
   - Chondroma
   - Giant cell tumor
- Local metastases
   - Nasopharyngeal tumor
   - Cylindroma
   - Adamantinoma
   - Squamous cell carcinoma
- Distant metastases
   - Lymphoma
   - Multiple myeloma
   - Carcinomatous metastases

Inflammation:
- Bacterial
- Sinusitis
   - Mucocele
   - Periostitis
- Viral
   - Herpes zoster
- Fungal
   - Mucormycosis
- Spirochetal
   - *Treponema pallidum*
- Mycobacterial
   - Mycobacterium tuberculosis
- Unknown cause
   - Sarcoidosis
   - Wegener's granulomatosis
   - Eosinophilic granuloma

painful ophthalmoplegia may be caused by either contiguous or metastatic spread of a neoplasm. Metastatic involvement of the cavernous sinus/superior orbital fissure is generally due to haematogenous dissemination of neoplastic cells. Occasionally, intracranial neoplastic invasion may occur by intraneural or perineural spread, as in the case of squamous cell carcinoma producing painful ophthalmoplegia many months after local excision of a facial skin tumor. Two things about neoplastic involvement of the cavernous sinus/superior orbital fissure require emphasis. Firstly, mode of onset and clinical course are not indicative of the type of lesion causing painful ophthalmoplegia. In their review of parasellar syndrome, Thomas and Yoss stated that "A sudden onset of symptoms does not weigh in favor of aneurysmal or against neoplastic origin, and gradual onset is not necessarily indicative of a neoplasm. Spontaneous single or multiple remissions of symptoms, even of years duration, are unreliable in predicting the nature of the underlying process". Secondly, high-dose corticosteroid therapy may initially improve signs and symptoms due to neoplasm. Inflammatory causes of painful ophthalmoplegia include those due to a specific infectious agent. It is essential that careful CSF examination be done and that cultures (bacterial, fungal, mycobacterial) be obtained. The potential role of a paranasal sinus as a cause of painful ophthalmoplegia requires attention. Sinus disease may lead to cavernous sinus involvement, either via contiguous spread of infection or due to sphenoid sinus mucocele.

OTHER CAUSES OF PAINFUL OPHTHALMOPLEGIA

Box 4 summarizes other etiologies of painful ophthalmoplegia in which there is no involvement of the cavernous sinus/superior orbital fissure. Various orbital diseases cause painful ophthalmoplegia. Typically, the patient presents with "orbital signs", including proptosis, conjunctival injection, chemosis, and resistance to retrodisplacement of the globe. In addition, the eye may be displaced within the orbit, and there may be abnormalities of the ocular adnexa (e.g., lids, lacrimal gland). Diabetic ophthalmoplegia typically produces an acute, often painful mononeuropathy in either a

Box 4: Additional causes of painful ophthalmoplegia

Orbital disease:
- Idiopathic orbital inflammation (pseudotumor)
- Contiguous sinusitis
- Mucormycosis or other fungal infection
- Metastatic tumor
- Lymphoma/leukemia

Diabetic ophthalmoplegia:
- Mononeuropathy
- Multiple cranial nerve palsies

Posterior fossa aneurysm:
- Posterior communicating artery
- Basilar artery

Giant cell arteritis

Ophthalmoplegic migraine

known or previously undiagnosed diabetic person. Invariably, there is recovery of ocular motor cranial nerve function, usually within 3 months.

In addition, there are reports of diabetic patients with simultaneous paralysis of multiple ocular motor nerves. Although multiple nerve involvement is rare in diabetes, these episodes are painful, often recurrent, and not particularly responsive to corticosteroid therapy. Posterior fossa aneurysms may produce either acute, painful ophthalmoplegia, or may present in a more subacute or chronic fashion. The acute presentation is most often due to an aneurysm in the anterior circulation, typically at the junction of the internal carotid-posterior communicating arteries, whereas the subacute presentation is caused by basilar artery aneurysms. In both, cerebral angiography is diagnostic. Giant cell arteritis may also produce painful ophthalmoplegia. The clinical picture may be one of single or multiple ocular motor nerve palsies. In the only pathological study of ophthalmoplegia occurring in giant cell arteritis, ischaemic necrosis of the extraocular muscles was demonstrated. Examination of the ocular and motor cranial nerves was unremarkable. Ophthalmoplegic migraine is a poorly understood and debatable form of complicated migraine. Typically, this clinical syndrome occurs in a child or young adult with periodic headache who develops an ocular motor cranial nerve palsy at the height of an attack of cephalgia, which is primarily unilateral and in the orbital region. Most often involved is the oculomotor nerve in children, the abducens nerve is commonly involved in adults, and rarely the trochlear nerve. The paresis lasts for days to weeks after cessation of a headache. Steroids often hasten recovery making differentiation from THS difficult.

Family history of migraine may be helpful. There are reports of enhancement of the extra-axial portion of the oculomotor nerves of patients with ophthalmoplegic migraine when evaluated with contrast-enhanced MRI which leads to the debate—migraine or neuropathy?

Miller Fisher Syndrome

Miller Fisher syndrome (MFS), also called Fisher's syndrome, was first recognized by James Collier in 1932 as a separate clinical trial of ophthalmoplegia, ataxia, and areflexia. Later, MFS was named after Charles Miller Fisher who reported it in 1956 as a limited variant of Guillain–Barré syndrome (GBS). The degree of ophthalmoparesis is variable, but certain patterns of involvement occur that might suggest involvement of the central nervous system. For example, the ophthalmoplegia may resemble a horizontal or vertical gaze palsy or internuclear ophthalmoplegia. Ptosis is often absent even in the presence of significant ophthalmoparesis. Bell's phenomenon may also be preserved even when vertical eye movements are otherwise absent. Rebound nystagmus, impairment of smooth pursuit, optokinetic nystagmus, and suppression (cancellation) of the vestibulo-ocular reflex point to cerebellar dysfunction. As with myasthenia gravis (vide infra), some of these findings might be due to the effects of central adaptation to peripheral weakness. Other findings, such as the confusion that some patients suffer, the dissociated involvement of the levator palpebrae superioris and superior rectus, and the MRI findings in some cases, point to central involvement—an encephalitic component. Fisher himself was impressed by the symmetry of the ocular motor deficit and by ataxia unaccompanied by sensory loss, and "reluctantly interpreted" the clinical signs "as manifestations of an unusual and unique disturbance of peripheral neurons".

It is clinically important to differentiate MFS from GBS. Many MFS patients go on to develop the prominent, widespread weakness of GBS. It is noted that neurological deficit in MFS follows a descending pattern starting with external ophthalmalgia causing diplopia in the eyes. However, GBS characteristically presents with the ascending weakness or paralysis. Miller Fisher syndrome may also be mistaken for an acute cerebellar stroke with an unsteady gait, dizziness, headache, eye movement dysfunction, as well as nausea and vomiting.

Most cerebellar strokes show lateralization of ataxia while MFS patients typically lack lateralization of ataxia helping the differentiation. However, ataxia can also be seen in conditions involving spinocerebellar tracts, or the proprioceptive fibers in peripheral nerves and dorsal columns. Toxins and medications such as phenytoin and some chemotherapeutic agents such as fluorouracil can precipitate ataxic episodes. Ataxia secondary to alcoholic intoxication (drunken gait), mostly affects the lower extremities and but may be associated associated with poor motor control of the hands, slurred speech, and impaired vision and very importantly areflexia. It can be differentiated from ataxia in MFS patients as the progression of weakness in MFS follows a "top to down" fashion.

Immunological evidence has clarified the relationship of MFS to GBS and involvement of the central nervous system. First, antibodies against the ganglioside GQ1b have been detected in over 90% of patients with MFS. Anti-GQ1b antibodies have also been detected in those patients with Guillain–Barré syndrome who have involvement of their eye movements, and also in patients with the brainstem encephalitis described by Bickerstaff. The latter is characterized by ophthalmoplegia and ataxia, but also by pyramidal and sensory tract findings and cerebrospinal fluid pleocytosis. Consistent with this immunopathological hypothesis, plasmapheresis is reported to improve both Bickerstaff's encephalitis and MFS. Neuropathologic examination of two patients with MFS has shown a normal central nervous system. Autopsy of a patient who had Bickerstaff's encephalitis in association with GBS and anti-GQ1b antibodies showed a normal brainstem but demyelination of the ocular motor and spinal nerves. Other studies have shown staining of the molecular layer of the cerebellum by anti-GQ1b antibodies, which is evidence for a central origin of the ataxia—and probably some of the eye movement disorders in MFS.

Thus, present evidence suggests that anti-GQ1b antibodies play a key role in producing the disturbance of eye movements in MFS, GBS, and Bickerstaff's encephalitis. As in GBS *Campylobacter jejuni* may be the responsible trigger, since anti-GQ1b antibodies bind to surface epitopes on this organism. *Haemophilus influenzae, Mycoplasma pneumonia,* and cytomegalovirus are also found to be associated. Patients presenting with unexplained ophthalmoplegia may benefit from testing for anti-GQ1b antibodies.

Miller Fisher Syndrome to Guillain–Barré Syndrome and Involvement

Miller Fisher syndrome is essentially a benign self-limiting disease. Cardiac arrhythmia and respiratory failure very rarely occur. Immunomodulatory agents may be used to hasten recovery and to prevent development into more serious GBS. In MFS, areflexia may persist even after full motor recovery.

EVALUATION OF FOURTH CRANIAL NERVE PALSY

In contrast to the much higher frequency that brain tumors cause third or sixth cranial nerve palsies, mass lesions, including cerebral aneurysms, are far less likely to present as fourth cranial nerve palsy. When they do, tumors are often located in the posterior fossa or region of the sella turcica while aneurysms are most often giant ones of the intracavernous carotid artery (Box 5). These lesions typically injured neighboring structures so that other signs of posterior fossa or parasellar dysfunction are present.

The vast majority of isolated fourth cranial nerve palsies in adults will be due to either infarction of the peripheral trochlear nerve or congenital palsy (or decompensation of long-standing phoria).

Since ocular ductions usually appear full in patients with fourth cranial nerve palsy, it can be a very difficult diagnosis to establish. Here is a situation where an ophthalmologist can help because of their training in diplopia and squint assessment (e.g., cover testing) to test extraocular muscle balance.

The superior oblique, the target muscle of the fourth cranial nerve, depresses the eye

> **Box 5: Causes of fourth nerve palsy by location of the responsible lesion**
>
> **Brainstem/posterior fossa:***
> - Trauma—nonsurgical and neurosurgical
> - Congenital
> - Hydrocephalus
> - Hemorrhage
> - Tumors
> - Infarction
>
> **Subarachnoid:**
> - Trauma—nonsurgical and surgical
> - Tumors—parasellar, middle fossa
> - Hydrocephalus
> - Meningitis
>
> **Cavernous sinus/superior orbital fissure:**
> - Aneurysm—giant intracavernous carotid artery
> - Carotid—cavernous fistula
> - Tumors
> - Inflammation—Tolosa–Hunt syndrome
> - Infection—Herpes zoster
>
> **Uncertain or variable location:**
> - Peripheral nerve infarction
> - Congenital
> - Infections
> - Trauma
>
> *Posterior fossa included due to its close proximity with fourth nerve fascicles and extra axial course around midbrain.

in adduction and in cyclodeviates the globe. Accordingly, the affected eye of a patient with acute trochlear nerve palsy is relatively hyperdeviated and excyclodeviated. One would suspect acute fourth nerve palsy based on the patient's complaint of vertical and torsional diplopia. They typically describe that their double vision is worse when looking down, better when looking up, and better when tilting their head to the side opposite the paretic eye (head tilt to opposite side). Their double vision is usually maximum when they gaze down and in with their paretic eye.

Decompensation of a congenital or longstanding superior oblique phoria is a common cause of "acute" symptomatic trochlear nerve palsy. There are three reasons why patients with this condition, even though presumably congenital or long-standing in nature, may not have experienced double vision earlier in life:

1. Many patients have amblyopia, a condition that prevents normal binocular vision
2. Adoption of an anomalous head tilt to the opposite side minimized their perception of double vision. Inspection of available photographs in a patient with an unexplained superior oblique palsy may reveal that the patient has had a long-standing contralateral head tilt, providing a supportive clue that decompensation of an old phoria is the mechanism of their "acute" presentation
3. A patient with a longstanding vertical phoria often develops greater than normal ability to fuse misaligned images using vergence mechanisms, a sign that can be measured as vertical fusion amplitude. An ophthalmologist can help provide this information. Demonstrating that the patient has greater than normal vertical fusion strength is strong evidence that they have developed this over a long period, supporting the longstanding or congenital nature of their vertical ophthalmoplegia. Common situations that precipitate double vision (i.e., produce loss of fusion) in an adult with previously asymptomatic superior oblique phoria include:
   - Head trauma
   - Intercurrent systemic illness (e.g., pneumonia)
   - Exposure to new medication with anticholinergic or sedative side effects
   - A new pair of glasses
   - Change in refractive needs (e.g., presbyopia).

Neuroimaging is generally not needed in a patient with neurologically isolated acute fourth cranial nerve palsy, especially if they have the vasculopathic clinical profile previously discussed or features supporting decompensation of a longstanding superior oblique phoria.

These patients can generally be followed without the need for further neurodiagnostic investigation. One should anticipate that their ophthalmoplegia will not worsen or demonstrate a variable pattern and that recovery will ensure during the following few months, as expected if they had infarcted their fourth cranial nerve. Any deviation from this expected natural history should suggest that the original suspicion was in error. In that setting, other causes of fourth cranial nerve palsy (e.g., cavernous sinus or posterior fossa mass) and the differential diagnosis of vertical ophthalmoplegia (Box 6) must be considered.

> **Box 6: Differential diagnosis of vertical ophthalmoplegia**
> - Fourth cranial nerve palsy
> - Third cranial nerve palsy
> - Skew deviation
> - Ocular myasthenia
> - Graves' ophthalmopathy
> - Orbital trauma
> - Orbital tumor
> - Orbital pseudotumor (myositis)
> - Brown's superior oblique tendon sheath syndrome

In patients with neurologically isolated acute fourth cranial nerve palsy who do not have clinical features suggestive of decompensated superior oblique phoria or the clinical profile of fourth cranial nerve infarction, the decision to obtain neuroimaging is determined on an individual case basis. Neuroimaging, preferably using MRI with special attention to the posterior fossa and cavernous sinus, should be done in patients with the following characteristics:
- Ophthalmoplegia that follows seemingly minor head trauma
- Age younger than 45 years
- Documented progression of ophthalmoplegia
- Unexplained bilateral fourth cranial nerve palsy.

Examination of cerebrospinal fluid is generally not needed to evaluate patients with unilateral fourth cranial nerve palsy, unless there are other clinical symptoms or signs that suggest a meningeal process (e.g. "chronic" meningitis). The index of suspicion of leptomeningeal infiltration or infection should be heightened in patients with unexplained bilateral palsy, those with known or suspected systemic malignancies, or those who are immunocompromised.

Two interesting neuro-ophthalmic syndromes related to fourth cranial nerve supplied superior oblique muscle dysfunction may be discussed in this section.

Brown's Syndrome

Brown's syndrome is characterized by limited elevation of the adducted eye because the movements of the superior oblique tendon are restricted in the trochlea. When congenital, the superior oblique tendon may be short or tethered. When acquired, the tendon may be prevented from passing through the trochlea by tenosynovitis, adhesions, metastases, or trauma which may cause the muscle itself to become entrapped in the roof of the orbit. Paradoxically, sometimes trauma to the trochlea leads to hypertropia rather than impaired elevation in adduction. When Brown's syndrome occurs in association with rheumatological disorders, anti-inflammatory drugs are usually effective. The "click" syndrome is a variation of Brown's syndrome in which the tendon can slide through the trochlea but because of the mechanical hindrance it may transiently get held up as the patient tries to look up. There may be an audible or palpable "click" when the obstruction is overcome.

Superior Oblique Myokymia

With superior oblique myokymia patients typically complain of brief, recurrent episodes of monocular blurring of vision, or tremulous sensation in one eye. Some also report vertical or torsional diplopia or oscillopsia. Attacks usually last <10 seconds, but may occur many times per day. Looking downward, tilting the head towards the side of the affected eye, blinking may bring on the attacks. Most cases are idiopathic. The condition may follow fourth nerve palsy, brain stem stroke, or demyelination. Uniocular oscillations of eye ball should always raise suspicion of superior oblique myokymia.

Measurement of the movements of superior oblique myokymia using the magnetic search coil technique has demonstrated an initial intorsion and depression of the affected eye, followed by irregular oscillations of small amplitude.

Electromyographic recording from superior oblique muscles affected by the disorder have revealed abnormal discharge from some muscle fibers that occur either spontaneously or following contraction of the muscle. These findings have been interpreted as indicating neuronal damage and subsequent regeneration, leading to desynchronized contraction of muscle fibers. Patients with superior oblique myokymia usually do not report a prior episode of diplopia, but MM studies show atrophy of the superior oblique muscle. Occasionally, demyelinating or compressive (e.g., microvascular compression) lesions may be the cause.

There are no consistently effective treatments for superior oblique myokymia but individual patients may respond to gabapentin, carbamazepine, baclofen, and systemically or topically administered beta-blockers. In some patients, superior oblique myokymia spontaneously resolves but in others the symptoms are so troublesome that surgical treatment is considered, and either a weakening procedure (superioroblique tenectomy plus inferior oblique myectomy) or a modification of the Harada-Ito procedure (nasal transportation of the anterior portion of the superior oblique tendon) to weaken cyclorotation, can be beneficial.

Evaluation of Sixth Cranial Nerve Palsy

It is tempting to jump to the conclusion that a patient who cannot rotate their eyes laterally has a sixth nerve palsy. However, doing so will limit one's thinking and may prevent one from considering the other important causes of abduction deficit (pseudo-sixth nerve palsy) (Box 7). Most patients with an abduction deficit will have one of three mechanisms of ophthalmoplegia.

Neurogenic

Sixth cranial nerve palsy may be acquired (Box 8) or congenital. Of congenital disorders, Duane's retraction syndrome is the most common, and is often confused with acquired ophthalmoplegia (vide infra).

> **Box 7: Causes of abduction deficit (pseudo-sixth nerve palsy)**
>
> - Neurogenic palsy:
>   - Sixth cranial nerve palsy
>   - Duane's retraction syndrome
> - Ocular myasthenia
> - Restrictive ophthalmoplegia:
>   - Graves' ophthalmopathy
>   - Orbital trauma
>   - Orbital tumor
>   - Orbital pseudotumor
> - Others:
>   - Spasm of the near reflex

Box 8: Causes of sixth nerve palsy by location of the responsible lesion

Brainstem:
- Infarction
- Hemorrhage
- Tumors
- Demyelination
- Congenital—Duane's retraction syndrome
- Trauma—nonsurgical
- Wernicke's encephalopathy

Subarachnoid:
- Tumors—parasellar region, clivus, nasopharynx, cerebellopontine angle
- Trauma—nonsurgical and surgical
- Aneurysms—dolichoectatic vertebrobasilar artery, berry aneurysms of the anterior or posterior inferior Cerebellar and basilar arteries
- Leptomeningeal carcinomatosis
- Inflammation—Guillain-Barré syndrome, Miller Fisher variant
- Meningitis—tuberculosis, bacterial
- Infection of the petrous apex/mastoiditis

Cavernous sinus/superior orbital fissure:
- Tumors—pituitary adenoma, meningioma, other parasellar malignancies
- Aneurysm—giant intracavernous carotid artery
- Carotid—cavernous fistula
- Cavernous sinus thrombosis
- Inflammation—Tolosa-Hunt syndrome
- Infection—herpes zoster

Uncertain or variable location:
- Peripheral nerve infarction
- Congenital
- Infections
- Post-viral or benign sixth nerve palsy of childhood
- Trauma
- Ophthalmoplegic migraine
- Intracranial hypertension—tumors, pseudotumor cerebri, meningitis, intracranial hemorrhage, hydrocephalus
- Intracranial hypotension—following lumbar puncture, myelography, spinal anesthesia, shunting
- Not including gaze palsies due to nuclear involvement

Myasthenia

The hallmark of this condition is variable ophthalmoplegia and ptosis, typically improved with rest and worsened with fatigue. Ocular myasthenia can mimic nearly all types of ophthalmoplegia, except for those associated with significant pain or pupil involvement. Comparing quantitative assessment of eye movement during serial examinations at different times of the day will usually uncover the variable nature inherent in this condition. Since ancillary diagnostic tests, such as acetylcholine receptor antibody assay and repetitive stimulation electromyography (EMG), are often normal in ocular myasthenia, serial neuro-ophthalmologic examination is one of the preferred diagnostic tests in patients suspected as harboring this condition. This is discussed in detail later in this chapter.

Restrictive

The two diagnostic features of disorders producing restrictive ophthalmoplegia are: (i) additional symptoms and signs of orbital disease and (ii) positive results of forced duction testing. Important symptoms and signs suggestive of orbital disease include pain, visual loss, proptosis, redness, and swelling of the eye. An ophthalmologist can assist in identifying these signs, and in performing forced duction testing. Graves' ophthalmopathy is the commonest orbital disorder in adults associated with ophthalmoplegia. In particular, it may be associated with pseudo-sixth nerve palsy due to fibrosis of the medial rectus muscle. Other orbital disorders to consider include muscle entrapment due to trauma, tumors, and inflammatory pseudotumors (e.g., orbital myositis).

Another condition deserves mention because it can often fool the unwary examiner that the patient may be harboring a sixth nerve palsy and result in unnecessary neurodiagnostic work-up. Voluntary adduction with convergence, miosis, and accommodation is called spasm of the near reflex. This is often asymmetrical and intermittent. The condition need to be distinguished from bilateral sixth nerve palsy by involvement of the pupil and covering one eye when the "spasm" disappears. Normal eye movement is observed when one eye is patched.

As with third and fourth cranial nerve palsies, the commonest cause of neurologically isolated and acute sixth nerve palsy in adults infarction of the extra-axial segment (Box 8).

Since, the vast majority of patients with infarction of the sixth nerve recover by three months, persistence of ophthalmoplegia beyond

that point is a warning that a mass lesion may be the true culprit. Notorious offenders in this setting include:
- Cavernous sinus meningioma
- Cavernous sinus giant internal carotid artery aneurysm
- Cavernous sinus metastasis
- Cavernous sinus invasion by pituitary adenoma
- Other tumors of the parasellar region, clivus, and nasopharynx
- Pontine gliomas
- Multiple sclerosis.

These lesions are often missed using CT, and are even often missed using routine MRI sequences that are not targeted specifically for the region of interest (i.e., skull base and cavernous sinus). Cavernous sinus lesions, especially meningiomas and other tumors, are easily missed using MRI if the study is performed without contrast administration.

The frequency profile of disorders associated with bilateral sixth nerve palsy differs in a few important ways from that associated with unilateral sixth nerve palsy. Simultaneous infarction of both peripheral sixth cranial nerves does not occur. Tumors capable of producing bilateral sixth nerve palsy include brainstem gliomas, clival chordomas, nasopharyngeal carcinomas, and pituitary adenomas, in particular those that have rapidly expanded due to apoplexy. Leptomeningeal disorders are encountered more often in a patient "with bilateral sixth nerve palsy than in a patient with unilateral sixth nerve palsy. These conditions include CNS tuberculosis, carcinoma meningitis, GBS (or the Miller Fisher variant), and other infections, such as Lyme disease, syphilis, fungal meningitis, and other opportunistic agents. Wernicke's encephalopathy is a treatable condition that may cause bilateral sixth nerve palsy in addition to other features of that disorder (e.g., encephalopathy and ataxia). Lastly, unilateral or bilateral sixth nerve palsy as a nonlocalizing sign of raised intracranial pressure from any cause must not be forgotten. A careful fundoscopy should always be performed.

In all such situations, if neuroimaging study with contrast is negative, a detailed CSF analysis is mandatory.

Duane's Syndrome

Congenital absence of innervation to the lateral rectus muscle is the cause of most cases of Duane's retraction syndrome. Three types are known:
- Type 1: Limitation of abduction but full adduction with narrowing of palpebral fissure on adduction due to retraction of the globe
- Type 2: Full abduction but limited adduction
- Type 3: Limitation of both adduction.

Diagnostic confirmation is by identification of retraction of the eyeball with narrowing of the palpebral fissure, on adduction brought out doing horizontal saccades, or by observing the affected eye from the side during optokinetic nystagmus with the help of a rotating striped drum.

Patients with Duane's syndrome seldom complain of diplopia and, in fact, usually have binocular vision with good stereopsis and fusion in the field of binocular single vision. Occasionally, diplopia may develop later in life, making differential diagnosis from abducens palsy difficult. In such patients, ocular retraction during adduction provides a useful diagnostic clue.

Most cases of Duane's syndrome are due to a congenital abnormality of innervation. This view was initially based on electromyographic evidence, and has been confirmed by clinicopathological studies. Neuropathologic examination of one patient with a unilateral left sided type-I Duane's syndrome showed an absent left abducens nerve; the left lateral rectus was innervated by aberrant branches from the inferior division of the oculomotor nerve. The brainstem of this patient showed a normal right abducens nucleus but the left abducens nucleus contained less than half as many neurons as the right; these remaining cells were thought to be abducens internuclear neurons, since the medial longitudinal fasciculus were intact. These findings are in accord with the observation that adducting saccades in the normal eye of patients with a unilateral type-I Duane's syndrome usually had normal velocities or only slight slowing. Similar autopsy findings were reported in a patient with familial, unilateral Duane's type-III syndrome, and another patient who had bilateral type-III Duane's syndrome lacked both abducens nuclei and nerves. Thus, the limitation of horizontal movement in most cases of Duane's syndrome can be ascribed to an agenesis of abducens motoneurons. Failure of abduction is due to lack of innervation of the lateral rectus by the abducens nerve. Retraction of the globe on adduction is brought about by cocontraction of the horizontal recti, which is the consequence of aberrant innervation of the lateral rectus muscle by the oculomotor nerve. When there is limited adduction of the eye, this could also be due to cocontraction of the lateral and medial recti.

Although most cases of Duane's syndrome are congenital, a similar clinical syndrome can occur with acquired disease of the extraocular muscles or of the orbit (e.g., fibrosis or inflammation of muscle or fascia).

Brain Stem Causes of Ophthalmoplegia (Fig. 5)

Patients presenting with strabismus from brainstem lesions often exhibit "neighborhood" symptoms and signs. The pattern of strabismus together with accompanying ocular motor signs, such as nystagmus and gaze paresis, may comprise brainstem syndromes that localize the lesion. Common causes are infarction, demyelination and hemorrhage (especially from cavernomas). Wernicke's encephalopathy is a rare cause but deserves consideration because it is treatable.

Fascicular and Nuclear Ocular Motor Nerve Syndromes

Lesions of the third nerve fascicle may also affect: the cerebral peduncle causing contralateral hemiparesis (Weber's syndrome), the red nucleus and crossed fibers of the superior cerebellar peduncle causing contralateral ataxia ± tremor (Claude's syndrome); or all three structures plus the substantia nigra causing contralateral hemiparesis and involuntary movements or tremor (Benedikt's syndrome). Nothnagel syndrome includes damage to one or both sided third cranial nerve and to the superior cerebellar peduncle by a tumor in the mesencephalic tectum or by a mesencephalic vascular accident. This may just be a variant of the Benedikt's syndrome. Contralateral facial hypoesthesia implicates involvement of the nearby ventral ascending trigeminal tract. Discrete lesions of the fascicle may cause subtotal paresis of the third nerve. Lesions of the rostomedial fascicle affect the pupil, inferior rectus and medial rectus whereas, caudolateral lesions affect the levator, superior rectus ± inferior oblique. Lesions of the third nerve nucleus may cause bilateral ptosis and impaired elevation of both eyes in addition to the impaired adduction and depression of the ipsilateral eye. Axons from the superior rectus subnucleus travel through the contralateral third nerve nucleus and innervate the contralateral superior rectus muscle. Partial lesions of the third nerve fascicle or nucleus may produce isolated palsies of the inferior rectus or inferior oblique muscle.

Lesions of the sixth nerve fascicle may involve the pyramidal tract and cause contralateral hemiparesis (Raymond's syndrome). A closely linked condition with a similar site of lesion is the Millard-Gubler syndrome which includes in addition an ipsilateral lower motor facial palsy as a constant feature. This syndrome described separately by Gubler and Millard referred to probable brainstem vascular lesions whereas Raymond noted association with a syphilitic gumma.

Foville's syndrome (anterior inferior cerebellar artery syndrome) includes ipsilateral paralysis of horizontal gaze, lower motor facial palsy, loss of taste in the anterior two thirds of the tongue, Horner's syndrome, facial analgesia, and deafness.

Infarction and demyelination may cause discrete fascicular lesions and present as isolated sixth nerve palsies.

Axons from the fourth nerve nucleus course dorsally around the aqueduct and cross in the superior medullary velum to supply the contralateral superior oblique. Signs that localize a

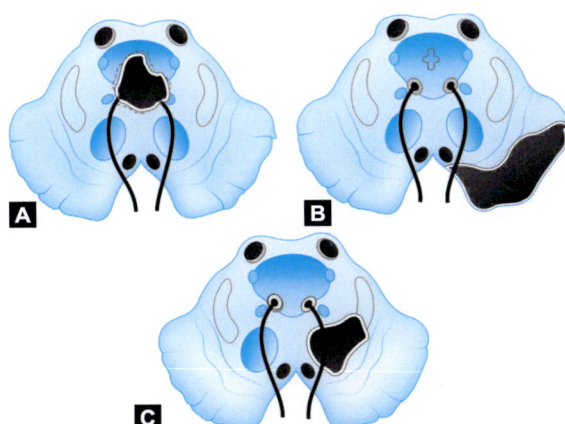

FIG. 5: Classic midbrain syndromes. A, Aqueductal blockage; B, Weber's syndrome; and C, Benedikt's syndrome.

fourth nerve palsy to the nucleus or to the fascicle before it crosses include Horner's syndrome or internuclear ophthalmoplegia (INO) on the side opposite the palsy, or a relative afferent pupil defect or facial hypesthesia on the same side. A lesion of the fascicle after it crosses may involve the nearby spinothalamic tract and cause hypalgesia of contralateral limbs and trunk.

Skew deviation is a vertical misalignment of the eyes due to a supranuclear lesion. The misalignment may be comitant (the same in all gaze positions) or incomitant and may mimic palsies of one or more vertical rectus or oblique muscles. The higher eye may reverse on gaze to either side. Skew deviation is attributed to interruption of vestibular signals travelling from the otolith organs to the vertical ocular motor nuclei. Lesions in the caudal portion of the pathway, which includes the vestibular nerve and nucleus (e.g., lateral medullary syndrome), often cause a contralateral hypertropia. The excitatory pathway crosses and ascends in the medial longitudinal fasciculus (MLF), projecting to the interstitial nucleus of Cajal in the rostral midbrain. Lesions affecting these structures (e.g., INO) often cause an ipsilateral hypertropia. Disruption of otolith inputs also may produce a "tilt reaction" comprising eye torsion and head tilt toward the lower eye. Skew deviation may occasionally result from cerebellar lesions. A combination of head tilt, skew deviation, and ocular counter roll (direction change of the skew on covering one eye) is referred to as ocular tilt reaction and is suggestive of a utricular lesion.

Internuclear Ophthalmoplegia

A lesion of the MLF causes impaired adduction of the ipsilateral eye and abducting nystagmus of the contralateral eye. Frequently, the range of adduction is normal. The diagnosis then depends on the detection of slowing of adduction during contralateral saccades, often with one or two beats of overshooting nystagmus in the abducting eye. Most patients with INO exhibit no misalignment in primary position and do not complain of diplopia. A subtle skew deviation (ipsilateral hypertropia) is often present. Rostral lesions affecting both MLFs near the third nerve nuclei may cause exotropia and bilateral loss of adduction, termed "well-eyed" bilateral INO. Caudal pontine lesions affecting both the MLF and the adjacent sixth nerve nucleus or the paramedian pontine reticular formation (PPRF) cause impaired adduction of the ipsilateral eye plus ipsilateral gaze palsy—the one-and-a-half syndrome. In some patients, unopposed activity in the normal PPRF may cause the eye contralateral to the lesion to deviate outwards, a syndrome called "paralytic pontine exotropia".

Neuromuscular Junction Disorder: Ocular Myasthenia

Myasthenia gravis is an autoimmune disease affecting nicotinic acetylcholine receptors that is characterized by fatigable muscle weakness. It commonly affects the extraocular muscles. Half of all patients present with ocular symptoms and more than 90% eventually develop eye movement abnormalities. Of those patients with ocular symptoms, less than half persist with purely ocular myasthenia and, of those that generalize, most do so within 2 years of the onset of the disease.

The fundamental process in myasthenia gravis is an autoimmune response against the acetylcholine receptor. Thus, over 80% of patients with generalized myasthenia and about 65% with the pure ocular form, have anti-acetylcholine receptor antibodies in their sera. It has been suggested that antibodies specifically directed against the fetal form of the acetylcholine receptor—which may be found at synapses on extraocular but not skeletal muscles—may be an important factor that predisposes the extraocular muscles to involvement by myasthenia. However, myasthenia also affects the levator of the lids, which does not have synaptic fetal acetylcholine receptors. This, and the report that a patient with antibodies directed against fetal acetylcholine receptors did not manifest ocular myasthenia, even though her baby developed transplacental, neonatal myasthenia, indicate the complexity of the issue. Rarely, pure ocular myasthenia may also be caused by presence of muscle specific kinase antibody (Muscle Nerve 2013).

Muscle fatigue is the hallmark of myasthenia gravis and may affect the lids, eye movements, or both. Lid abnormalities include progressive and often asymmetric ptosis, brought out by attempting sustained upward gaze. Ptosis in myasthenia may be improved by applying ice, wrapped in a towel, over the closed eye for 2 minutes. Transient eyelid retraction occurs during refixations from down to straight ahead. Cogan's eyelid twitch sign: this sign is not, however, pathognomonic and may occur with brainstem or oculomotor disorders. Attempted eyelid closure may be impaired. Ptosis is often relieved after a short nap (sleep test).

Myasthenia gravis characteristically causes intermittent diplopia, due to fluctuating extraocular muscle weakness. Such weakness is often asymmetric and may mimic third, fourth, or sixth nerve palsy, gaze paresis, internuclear ophthalmoplegia, one-and-a-half syndrome, or strabismus. The pseudo-internuclear ophthalmoplegia of myasthenia gravis is sometimes associated with depression or downshoot of the adducting eye. Fatigue, during sustained attempts to hold lateral or upward gaze, is manifest as centripetal drift or increasing gaze-evoked nystagmus that may be followed by rebound nystagmus (recall that cerebellar gaze-evoked nystagmus typically diminishes as eccentric gaze is held for longer period of time). Abnormalities of saccades and quick phases of nystagmus may be early signs of myasthenia gravis. Large saccades may be hypometric and small saccades may be hypermetric. For large saccades, the eye may start off rapidly, but slow in mid-flight and creep up to the desired eye position. A characteristic quiver movement consists of an initial, small saccadic movement followed by a rapid drift backward. During prolonged optokinetic nystagmus, quick phases may become slow. Injection of edrophonium (tensilon) often reverses extraocular muscle weakness and causes saccades to become hypermetric. Sometimes, the patient is not able to hold steady fixation because of repetitive hypermetric saccades that overshoot the target in both directions—macrosaccadic oscillations.

Two separate factors account for the various ocular motor findings in myasthenia gravis—failure of neuromuscular transmission and central adaptive mechanisms. During repetitive activation of motor nerves, the amount of acetylcholine released at the nerve terminals declines to a plateau value that depends upon the firing frequency. In myasthenia, neuromuscular transmission is tenuous, since the number of functioning postsynaptic acetylcholine receptors is reduced. A small decrease in the amount of released neurotransmitter reduces the probability that an end-plate potential will be generated and so predisposes to failure of neuromuscular transmission. Factors that may predispose the extraocular muscles to frequent involvement in myasthenia gravis include their higher discharge rates, chemical differences in the nature of the receptors, and the lack of action potentials in the tonic fibers. Though failure of neuromuscular transmission affects both global and orbital extraocular muscle fibers, the more constant activity of the latter makes them more susceptible to fatigue.

Saccades that start off at high velocities but slow in mid-flight and creep up to the target probably reflect intrasaccadic fatigue; muscle fibers are unable to sustain the vigorous muscular contraction required for the duration of the saccadic pulse. The step of innervation (which requires less muscle force) then carries the eye slowly to its final position. The peak velocity of such saccades may be normal but the duration is prolonged.

Later in the disease, patients with little residual motility may seem to make super-fast saccades within their limited range of motion. The peak velocity of these movements is often greater than would be expected for the size of the saccade. Though central adaptive changes may be partly responsible, this cannot be the whole explanation; adaptive increases in saccadic innervation that occur in other types of muscle palsies do not produce super-fast saccades. A more likely explanation is that the global (predominantly fast-twitch) fibers of the agonist muscle, which are relatively inactive and rested during fixation can start the saccade with a normal pulse of activity. So tenuous is neuromuscular transmission, however, that fatigue develops rapidly, aborting the pulse. Since the orbital (predominantly tonic) fibers may also become fatigued during the saccade, the eye stops and may even begin to drift backward. When the tonic fibers are completely fatigued, the step is absent. Then the mechanical forces of the orbit pull the eye rapidly back towards the central position. The combination of the aborted saccade and oppositely directed drift toward center constitutes the quiver movement. The presence of such rapid movements in patients with restricted ocular motility should always suggest myasthenia; such movements are absent in patients who have a low or restricted movements due to disease of the central nervous system. The quiver-like movements may be followed by a slow continuation of the saccade; presumably the fatigued pulse is followed, after a brief period of electrical silence, by either a renewed step from tonic fibers or another corrective saccadic pulse.

The ability to hold the eye steadily after a saccade may be affected by post-saccadic fatigue. Often sustained eccentric gaze will bring out nystagmus with slow-phase waveforms that follow a linear or negative exponential time course. This has been called muscle paretic nystagmus, and probably occurs when the orbital fibers are fatigued. The global fibers are relatively spared, since they only discharge vigorously during saccades or quick phases. Occasionally, when nystagmus develops with sustained eccentric gaze, the amplitude (and velocity) is more marked in the abducting eye. This dissociated nystagmus mimics internuclear ophthalmoplegia.

Not all features of myasthenic eye movements can be ascribed to neuromuscular block. The brain monitors the accuracy of saccades and makes adaptive changes of innervation to optimize ocular motor performance. When myasthenia causes paretic saccades, central adaptation is stimulated if the patient habitually views with the paretic eye. These mechanisms can be applied to the pulse-step pattern of innervation that normally produces fast, accurate saccades. Large saccades often fall short of the target; they are hypometric. Smaller saccades, however, made around the primary position, are often accurate or even overshoot the target. Why should saccades become hypermetric in myasthenia gravis? The answer is apparent from the observation of the effects of edrophonium (tensilon). During the edrophonium test, saccade size increases. Many saccades become too large, and occasionally an extreme degree of hypermetria produces continuous, to-and-fro saccadic movements about the target known as macrosaccadic oscillations. Saccade hypermetria occurs because the central nervous system had adaptively increased the size of the saccadic pulse in an attempt to overcome the myasthenic weakness. The central changes are revealed by edrophonium, which transiently removes the peripheral neuromuscular blockade, exposing the increased saccadic innervation. If the brain had been standing idly by, edrophonium would merely have caused refixations to become accurate. Similar findings are apparent with slower-acting anticholinesterase medications. Saccades can be fast and overshoot the target, 15–30 minutes after intramuscular neostigmine or 30–90 minutes after oral pyridostigmine.

When ocular motility is minimally affected, careful study of eye movements—preferably measurements of saccades—before and after edrophonium (tensilon) or neostigmine may be particularly useful. Edrophonium is best given in small (0.2 mg) increments to avoid missing a positive response, due to cholinergic excess. Neostigmine (0.5 mg, given intramuscularly with atropine, 0.5 mg) is also useful since it allows more time to make both clinical observations and quantitative measurements. One should examine and record at 15–20 minutes intervals for about 45 minutes to look for a positive response, which includes changes in saccadic accuracy and especially the production of hypermetria which are probably diagnostic of myasthenia gravis. Saccadic velocity, especially of larger saccades, tends to increase. In contrast, normal subjects or patients with ocular motor palsies show slowing and increased duration of saccades after edrophonium. These changes in normal subjects and in patients with nonmyasthenic strabismus illustrate the dangers in not measuring the nature of the changes produced by edrophonium. Furthermore, some nonmyasthenic ocular deviations get worse after edrophonium, if one muscle is more susceptible to the effects of the drug than the others. In particular, subjective tests such as the red glass or Maddox rods (see diplopia) must be interpreted cautiously as they may give misleading results. Only the direct observation of a weak muscle becoming stronger after edrophonium is reliable evidence of myasthenia. Even then, the diagnosis depends on the full clinical picture; false-positive test results have been reported with central structural lesions, and myasthenia can coexist with intracranial lesions. Neostigmine has the advantage of giving the examiner more time to detect a change in ocular alignment or saccade metrics, but has the disadvantage that its rate of absorption after intramuscular injection is variable. In patients with purely ocular manifestations, single fiber EMG of the superior rectus and levator muscles may contribute to the diagnosis by showing jitter. Single fiber studies of the facial muscles are useful too, but may not differentiate mitochondrial myopathy or oculopharyngeal dystrophy from myasthenia. Currently, of course the wide spread use of the acetylcholine receptor antibody test combined with repetitive nerve stimulation study makes edrophonium test somewhat redundant.

Late in the course of myasthenia gravis, all ocular motility may become restricted and the patient may be refractory to edrophonium or neostigmine testing. Imaging studies show atrophied extraocular muscles. If a clear history is unavailable, differentiation from the syndrome of chronic progressive external ophthalmoplegia may be difficult.

Therapeutic aspects of myasthenia is not discussed in this volume.

DISORDERS OF OCULAR MUSCLES

Mitochondrial Disease

Chronic Progressive External Ophthalmoplegia and Kearns–Sayre Syndrome

Kearns–Sayre syndrome, is due, in most cases, to deletions or duplications of mitochondrial deoxyribonucleic acid (DNA). Rare cases are reported in which there appears to be a defect of communication between nuclear and mitochondrial genomes. This multisystem disorder is characterized by progressive ophthalmoparesis beginning in childhood or adolescence, atypical pigmentary degeneration of the retina, and heart block. These patients rarely ever complain of diplopia. Both the cardiac and endocrine complications of Kearns–Sayre syndrome may be life threatening. The involvement of the eye muscle in mitochondrial myopathies probably reflects their high oxidative stress as functionally compromised mitochondria accumulate.

Patients have been described who show clinical features that overlap Kearns–Sayre syndrome and other mitochondrially inherited disorders—mitochondrial encephalopathy, lactic acidosis, and stroke-like episodes (MELAS) and myoclonic epilepsy and ragged red fibers (MERRF). An uneven distribution of deletions of mitochondrial DNA in different tissues may account for the different phenotypic expression. Pathologically, both limb and extraocular muscles often show ragged-red fibers with trichrome stains; this appearance is due to increased numbers of abnormal sarcolemmal mitochondria. The brain shows a spongy degeneration that results in cerebral and cerebellar atrophy, Therapy with coenzyme Q10 aims to improve respiratory chain activity, but its clinical efficacy is unproven.

Thyroid Ophthalmopathy

Thyroid disease is an important cause of restrictive ophthalmopathy. A number of orbital abnormalities are encountered in patients with thyroid disorders. These include chemosis, periorbital congestion, lid retraction and lid lag, proptosis (exophthalmos), ophthalmoparesis, and optic neuropathy. Exophthalmos and periorbital edema usually precede the development of impaired ocular motility, though diplopia may be the first symptom. Patients with thyroid ophthalmopathy often complain of diplopia, unlike most forms of chronic progressive external ophthalmoplegia. In contrast to myasthenia, symptoms are usually worse in the morning. Lid retraction and lid lag on downward gaze are common signs.

The most common abnormalities of eye movements are impaired elevation, and extorsion of the eye on abduction. Abduction and downward movements may also be affected. Thus, the limitation of movement reflects a restrictive ophthalmopathy, which can usually be confirmed by the forced duction test. The velocity and amplitude of saccadic eye movements is reduced in some patients, and the development of these abnormalities may correlate with progression of orbital disease. Thyroid ophthalmopathy is discussed in detail later in the volume (see chapter no. 19 on Proptosis).

Orbital pseudotumor and orbital myositis comprise two variants of idiopathic orbital inflammation, the first involving the orbit diffusely and the second localized to eye muscles. The most common presentation of myositis is unilateral involvement of one eye muscle and its tendon but several eye muscles and both orbits may be involved.

Orbital pseudotumor has been discussed elsewhere in this volume (see chapter no. 19 on Proptosis).

Ocular cysticercosis is not very uncommonly seen in India (Fig. 6). Although mostly encountered by ophthalmologists, neurologists occasionally encounter these patients when extraocular muscles are involved and presentation is with an ophthalmoplegia. The present author has encountered only 6 such cases over a 15 years period. One of which had been reported. Neurologists practicing in Northern India seem to encounter more such cases (A Agarwal, Lucknow, Personal communication). Cysticerci can lodge in any part of the eye or its adenexae-anterior chamber, adherent to the extraocular muscle, vitreous cavity, subretinal space, optic nerve head, subconjunctival space, lids, lacrimal gland and anecdotally the lens. Adnexal location seem to be more common in India than in Latin America. Cysticercosis of the extraocular muscles present with recurrent inflammation, proptosis, restricted ocular motility and ptosis. The diagnosis can be made clinically in most cases (injected appearance with a cyst visible to the naked eye) but neuroimaging studies (contrast CT or MRI) are often needed for exact localization and cyst characterization. The appearance is similar to parenchymal cysts in the brain. Ultrasonography is helpful for diagnosing intraocular (e.g., vitreous) cysts. The present author's personal experience of treating extraocular muscle cysts with a combination of corticosteroids (prednisolone 40 mg/day for 7 days and then slow tapering over 14 days) along with a 3 weeks course of albendazole (15 mg/kg body weight/day) has been quite satisfactory in the small number of patients treated.

Orbital cellulitis usually causes acute chemosis, lid swelling, proptosis and pain, along with varying degrees of ophthalmoplegia and visual loss. Fever and leukocytosis are often absent, perhaps because many patients are partially treated with oral antibiotics when first seen. The most frequent cause of orbital cellulitis is spread of bacterial infection from adjacent sinuses, especially the ethmoid and frontal sinuses. In addition to sinus disease, imaging shows variable enhancement and swelling of orbital fat and muscle and occasionally orbital abscess. Bacterial orbital cellulitis is treated with intravenous antibiotics ± surgical drainage. In diabetic or debilitated patients, mucormycosis causes an aggressive cellulitis and local tissue necrosis due to septic vasculitis. Sino-orbital aspergillosis may produce fulminant disease in immunocompromised patients, or more slowly progressive disease in patients with normal immunity. These fungi may invade the internal carotid artery and cause stroke. Invasive fungal disease generally requires surgical debridement in addition to antifungal therapy (see chapter no. 19 on Proptosis).

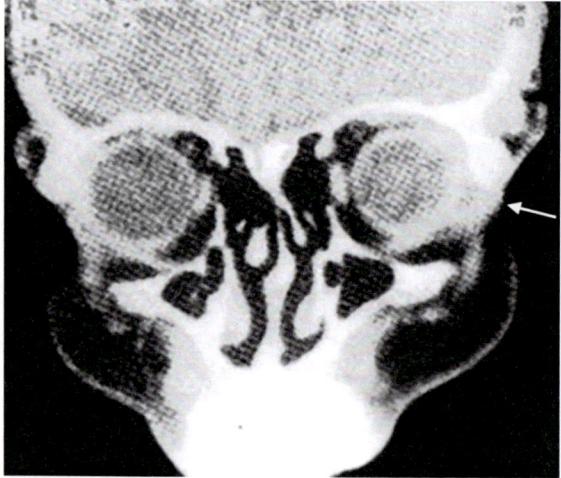

FIG. 6: Contrast-enhanced computed tomography showing a cysticercal lesion at the insertion of left lateral rectus muscle.

SUGGESTED READINGS

1. Alexandrakis G, Saunders RA. Duane retraction syndrome. Ophthalmol Clin North Am. 2001;14(3):407-17.
2. Asbury AK, Aldredege H, Hershberg R, et al. Oculomotor palsy in diabetes mellitus: A clinico-pathological study. Brain. 1970;93:555-66.
3. Barton JJ, Fouladvand M. Ocular aspects of myasthenia gravis. Semin Neural. 2000;29(1):7-20.
4. Barton JJ, Intriligator JM. Vertical saccades in superior oblique palsy and Brown's syndrome. J Neuroophthalmol. 2001;21(4):250-55.
5. Bergin DJ, Wright JE. Orbital cellulitis. Br J Ophthalmol. 1986;70:174-8.
6. Bickerstaff ER, Cloake PC. Mesencephalitis and rhombencephalitis. Br Med J. 1951;2:77-81.

7. Blau I, Casson I, Lieberman A, et al. The not so benign Miller Fisher syndrome: A variant of the Guillain-Barre syndrome. Arch Neurol. 1988;37:334-85.
8. Brazis PW. Palsies of the trochlear nerve: Diagnosis and localization - recent concepts. Mayo Clin Proc. 1993;68:501-9.
9. Breen LA, Hopf HC, Farris BK, et al. Pupil-spadng oculomotor palsy due to midbrain infarction. Arch Neurol. 1991;48:105-6.
10. Castro O, Johnson LN, Mamourian AC. Isolated inferior oblique paresis from brain-stem infarction: Perspective on oculomotor fascicular organization in the ventral midbrain tegmentum. Arch Neurol. 1990;47:235-7.
11. Chakravarty A, Mukherjee A. Ocular cysticercosis—Report of a case. J Assoc Neuroscienfists of Eastern India. 1999;4:49-50.
12. Crane TB, Yee RD, Baloh RW, et al. Analysis of characteristic eye movement abnormalities in internuclear ophthalmoplegia. Arch Ophthalmol. 1983;101:206-10.
13. Daroff RB. Chronic progressive external ophthalmoplegia: A critical review. Arch Ophthalmol. 1969;82:845-50.
14. Elliott D, Cunningham Jr ET, Mller NR. Fourth nerve paresis and ipsilateral afferent pupillary defect without visual sensory disturbance. Clin Neuroophthalmol. 1991;11:169-72.
15. Ellis FD, Hoyt CS, Ellis FJ, et al. Extraocular muscle responses to orbital cooling (ice test) for ocular myasthenia gravis diagnosis. J AAPOS. 2000;4(5):271-81.
16. Fisher CM. An unusual variant of acute idiopathic polyneuritis (syndrome of ophthalmoplegia, ataxia and areflexia). N Engl J Med. 1956;255:57-65.
17. Fisher CM. Some neuro-ophthalmological observations. J Neurol Neurosurg Psychiatry. 1967;30(5):383-92.
18. Ford FR, Walsh FB, King A. Clinical observations on the pupillary phenomena resulting from regeneration of the third nerve with especial reference to the Argyll Robertson pupil. Bull Johns Hopkins Hosp. 1941;68:309-18.
19. Galetta SL, Smith JL. Chronic isolated sixth nerve palsies. Arch Neurol. 1989;46:79-82.
20. Goldstein JE, Cogan DG. Diabetic ophthalmoplegia with special reference to the pupil. Arch Ophthalmol. 1960;64:592-600.
21. Green WR, Hackeft ER, Schlezinger NS. Neuro-ophthalmologic evaluation of oculomotor nerve paralysis. Arch Ophthalmol. 1964;72:154-67.
22. Gutowski NJ. Duane's syndrome. Bur Neurol. 2000;7(2):145-9.
23. Guy J, Day AL, Mckle JP, et al. Contralateral trochlear nerve paresis and ipsilateral Horner's syndrome. Am Ophthalmol. 1989;107:73-6.
24. Guy JR, Day AL. Intracranial aneurysms with superior division paresis of the oculomotor nerve. Ophthalmology. 1989;96:1071-76.
25. Jacobson DM, McManna TD, Layde PM. Risk factors for ischemic ocular motor nerve palsies. Arch Ophthalmol. 1994;112:961-66.
26. Jacobson DM, Trobe JD. The emerging role of magnetic resonance angiography in the management of patients with third cranial nerve palsy. Am Ophthalmol. 1999;128:9496.
27. Jacobson DM. Early progression of ophthalmoplegia in patients with ischemic oculomotor nerve palsies. Arch Ophthalmol. 1995;113:1535-37.
28. Jacobson DM. Progressive ophthalmoplegia with acute ischemic abducens nerve palsies. Am Ophthalmol. 1996;122:278-79.
29. Jacobson DM. Pupil involvement in patients with diabetes-associated oculomotor nerve palsy. Arch Ophthalmol. 1998;116:723-27.
30. Jacobson DM. Relative pupil-sparing third nerve palsy: Etiology and clinical variables predictive of a mass. Neurology. 2001;56:797-98.
31. Kaminski HJ, Ruff RL. Ocular muscle involvement by myasthenia gravis. Ann Neurol. 1997;41:419-20.
32. Kaminski HJ. Acetylcholine receptor epitopes in ocular myasthenia. Ann NY Acad Sci. 1998;841:309-19.
33. Keane JR. Aneurysms and third nerve palsies. Ann Neurol. 1983;14:696-97.
34. Keane JR. Bilateral sixth nerve palsy. Analysis of 125 cases. Arch Neurol. 1976;33:681-3.
35. Keane JR. Trochlear nerve pareses with brainstem lesions. J Clin Neuroophtahlmol. 1986;6:242-6.
36. Kearns TP, Sayre GP. Retinitis pigmentosa, external ophthalmoplegia and complete heart block: Unusual syndrome with histologic study in one of two cases. Arch Ophthalmol. 1958;60:280-9.
37. Kearns TR. External ophthalmoplegia, pigmentory degeneration of the retina and cardiomyopathy: A newly recognized syndrome. Trans Am Ophthalmol Soc. 1965;63:554-635.
38. Kim JS. Trigeminal sensory symptoms due to midbrain lesions. Eur Neurol. 1993;33:218-20.
39. Kissel JT, Burde RM, Klingele TG, et al. Pupil-sparing oculomotor palsies with internal carotid-posterior communicating artery aneurysms. Ann Neurol. 1983;13:149-54.
40. Kline LB, Hoyt WF. The Tolosa-Hunt syndrome. J Neurol Neurosung Psychiatry. 2001;71(5):577-82.
41. Ksiazek SM, Repka MA, Maguire A, et al. Divisional oculomotor nerve paresis caused by intrinsic brainstem disease. Ann Neurol. 1989;26:714-8.
42. Kumar A, Sharma N. Taenia solium cysticercosis: Ophthalmic aspects. In: Singh G, Prabhakar S, et al. Basic to clinical science. CABI Publishing Oxford; 2002. pp. 269-80.

43. Lee AG, Hayman LA, Brazis PW. The evaluation of isolated third nerve palsy revisted: An update on the evolving role of magnetic resonance, computed tomography, and catheter angiography. Surv Ophthalmol. 2002;47:137-57.
44. Lee AG, Tang RA, Wong GG, et al. Isolated inferior rectus muscle palsy resulting from a nuclear third nerve lesion as the initial manifestation of multiple sclerosis. Neuro-Ophthalmol. 2001;20(4):246-7.
45. Leigh RJ, Zee DS. The neurology of eye movements. New York: Oxford University Press; 1999.
46. Linskey ME, Sekhar LM, Hirsch W, et al. Aneurysms of the intracavemous carotid artery: Clinical presentation, radiographic features, and pathogenesis. Neurosurg. 1990;26:71-9.
47. Liu GT, Crenner CW, Logigian EL, et al. Midbrain syndromes of Benedikt, Claude, and Nothnagel: Setting the record straight. Neurology. 1992;42:1820-2.
48. Lustbader JM, Miller NR. Painless, pupil-sparing but otherwise complete oculomotor nerve paresis caused by basilar artery aneurysm. Arch Ophthalmol. 1988;106:582-83.
49. Mathew NT, Chandy J. Painful ophthalmoplegia. Neurol Sci. 1970;11:243-56.
50. Mathew NT. Painful ophthalmoplegia. In: Spillaine JD, editor. Tropical Neurology. London: Oxford University Press; 1972. pp. 120-23.
51. McGettrich P, Eustace P. The WEBINO syndrome. Neuro-ophthal. 1985;5:109-15.
52. Odaka M, Yuki N, Hirata K. Anti-GQlb IgG antibody syndrome: Clinical and immunological range. J Neurol Neurosurg Psychiatry. 2001;70(1):50-5.
53. Plager D. Superior oblique palsy and superior oblique myokymia. In: Rosenbaum AL, Santiago AP, editors. Clinical strabismus management. Philadelphia: WB Saunders; 1999. pp. 219-29.
54. Pusateri TJ, Sedwick LA, Margo CE. Isolated inferior rectus muscle palsy from a solitary metastasis to the oculomotor nucleus. Arch Ophthalmol. 1987;105:675-7.
55. Raffelsberger T, Rossmanith W, Thaller-Antlanger H, et al. CPEO associated with a single nucleotide deletion in the mitochondrial tRNA(Tyr) gene. Neurology. 2001;57(12):2298-301.
56. Richards BW, Jones FR Younge BR. Causes and prognosis in 4,278 cases of paralysis of the oculomotor, trochlear and abducens cranial nerves. Am J Ophthalmol. 1992;113:489-96.
57. Scharwey K, Krzizok T, Samii M, et al. Remission of superior oblique myokymia after microvascular decompression. Ophthalmologica. 2000;214(6):426-28.
58. Sharpe JA, Resenberg MA, Hoyt WF, et al. Paralytic pontine exotropia. A sign of acute unilateral pontine gaze palsy and internuclear ophthalmoplegia. Neurology. 1974;24(11):1076-81.
59. Shasimoto M, Ohtsuka K, Hoyt WF. Vascular compression as a cause of superior oblique myokymia disclosed by thin-slice magnetic resonance imaging. Am Ophthalmol. 2001;131(5):676-77.
60. Tomsak RL, Kosmorsky GS, Leigh RJ. Gabapentin attenuates superior oblique myokymia. Am Ophthalmol. 2002;133:721-23.
61. Vanooteghem P, Dehaene I, Vanzandycke M, et al. Combined trochlear nerve palsy and internuclear ophthalmoplegia. Arch Neurol. 1992;49:108-9.
62. White VA, Cline RA. Pathologic causes of the superior oblique click syndrome Ophthalmology. 1999;106:1292-95.
63. Yuki N. Acute ophthalmoparesis without ataxia. Ophthalmology. 2001;108:196-200.

15 CHAPTER
Squint, Phoria, and Diplopia

Pushpita Sahu, Ambar Chakravarty

SQUINT AND PHORIAS

Binocular vision is the coordinated use of two eyes to produce a single (mental) visual impression. It goes without saying that, therefore, it depends on proper structural development of the two eyes linked by a strong physiological bondage between them. This is not fully developed at birth but normally develops within the first few years so that binocular single vision is maintained in all positions and in different directions of gaze.

ADVANTAGES OF BINOCULAR VISION

- Binocular visual field is larger than mono-cular visual field.
- Blind spot of one eye is compensated by the other so that an individual is not usually aware of it.
- The combined binocular visual acuity is slightly greater than the uniocular acuity.
- Depth perception.

CERTAIN FACTS TO REMEMBER

- The retina and fovea are not fully developed at birth so perception is poor. This develops rapidly. The visual acuity is roughly 6/60 at less than 1 year, by the age of 2 years, it is about 6/12, by the age of 3 years, it is about 6/9, and 6/6 is achieved by 5 years approximately.
- The eyeball is 75% of adult size at birth resulting in physiological hypermetropia.
- The ciliary muscle is not fully developed till age 3 years.
- The medial recti are structurally more developed than the other extraocular muscles.

REFLEXES

At Birth

The compensatory fixation reflex—enabling fixation of an object to be maintained, in spite of movement of head and neck.

At 2–3 Months

- The orientational reflex—enabling conjugate movement of the eyes to maintain fixation of an object moving across the field of vision.
- Refixation reflex—enabling fixation of a new object of interest in space.
- The pupillary reflex—direct and consensual.
- The vergence reflex—enabling disconjugate movement of eyes to maintain fixation of an approaching object. This is strongly developed by 6 months.

At 2–3 Years

- The accommodation reflex
- The fusional vergence reflex—governing the coordination between vergence and accommodation reflex.

Accommodation and convergence are closely linked and exertion of one will automatically induce the other.

To understand binocular vision properly, we must be familiar with two terms: (1) *corresponding retinal points* and (2) *Panum's area*. Corresponding retinal points are those points in each retina which when stimulated project to the same point in space—thus giving rise to a single visual impression. However, there is not only a strict point-to-point correspondence between the two retinae. Around each corresponding point, there is an elliptical area which when stimulated by an object also project to the same point in space—this is the *Panum's area*. So, two slightly dissimilar images can be fused to produce a single visual impression. This is the basis of stereoscopic vision—the highest grade of binocular vision which enables us to perceive depth.

GRADES OF BINOCULAR VISION

- *Simultaneous macular perception*: This is the ability to see two images, one formed on each macula simultaneously and to superimpose them.
- *Fusion*: This is the ability to see two similar images one formed on each retina and to blend them as one. Visual sensation is constantly moving and there is always a tendency for latent deviation. This is constantly compensated and corrected in order to maintain binocular single vision. The power which regulates this compensatory corrective movement is the power of fusion.
- *Stereopsis or depth perception*: This is the ability to see two slightly dissimilar images one formed on each retina simultaneously, blend them as one, and to perceive depth. As explained in the previous paragraph, there is not only a strict point-to-point correspondence between the two retinae, but around each corresponding point there is an elliptical area (Panum's area) which when stimulated also project to the same point in space. Thus, slightly dissimilar images, one formed from each retina can be blended and fused with the perception of depth.

Thus, by gradual perfection of anatomical and physiological development, the coordination of the two eyes in binocular single vision is maintained in all positions of gaze and in different directions so that a clear retinal image is formed. This is achieved by the strength of the binocular fusion reflex enabling constant fusion of the two monocular retinal images and not by simple fixed parallel arrangement of the two visual axes. In fact, perfect balance of the two visual axis or orthophoria is a rarity. There if often a latent tendency for the visual axis to deviate from the parallelism, but this latent deviation or heterophoria is controlled by the strength of fusion, so that a manifest deviation with the loss of binocular vision resulting in squint or strabismus does not happen.

It is important to be familiar with certain terminologies commonly used to describe ocular movement. They are duction, version, and vergence. *Duction* is movement of each eye depending on primary action of individual muscle. There are six such positions for each eye. These are: (1) adduction (looking in toward the nose), (2) abduction (looking out away from the nose), (3) sursumduction (looking up), (4) deorsumduction (looking down), (5) incycloduction (where the 12 o'clock is rotated toward the nose), and (6) excycloduction (where it is rotated away from the nose).

Ocular version is the conjugate binocular movement of the two eyes in the same direction. There are nine such positions of gaze—(1) dextroversion, (2) dextroelevation, (3) dextrodepression, (4) laevoversion, (5) laevoelevation, (6) laevodepression, (7) primary position, (8) direct elevation, and (9) direct depression. Ocular vergence is disconjugate movement of the two eyes in order to view approaching object and can be convergent or divergent.

As already stated, strict parallelism of the two visual axes is a rarity and small deviations are common. If this deviation is latent—it is called phoria, and if it is manifest, it is tropia or squint.

Phoria or latent squint is a common occurrence and in most cases, it is easily controlled and asymptomatic. However, large phorias may give rise to asthenopic symptoms of eye strain due to the constant effort made by the eye muscles to overcome it in order to maintain binocular single vision.

Decompensating phorias can give rise to symptoms of headache, blurring of vision, intermittent diplopia, photophobia, small inaccuracies in judging distances, and even nausea and dizziness.

Phoria may be esophoria where the latent deviation is inward toward the nose, exophoria where the latent deviation is outward, hyperphoria and hypophoria where the latent deviation is respectively upward and downward, and cyclophoria which can be incyclophoria or excyclophoria depending on whether the 12 o'clock position is turned in toward the nose or out.

The *cover test*—is the single most important test that can and should be performed at the clinic. It is performed both with and without glasses. It should be performed at near point of 33 cm, and distant point of 6 meters, and in some cases for far distance.

Target for near can be an accommodative target like a small picture on a stick or a light. Target for distance can be 6/60 on Snellen's chart.

The examiner should be at eye-to-eye level with the patient, and should use an occluder for testing.

If there is a head posture, then the test should be done in that position first, before straightening the head.

- First look for bifoveal fixation. The patient is asked to look at the fixation target and then one eye is covered. Any corrective movement in the other eye to take up fixation shows that the eye was deviated and has a manifest squint or tropia. If the eye turns into fix, then there is exotropia, if it goes out to fix, it is esotropia; similarly, hypertropia and hypotropia. The test is repeated covering the other eye. This is *cover–uncover* test (Fig. 1).
- For the latent squint to become manifest, the eyes must be dissociated. This is the *alternate cover* test. One eye says the right eye is occluded. The target is then moved from side-to-side to make dissociation complete. The phoria or latent squint occurs behind the occluder. Now on removing the cover, any corrective movement of the right eye is noted. Moving in shows the eye was exophoric, moving out shows the eye was esophoric; similarly, hyper- and hypophoric (Fig. 2).

Each eye should be tested in similar way. While describing phorias, we must note the direction of phoria, e.g. exophoria, esophoria, and hyper- or hypophoria, whether it is small medium or large and rate of recovery.

TROPIA/STRABISMUS/SQUINT

Tropia or squint is a condition where one visual axis is directed toward the fixation object and the other deviating from it. So, there is a manifest deviation. This may be *concomitant* or nonparalytic and *inconcomitant* or paralytic.

In a concomitant or nonparalytic squint, the angle of the squint remains the same in different

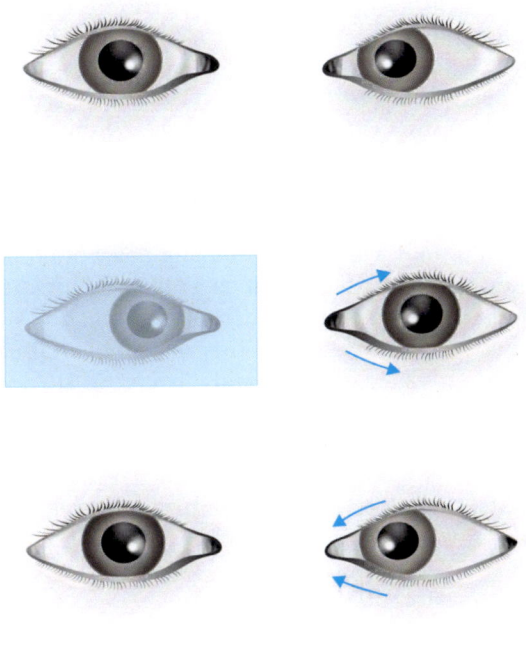

FIG. 1: Left convergent squint: Cover test.

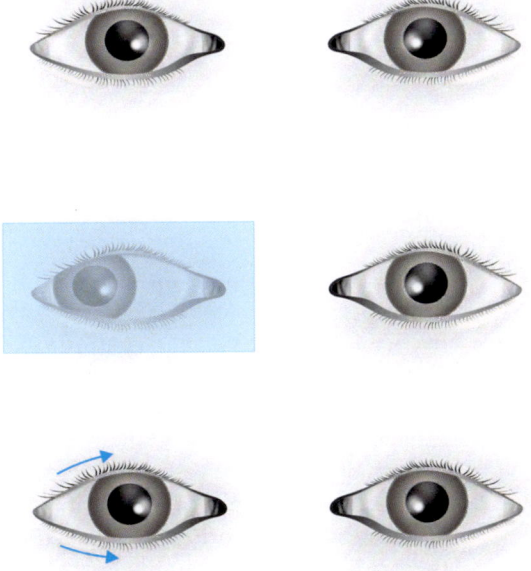

FIG 2: Latent divergent squint: Cover test.

positions of gaze whereas in a paralytic or inconcomitant squint, the angle varies in different positions of gaze and the secondary angle is greater than the primary angle. In a paralytic squint, say left lateral rectus palsy, there will be overaction of the left medial rectus (direct antagonist) so, the left eye will be slightly convergent in the primary position—this is the primary angle. At the same time, if the right eye is covered and the left eye is made to take up fixation in the primary position, then a larger effort has to be exerted by the lateral rectus of that eye, and by Herring's law of equal innervation, a larger stimulus goes to the medial rectus of the right eye which therefore, shows a larger inward deviation—this is the secondary angle. So, as a result of paralytic squint, say left lateral rectus palsy, the following happen—there is overaction of direct antagonist—left medial rectus, overaction of contralateral synergist—right medial rectus, and underaction of contralateral antagonist—right lateral rectus.

Causes and Effects of Squint

Causes of squint can be broadly classified under three heads—(1) sensory, (2) motor, and (3) central factors.

Sensory Factors

- Dioptric factors interfering with the formation of a clear retinal image.
  - Any opacity in the media preventing the formation of a clear retinal image, e.g. central corneal opacity, congenital cataract, retrolental fibroplasia, tumors, etc.
  - *Refractive error if uncorrected*:
    - If insuperable, i.e., cannot be corrected by any corrective accommodative movement of the eye—the image formed is blurred making fusion difficult, especially if there is a high refractive error in one eye.
    - If superable, i.e. can be corrected by accommodative effort of the eye—then the individual will make corrective effort to overcome it putting a strain on accommodation and convergence.
- Retinoneural disturbances, e.g. birth hemorrhage, or other retinal defects will reduce the strength of visual sensation.
- Prolonged monocular patching, especially before the reflexes are fully developed.

Motor Factors

This may affect the orbits, extraocular muscles, nerve pathway myoneural junction, or the nerve nucleus.

- *Developmental anomalies*:
  - *Affecting orbit*:
    - Narrowly or widely spaced orbits
    - Facial asymmetry, oxycephaly, or telencephaly.
  - *Affecting muscle*:
    - Aplasia or incomplete differentiation
    - Abnormal insertion, abnormal check ligament
    - Abnormal sheath structure
    - Fibrosis of a muscle.
- *Nerve pathway*:
  - Anomalous connection or aplasia
  - Nerve nucleus—usually associated with widespread anomalies and cerebral defects: Mobius syndrome
  - Birth trauma, e.g. damage to lateral rectus during forceps delivery, hemorrhage in the orbit leading to fibrosis.
  - Various neurological diseases affecting ocular cranial nerves, myoneural junctions, and ocular muscles—as discussed in details in different chapters of this book.

Central Factors

- Physical and mental illness can lead to decompensation of heterophoria or a manifest deviation.
- Hyperexcitability can lead to overconvergence.
- Hypoexcitability can lead to a divergent squint.
- *Developmental delay and low IQ*: About a third of children with cerebral palsy have nonparalytic squint.

Long-term Effects of Nonparalytic Squint

At the onset of squint, there is often a brief period of double vision leading to confusion. This in turn leads to *suppression* of an image from one eye followed by *amblyopia* in that eye. *Fusion* rapidly deteriorates and abnormal retinal correspondence or eccentric fixation may develop.

Abnormal retinal correspondence is a binocular condition, where the fovea of one eye is used in conjunction with a point other than the fovea of the deviating eye. This is a binocular condition, so some grade of binocular vision is present. When one eye is covered, then the fovea of the deviating eye automatically takes up fixation.

Eccentric fixation is a monocular condition where a peripheral retinal element other than fovea takes up fixation.

Amblyopia or lazy eye is a condition where there is diminished vision in one eye without any structural abnormality of the afferent visual pathway. It is usually unilateral but may be bilateral. Acuity of vision develops as a condition reflex and any interruption in its development leads to arrest and then degeneration toward extinction. There are basically three types of amblyopia:
1. Stimulus deprivation amblyopia, e.g. corneal opacity, congenital cataract, early traumatic cataract, prolonged uniocular patching, and interrupting formation of a clear retinal image.
2. Anisometropic amblyopia—where there is high refractive error in one eye—resulting in a poor retinal image from that eye.
3. Strabismic amblyopia as explained earlier.

Paralytic Squint and Diplopia

Diplopia results from acquired misalignment of the eyes caused by weakness of one or more extraocular muscles, i.e. paralytic strabismus. When a patient with diplopia presents to the clinic, the neurologist needs to answer *four* questions:
1. Is the diplopia monocular?
2. Which eye muscles are weak?
3. Where is the lesion that is causing the eye muscle weakness?
4. What are the most likely causes and the appropriate investigations?

1. Is the diplopia monocular?

The first question is often overlooked because diplopia is assumed to be due to ocular misalignment. Monocular diplopia becomes obvious during the examination if the cover test or alternate cover tests are performed (see here). The cause is usually defects of ocular media, such as cataracts, less often macular disease, and very rarely cerebral lesions. Cerebral monocular diplopia (or polyopia) affects both eyes and usually results from lesions of occipital cortex or central visual pathways.

2. Which eye muscles are weak?

Analysis of eye muscle weakness is often a crucial step in the diagnosis of diplopia and will be reviewed here in some detail. Analysis depends on a basic understanding of the topography and kinematics of eye muscles and on clinical skills that identify the weak eye muscles. Also, it is important to use strabismus terminology as it represents important concepts and enables precise, "shorthand" descriptions of findings (*see* Appendix 2).

Which eye muscles are weak?—Eye muscle topography and kinematics

Six extraocular muscles act on each eye. When the eye is in primary position, the main pulling action (primary action) of each muscle corresponds to each of the six ocular ductions, as outlined in table 1, figure 3, and appendix 3.

The horizontal rectus muscles move the eye purely in the horizontal plane. The lateral rectus abducts the eye whereas the medial rectus adducts the eye. The vertical rectus muscles have primary vertical actions and these predominate over their secondary torsional actions. The oblique muscles have primary torsional actions and secondary vertical actions. When the eye is adducted, the major actions to the oblique muscles change from rotating the eye in its torsional plane to rotating in its vertical plane. Since intorsion cannot be

Table 1: The actions of the extraocular muscles in primary position

Muscles	Primary action	Secondary action	Tertiary action
Medial rectus	Adduction	–	–
Lateral rectus	Abduction	–	–
Superior rectus	Elevation	Intorsion	Abduction
Inferior rectus	Depression	Extorsion	Abduction
Superior oblique	Intorsion	Depression	Adduction
Inferior oblique	Extorsion	Elevation	Adduction

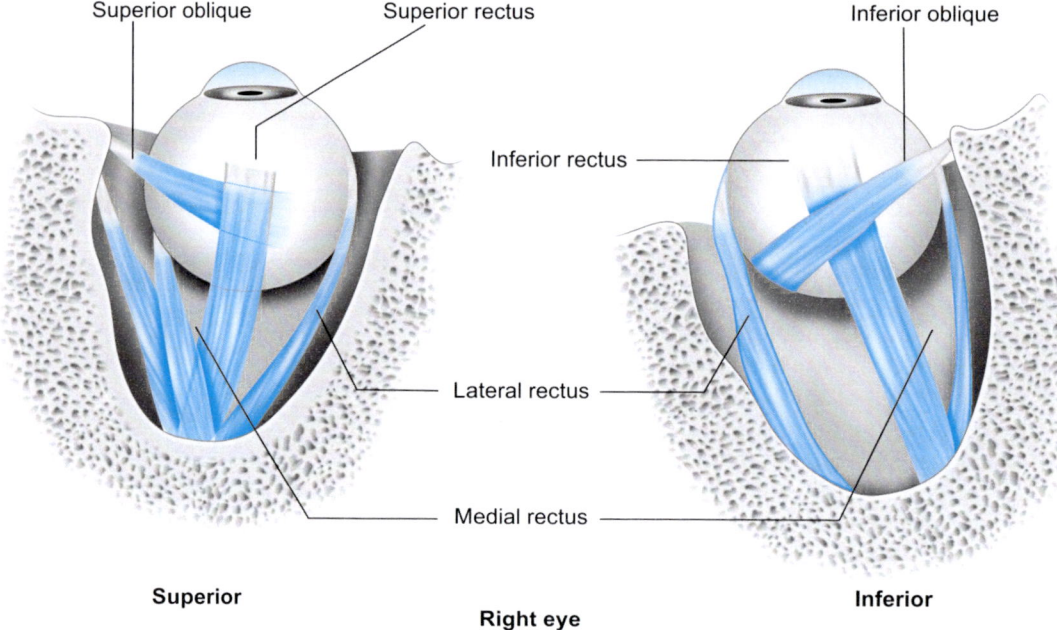

FIG. 3: Six extraocular muscles of the right eye viewed from above (superior) and below (inferior).

tested easily at the bedside, superior oblique (SO) function is tested by the ability to depress the eye in the adducted position (but see here). The tertiary horizontal actions of the obliques and vertical recti are minor and irrelevant to neurological diagnosis. For routine clinical bedside examination, it is important to remember the simple rule that the *recti (superior or inferior) are pure elevators and depressors of the eye in the abducted position (respectively) and the obliques (superior and inferior) are pure depressor and elevators (respectively) of the eye in the adducted position* (Fig. 4).

Which Eye Muscles are Weak?—History

Answers to *six* questions prove extremely useful:
1. Does the double vision go away when closing one eye?
2. Are the two images separated vertically, horizontally, obliquely, or torsionally?
3. Is the diplopia worse at distance or at near?
4. In which direction is the double vision worse?
5. Is there a history of congenital strabismus or abnormal head position?
6. Are associated pains, headache, or neurologic symptoms present?

Answers to these questions and their explanations would be found in the following section.

Patients with incipient diplopia occasionally complain of visual blurring, which clears when one or other eye is covered. Conversely, patients with widely separated images may complain of visual "confusion" rather than diplopia. Dizziness or vertigo may accompany diplopia but it clears when one eye is covered, indicating that it is not a symptom of vestibular dysfunction.

The most important question is whether the diplopia is horizontal or vertical (or oblique). A significant vertical component excludes an isolated horizontal rectus palsy. Horizontal diplopia excludes a vertical rectus or oblique palsy. For horizontal diplopia, greater image separation with gaze to one side suggests weakness of the ipsilateral lateral rectus or contralateral medial rectus. Relief of diplopia from turning the head to one side implicates the ipsilateral lateral rectus or contralateral medial rectus. Improvement when viewing near targets (e.g. reading) suggests lateral rectus weakness. For vertical diplopia, the effect of vertical gaze also is helpful. For example, greater image separation on downgaze suggests

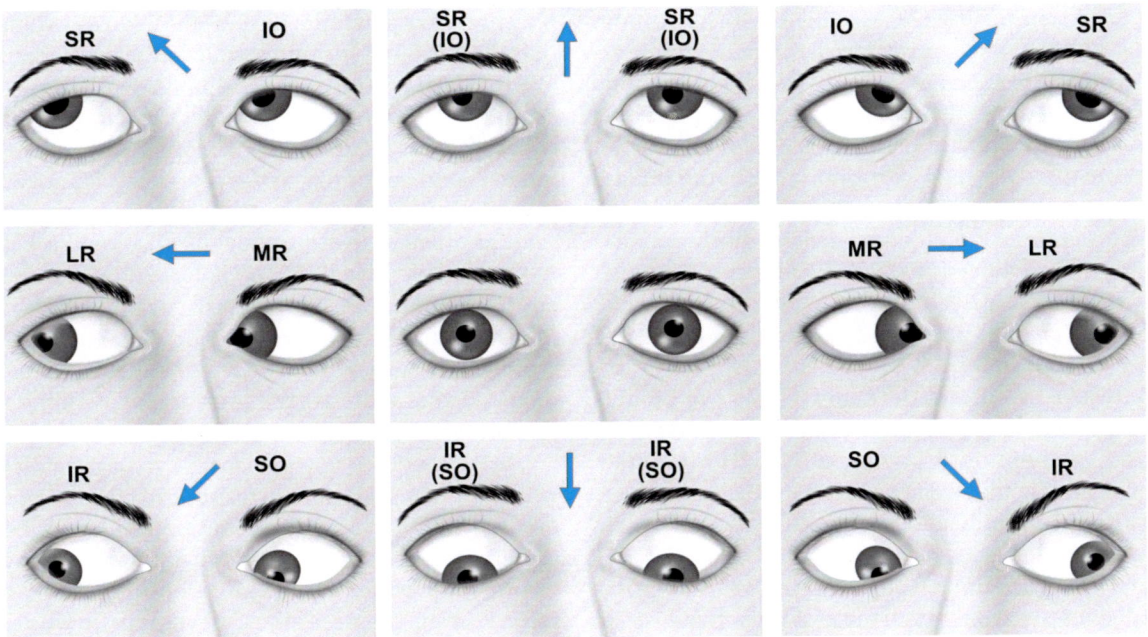

FIG. 4: Diagnostic eye positions illustrating the main field of action of each extraocular muscles. (IO, inferior oblique; IR, inferior rectus; LR, lateral rectus; MR, medial rectus; SO, superior oblique; SR, superior rectus)

weakness of a SO or inferior rectus muscle. Tilting of one image relative to the other usually signifies a paretic SO muscle, related to loss of intorsion and the resulting excyclotropia. *Improvement of diplopia with head tilt to one side suggests a SO palsy on the opposite side.*

Which Eye Muscles Are Weak?—Examination

A few basic measures optimize the examination of diplopia, including good illumination of the eyes (with a lamp if necessary) and sitting the patient up, eye-to-eye, with the examiner. Using a distant fixation target allows the examiner to observe the eyes without the distraction of holding a near target. The examiner simply turns the patient's head to observe different gaze positions. The exclusive use of a handheld near target risks missing a mild lateral rectus palsy since the eyes may still align normally at close range (i.e. converge). The results of the examination should be recorded concisely, employing standard terminology (*see* Appendix 2).

Two types of testing are used to localize weak eye muscles: (1) *ocular ductions* and (2) *ocular versions*. Testing ocular ductions assesses the range of movement of each eye in different gaze positions. Traditionally, six cardinal positions are tested. These six positions are determined by the primary actions of the extraocular muscles as mentioned earlier. Movement in the horizontal plane tests the action of the medial and lateral recti. Asking the patient to look to one side and then testing for elevation of the eyes, tests the superior rectus (SR) of the ipsilateral eye (abducted eye), and inferior oblique of the contralateral (adducted) eye.

At this position, asking the patient to look down (depression) would test the inferior rectus of the ipsilateral (abducted) eye and SO of the contralateral (adducted) eye. It is advisable to avoid testing for elevation and depression with the eyes looking straight ahead as several muscles may participate and isolating the weak muscles becomes difficult. Moderate or severe paralysis of a horizontal or vertical rectus muscle usually produces a limited duction in its main field of action. Mild paresis of a rectus muscle or more severe paresis of an oblique muscle may not produce a limited duction. For example, patients with diplopia caused by traumatic fourth nerve palsies often exhibit a full range of ocular ductions. When a muscle is incompletely paralyzed, a full duction may be achieved by driving the muscle (or nerve) with more intense central neural discharge. An assessment of ocular versions is then required to identify the weak muscle.

Version testing assesses ocular misalignment in different gaze positions, using the patient's verbal (*subjective*) responses or the examiner's (*objective*) observations. The basis of version testing is that diplopia and ocular misalignment worsen in the gaze direction corresponding to the pulling direction of the weak muscle and improve in the opposite direction. "Incomitance" of the deviation is a cardinal feature of paralytic strabismus, although it may lessen over time. To identify the weak muscle(s), both the type of ocular misalignment—an esotropia, exotropia, or hypertropia (i.e. inward, outward, or upward deviation of one eye relative to the other) and the effect of gaze direction on the misalignment must be determined. For example, an esotropia that worsens in left gaze and improves in right gaze indicated weakness of the left lateral rectus (or tethering by the left medial rectus).

The *cover test* and the *alternate cover* (cross-cover) tests are the most useful objective tests of versions. When an extraocular muscle is weak, the "paretic" eye deviates in the direction of the tonically active antagonist muscle (Fig. 5). This deviation is called the *primary deviation*. If the nonparetic eye is covered, the patient is obliged to "take up fixation" with the paretic eye (Fig. 6). The weak muscle requires a higher level of innervation to achieve the force necessary to allow foveal fixation. The yoke muscle of the other eye receives the same increment of innervation (Hering's law), which causes the nonparetic eye to deviate. This is called the *secondary deviation* (Figs. 5 and 6). The cover test and the alternate cover tests are very useful when the type of deviation is not obvious.

In a patient with horizontal diplopia due to mild paresis of the right lateral rectus, simple inspection may not show a definite deviation. When a cover is placed in front of his nonparetic left eye, the right eye is forced to move outward to fixate the target. The outward "movement of redress" elicited by the cover test reveals the small primary deviation and indicates an esotropia. When the cover is moved from the left eye to the right eye, the left eye is also seen to move outward to take up fixation. This is the secondary deviation. The right eye, now under cover, again resumes its primary deviation. This is the alternate cover (or cross-cover) test. The cover is alternated several times during the test to allow repeated observation of the "movement of redress" and bring out the maximal deviation.

The spontaneously deviating eye of a patient with diplopia may not correspond to the paretic eye. For example, if the patient referred to earlier, preferred to fixate with his right eye, the left eye would maintain an inward turn (a *turn* esotropia), representing the secondary deviation. It would be a mistake to diagnose a left lateral rectus palsy from this appearance. To determine the affected side, the examiner repeats the alternate cover test in right gaze and left gaze. In this patient with esotropia, a larger deviation (large movements of redress) would be seen in right gaze, indicating a right lateral rectus palsy. Also, recall that patients with lateral rectus weakness may have no diplopia or misalignment when viewing a near target. A distant target (at 2 or 3 meters) should be used to avoid false-negative results.

For horizontal diplopia, there are only four candidate muscles. Simply distinguishing an esotropia from an exotropia and determining the effect of lateral gaze identifies the weak muscle. For vertical or oblique diplopia, there are eight

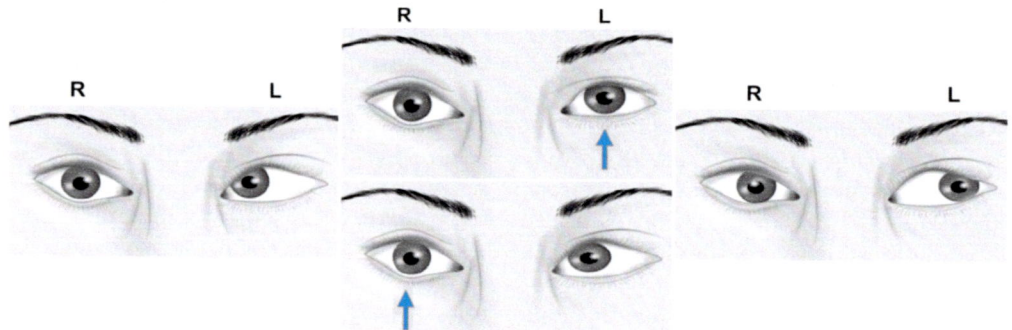

FIG. 5: Primary and secondary deviation. There is a right abduction defect on right gaze, but full duction on left gaze. The esotropia is small with the left (nonparetic) eye fixating (primary deviation, top) and much larger with the right (paretic) eye fixating (secondary deviation, bottom).

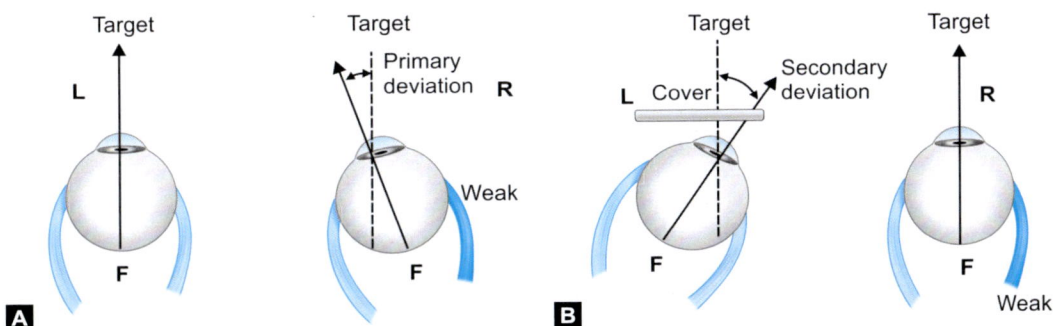

FIG. 6: Cover Test. Weakness of right lateral rectus muscle. **A,** When left eye fixates on distant target normal unopposed activity of right medial rectus muscle causes primary deviation of right eye; **B,** When left eye is covered, a higher level of innervation drives the right lateral rectus to allow the right eye to take up fixation. The same level of innervation is sent to its yoke muscle, the left medial rectus, causing secondary deviation of the left eye. (F — fovea)

candidate muscles. And hence, it is difficult often to isolate the weak muscle in routine clinical neurologic practice. Subjective version testing may at times be helpful.

Subjective version testing requires that the patient describes the direction and relative degree of separation of the two images in different gaze positions. There are two underlying principles of subjective testing:

The separation of images increases as the fixation target moves into the field of action of the paretic muscle, and

The more peripheral image is from the "paretic" eye. The examiner assigns the images to each eye simply by covering one eye and asking the patient to report the image that disappears.

Unfortunately patients very often fail to identify which image (the peripheral or the nearer) disappears on covering a particular eye. Using a red glass in front of one eye may be helpful. If the outer (peripheral) image at the diplopia position is red, then the eye with the red glass muscle is the offending eye. The particular weak muscle can then be identified from the position at which diplopia is maximum. For example, with the red glass in front of the left eye and diplopia on looking upward and to the right, if the red image is peripheral, the left inferior oblique is the weak muscle (inferior oblique is pure elevator of the adducted eye).

Such maneuvers even when meticulously performed by a neurologist, often fails to identify the weak muscle in some patients with diplopia as the paresis and resultant misalignment may be very subtle. An ophthalmologist's help may need to be sought at times. Use of Hess chart, the Maddox rod, and the Bielschowsky head tilt test are often resorted to by ophthalmologists. Only the head tilt test will be detailed as it is easy to perform at the bedside.

Head Tilt Test

The *Bielschowsky head tilt* was designed to determine the paretic muscle responsible for vertical misalignment and is an enormously valuable test. This is a three step test.

Step 1: Note the deviation in the primary position. Take for example, a patient with a right fourth nerve palsy. The individual will have a right hypertropia in primary position. This pattern could be due to underaction of the SO or inferior rectus muscle in the right eye (not pulling the right eye down sufficiently) or to underaction of the inferior oblique or SR muscle in the left eye (not pulling the left eye up).

Step 2: Record the deviation on gaze on either side. In this case, the deviation should be greater on left gaze, indicating that it must be due to a muscle that has its greatest action in that direction of gaze, either the right SO or the left SR.

Step 3: Compare the deviation with tilt to either side. In this case, the deviation is worse with right head tilt. A right head tilt demands an intorsion movement of the right eye, normally accomplished by the SO and SR muscles. The vertical actions of these two muscles normally cancel each other out but, in the face of a right weak SO, contraction of the unopposed SR elevates the eye.

The authors feel that disappearance of the outer blurred image, which comes from the affected eye, is an easier way to locate the eye at fault. However, many subjects tend to confuse which one is the clearer image and which is the blurred image when one eye is shut. An easy solution is to use a spectacle with a red glass for one eye and a green glass for the other. The outer image is always the false image from the affected eye and its color is noted. When one eye is closed, one of the images disappears. By noting the color of the disappearing image, the affected eye can be deduced. Furthermore, an abnormal torsional movement of the eyeball while looking down in the adducted position also suggests a trochlear nerve dysfunction causing vertical diplopia.

Forced Duction Test

Diplopia also may result from restriction of movement due to tethering of a normal muscle by its antagonist. When restriction is suspected, forced duction testing is used to confirm the diagnosis. First, the conjunctiva is anesthetized. The patient is asked to look in the direction of restricted movement. The examiner then tries to force the eye further in the same direction, either by pushing with a cotton-tipped applicator applied to the conjunctiva behind the limbus or by pulling on the same area with fine-toothed forceps. Resistance to movement signifies tethering. When voluntary ductions are mildly limited, forced ductions often produce equivocal results. *This test must always be performed by an ophthalmologist.*

Where is the lesion that is causing the eye muscle weakness?

What are the most likely causes and the appropriate investigations?

The major sites of disease responsible for diplopia in the clinic are the oculomotor, trochlear and abducens nerves, the neuromuscular junction, and the brainstem. Analysis of eye muscle weakness often identifies the involved site. The chronology, modifying factors, and symptoms and signs associated with diplopia help to refine the localization and determine the most likely cause. For example, a long history of intermittent or transient diplopia that can be controlled with effort suggests a benign process, such as a decompensated congenital palsy or phoria. Convergence insufficiency may cause variable horizontal diplopia that occurs only with reading.

Ocular myasthenia may mimic any type of ophthalmoplegia but typically produces fluctuating diplopia and ptosis, and both symptoms resolve for a short period after sleep.

"Neighborhood" symptoms that help localize the lesion include orbital symptoms such as local pain, swelling, eye redness, proptosis, or visual loss; cavernous sinus symptoms, such as headache or symptoms of multiple cranial nerve dysfunction; and brainstem symptoms, reflecting impairment of long tract or local brainstem functions. It may also be important, depending on the clinical setting, to screen for symptoms of increased intracranial pressure, generalized myasthenia, peripheral neuropathy, temporal arteritis or other systemic inflammatory disease, or a history of neoplasm or vascular risk factors. Head trauma is a common and obvious cause of diplopia but nerve palsies induced by minor head trauma may signal an underlying compressive lesion.

Detecting Infantile Strabismus

Patients with a strabismus of infantile onset may manage to fuse for years and do not complain of diplopia, until age, disease, or drug exposures lead to an eventual decompensation and associated diplopia. Determining when this is the case is crucial in preventing unnecessary workups and anxiety. A close look at early photographs is probably the easiest way to diagnose early onset of strabismus. A forced duction test may be needed in an occasional case of gaze restriction due to fibrosis of an extraocular muscle.

Detailing of clinical aspects of nuclear and infranuclear ophthalmoplegias had been done in the previous chapter (Chapter 14: Nuclear and Infranuclear Ophthalmoplegias). These two chapters are complementary to each other and should be read together.

SUGGESTED READINGS

1. Cornblath WT. Diplopia due to ocular motor cranial neuropathies. Continuum (Minneap Minn). 2014;20(4 Neuro-ophthalmology):966-80.
2. Dinkin M. Diagnostic approach to diplopia. Continuum (Minneap Minn). 2014;20(4 Neuro-ophthalmology):942-65
3. Gräf M, Lorenz B. How to deal with diplopia. Rev Neurol (Paris). 2012;168(10):720-8..

Gaze and Supranuclear Oculomotor Disorders

CHAPTER 16

Angshuman Mukherjee, Ambar Chakravarty

INTRODUCTION

The ocular motor system has two principal tasks—firstly to place the image of a viewed object on the fovea (gaze shifting) and secondly to keep the image on the fovea as the viewed object or the viewer's head moves in space (gaze holding). These objectives are achieved by means of four subsystems: Saccades, pursuit, vestibular, and vergence. The first three of these systems generate conjugate movements, called version, but the fourth system generates disconjugate or disjunctive horizontal movements, called vergence. The vergence system achieves binocular vision by generating disjunctive eye movements that align the two foveae on an object as it approaches the head.

Gaze disturbances are pathologic alterations in versional and vergence eye movements. Disturbances of versional eye movements consist of gaze deviations (displacement of the eyes into the extremes of the orbit) and gaze deficits (abnormalities in the latency of initiation, speed, amplitude, or accuracy of conjugate eye movements). Disturbances of vergence eye movements always lead to ocular misalignment.

SACCADIC SUBSYSTEM

Saccades are used to rapidly bring an image of interest onto the fovea for high resolution visual examination. It is now recognized that different cognitive intentions and different visual and motor properties of the stimulus for a saccade can, in turn, give rise to a number of different types of saccades.

- Spontaneous saccades are internally triggered but without a goal, and usually occur during another motor activity (e.g., speech), at rest in darkness and during rapid eye movement sleep
- Reflexive saccades are externally driven by the sudden appearance of a novel stimulus, e.g., a visual target on the peripheral retina (visually guided reflexive saccades) or a sudden noise (auditory reflexive saccades). Reflexive saccades also occur as corrective fast phases in nystagmus
- Volitional (intentional) saccades are internally triggered, and have a goal or intentional purpose.
    - Simple visually guided saccades purposively or on command move the eyes to look at a visual target. These are the usual saccades generated during clinical examination of eye movements
    - Antisaccades are saccades made deliberately to a mirror location (in darkness/without a target) in the hemifield opposite to that of a suddenly appearing visual target. Successful generation of antisaccades requires the subject to suppress the tendency to look at the visual target, while using its visual information to calculate and execute an eye movement of equal but opposite direction. Testing of antisaccades has assumed growing clinical importance because it particularly examines inhibitory processing, frontal lobe function, fixation, and saccadic distractibility
    - Memory-guided saccades are made towards the remembered position of one or more visual or vestibular derived targets, and allow clinical examination of spatial working memory, and chronological sequencing
    - Predictive saccades are made to a known location (spatial predictability)

at which a target is expected at a known time (temporal predictability). They are particularly susceptible to impairment with disorders such as Parkinson's disease and frontal lobe lesions.

Anatomy (Figs 1 and 2)

Saccadic control can be considered in terms of:
- Cortical areas capable of preparing saccades (e.g., dorsolateral prefrontal cortex, posterior parietal cortex, hippocampus and anterior cingulate cortex)
- Cortical areas capable of triggering saccades (e.g., frontal eye field, supplementary eye field, parietal eye field, intraparietal sulcus)
- Brainstem areas capable of generating horizontal and vertical saccades
- Subcortical areas capable of modulating saccade performance (e.g., thalamus, caudate, substantia nigra pars reticulata).

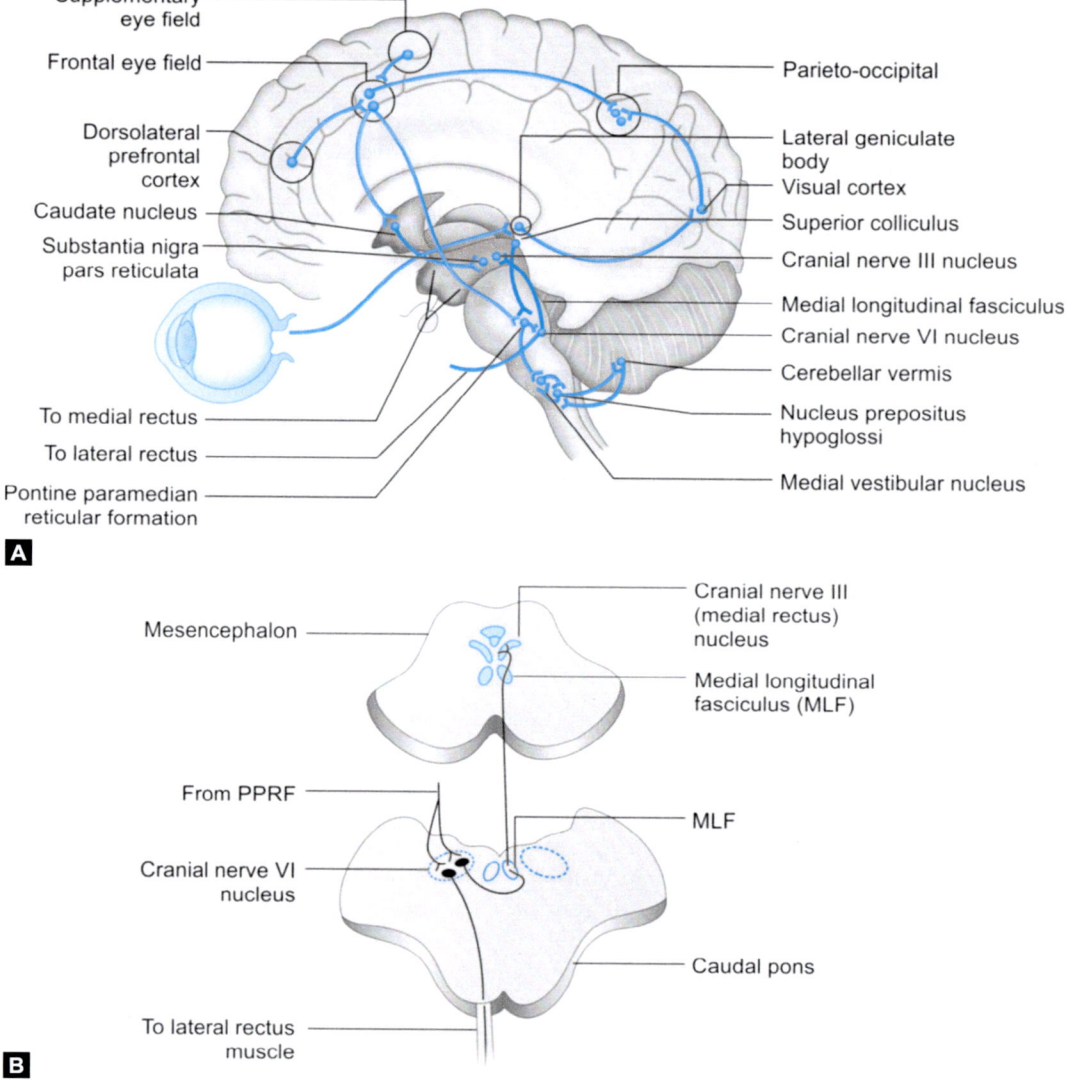

FIG. 1 : Control of horizontal saccades. **A,** Generation: Signals are generated in frontal and occipitoparietal centers and conveyed to the superior colliculus and pontine paramedian reticular formation (PPRF) via several descending pathways; **B,** Brainstem mechanism: Signals from PPRF travel to cranial nerve VI nucleus and then via the cranial nerve VI axons to the lateral rectus muscle and via the medial longitudinal fasciculus to the contralateral cranial III nucleus and then to the medial rectus.

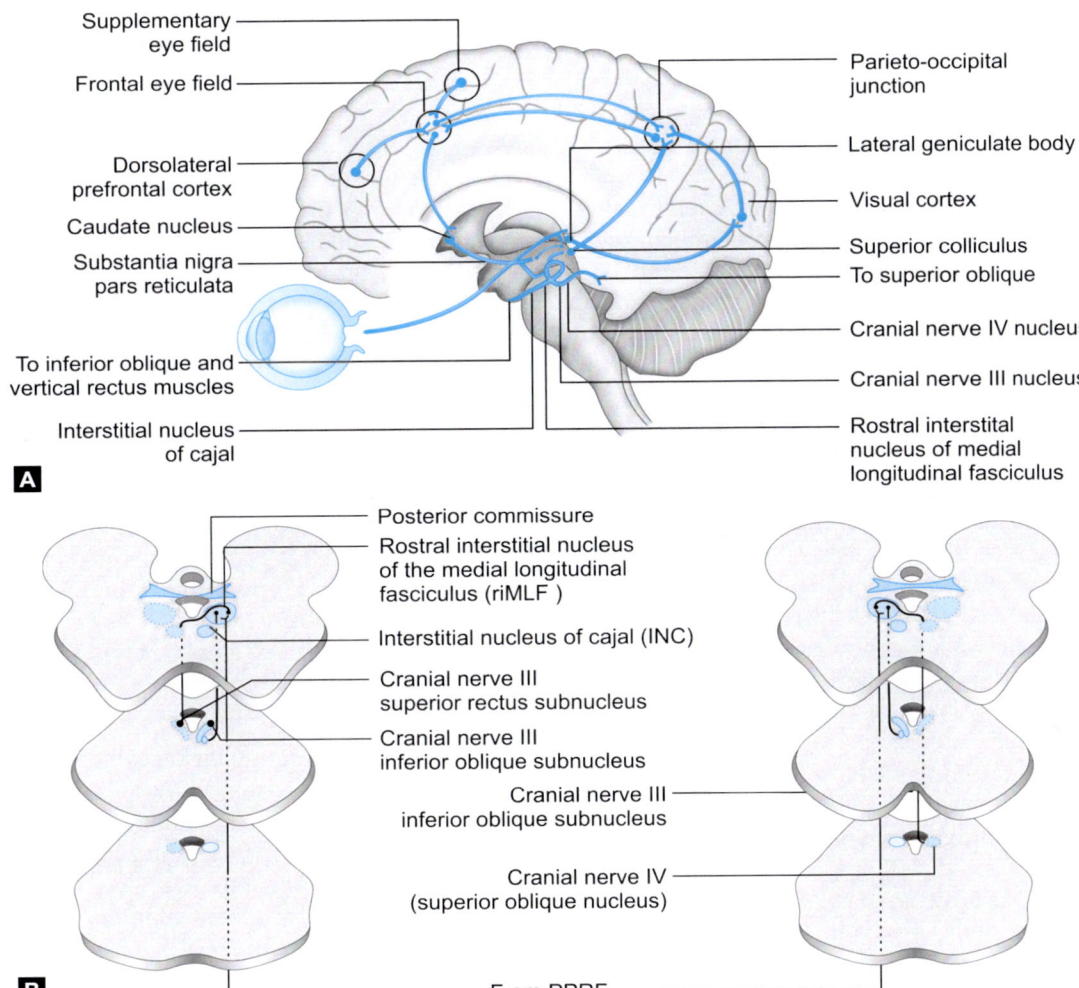

FIG. 2: Control of vertical saccades. **A,** Generation: Signals from frontal and parieto-occipital junction and frontal eye fields travel to the superior colliculus and then to the rostral interstitial nucleus of the medial longitudinal fasciculus. Signals then travel to the interstitial nucleus of Cajal and to the nuclei of cranial nerves III and IV. Torsional saccades are probably mediated by a similar pathway; **B,** Brainstem mechanism: Pathways for upward gaze pass dorsal to the aqueduct in the posterior commissure, where they are vulnerable to dorsal midbrain lesions or extrinsic compression by pineal masses or third ventricular pressure. Pathways for downward gaze pass ventral to the aqueduct in the midbrain tegmentum. They may be spared by dorsal midbrain lesions but selectively damaged by tegmental lesions.

Nonvisually guided saccades are initiated mainly by frontal eye fields (Brodmann's area 8), with contributions from supplementary motor cortex and prefrontal eye field regions. Visually guided voluntary saccades are initiated both frontally and at the cortical parieto-occipital junction with input from visual cortex. The frontal eye field and parieto-occipital junction are heavily interconnected; however, each activates both kinds of voluntary saccades.

The saccadic system has crossed innervation—the right cerebrum activating leftward gaze and the left cerebrum activating rightward gaze. Each hemisphere can however rapidly compensate for a lesioned contralateral side. Therefore, unilateral cerebral disease does not cause enduring saccadic dysfunction. Bilateral disease that affects the posterior cerebrum tends to interfere with visually guided saccades. Bilateral disease that involves the anterior cerebrum may reduce nonvisually guided saccades and allow involuntary saccades that intrude upon fixation to emerge.

For horizontal voluntary saccades, the cerebral signal travels downward to the omnipause cells of the contralateral pontine paramedian reticular formation (PPRF) through two pathways from the frontal region and one from the parietal region. One of the two frontal pathways goes directly to the PPRF; the other goes first to the caudate nucleus, then to the substantia nigra pars reticulate, then to the superior colliculus (SC), and finally to the PPRF. The pathway through the basal ganglia controls the balance between voluntary and involuntary saccades. The parietal pathway goes directly to the SC and finally to the PPRF.

Signals from the cerebral gaze centers turn off the omnipause (or pause) cells of the PPRF, which are inhibiting the firing of neighboring burst cells. The burst cells are responsible for a high-potency discharge (pulse) that gets the eyes moving. These cells mediate all horizontal saccades and disease in this region slows or abolishes horizontal saccades.

Following the pulse of innervation that starts the saccade, another neural network generates a lower-potency sustained discharge (step) that holds the eyes in an eccentric gaze against the elastic drag of the orbital soft tissues that otherwise would pull the eyes back towards the center of the orbit. Used by all four eye movement subsystems, this "neural integrator for horizontal gaze" is located in two medualllary centers, the medial vestibular nucleus (MVN) and the nucleus prepositus hypoglossi (NPH). These centers have prominent cerebellar dorsal vermis and flocculus connections. Lesions in these medullary or cerebellar regions result in dysmetric saccades and in eccentric gaze-evoked nystagmus.

The burst and step signals are conveyed to the cranial nerve VI (abducens) nucleus, where they form synapses with abducens motor neurons and interneurons. The signal is sent from abducens motor neurons to the lateral rectus muscle and via abducens interneurons through the medial longitudinal fasciculus (MLF) to the contralateral medial rectus subnucleus of cranial nerve III. A lesion within the abducens nucleus thus impairs all ipsilateral horizontal eye movements, not merely saccades.

For vertical and torsional voluntary saccades, the signal goes from cerebrum to omnipause cells in the rostral interstitial nucleus of the MLF (riMLF) in the rostral midbrain. As in the PPRF, signals sent to the omnipause cells disinhibit burst cells, which initiate vertical and torsional saccades. The neural integrator for all vertical and torsional eye movements is the neighboring interstitial nucleus of Cajal (INC). It holds the eyes in the eccentric position achieved by the burst cells of the riMLF.

The riMLF and INC mediate upward and downward gaze through separate pathways. For upward gaze, the signal travels through the posterior commissure (PC) to end on the contralateral superior rectus subnucleus and ipsilateral inferior oblique subnucleus of cranial nerve III. For downward gaze, the signal travels by means of a ventral pathway that does not go through the PC. The signals reach the ipsilateral inferior rectus subnucleus and contralateral superior oblique nucleus (cranial nerve IV).

Testing for Saccadic Dysfunction

The first step in examining for saccadic disorders is to observe patients as they fixate on a stationary target. Normally, the eyes should remain still. Fast eye movements that take the eyes off target represent saccadic intrusions.

The second step is to elicit voluntary saccades by having the patient move the eyes back and forth from a visible target displayed in straight-ahead gaze to one displayed in the peripheral field. Normally saccades should begin within 250 msec. A undershoot of 10% of the amplitude of a centrifugal saccade and an overshoot of 10% of a centripetal saccade are normal but should disappear after four or five repetitions.

The third step is to elicit involuntary saccades by rotating optokinetic stripes (right, left, up, down) and comparing the amplitude and velocity of the quick phases.

PURSUIT SUBSYSTEM

The pursuit subsystem tracks an object moving in a plane equidistant from both eyes. Pursuit is a vision-dependent slow conjugate eye movement always under voluntary cerebral control.

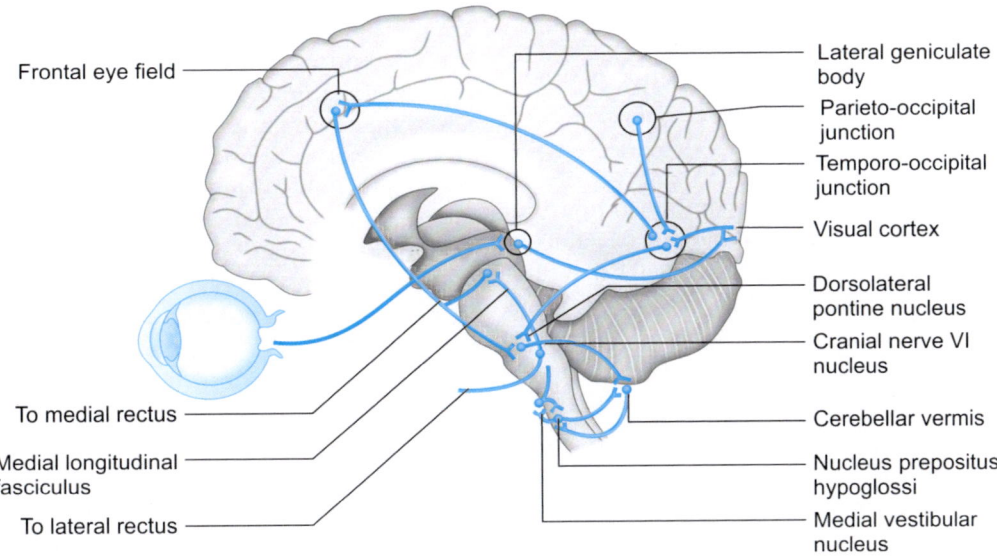

FIG. 3: Control of horizontal pursuit. Cerebral control is dependent on visual input and involves primarily the posterior hemisphere. However, a frontal lobe center contributes. Signals pass through the brainstem and cerebellum to reach the cranial nerve VI nucleus but do not synapse in the pontine paramedian reticular formation. Vertical pursuit pathways are less well known.

Anatomy (Fig. 3)

The anatomy of the pursuit pathway is less well understood than for saccades. Two major differences are:
- Hemisphere control is ipsilateral
- The PPRF and riMLF burst centers are not involved.

Visual cortex input projects to the temporo-occipital region, where attentional centers in the posterior parietal and superior temporal cortex make important contributions. An important output is to frontal eye fields. Descending signals from frontal and temporo-occipital centers go through internal capsule and pulvinar, respectively, to the ipsilateral dorsolateral pontine nucleus. They then travel to the cerebellar vermis, NPH, MVN, and then for horizontal pursuit movements, to the cranial nerve VI nucleus. To initiate vertical pursuit movements, signals travel to the INC through certain ascending pathways in the brainstem tegmentum including the MLF.

Testing for Pursuit Dysfunction

Pursuit is measured most precisely in the laboratory but can be practically assessed by having the patient follow a light moving at 40°/sec or slower. Movement of optokinetic stripes assesses pursuit as the initial phase of the evoked nystagmus.

VERGENCE SUBSYSTEM

The vergence subsystem is designed to keep the foveae on track as an object moves closer or further away. Unlike the saccadic and pursuit systems, which use conjugate eye movements (versions), the vergence subsystem uses disconjugate movements that move the eyes toward each other (convergence) or apart (divergence).

Anatomy

Vergence eye movements are generated bi-hemispherically in the parieto-occipital regions and prefrontal regions. Two types of visual conditions stimulate parieto-occipital regions: (i) Image blur or loss of image sharpness, and (ii) Image disparity, or images of a viewed object falling on noncorresponding retinal areas.

Image blur evokes accommodation, convergence, and miosis (the near triad), whereas image disparity evokes only convergence.

The parieto-occipital and frontal centers project to the midbrain reticular formation, where burst and tonic cells fire in relation to convergence, divergence, and accommodation. Signals travel from the convergence neurons to the medial rectus subnuclei and from the accommodation neurons to the Edinger–Westphal subnuclei.

Testing for Vergence Dysfunction

Vergence function is assessed by comparing ocular alignment in two gaze conditions: Fixing on a discrete symbol at far distance (ideally 20 ft or 6 m), and on symbols placed at reading distance (14 inches or 1/3 m).

VESTIBULAR SUBSYSTEM

The vestibular subsystem maintains posture and keeps the foveae on the viewed target when the viewer's head or body moves laterally or rotationally. Unlike saccadic, pursuit, and vergence subsystems, the vestibular subsystem is entirely reflexive (involuntary) and confined to the brainstem. A short loop, fast reacting circuit, maintains the eyes constant in space by causing an eye movement equal and opposite to the head or body movement, the vestibulo-ocular reflex (VOR).

Anatomy (Fig. 4)

For horizontal vestibulo-ocular movements, the signal generated in horizontal semicircular canals travels to multiple vestibular nuclei. From there it goes to the contralateral cranial nerve VI nucleus and to the ipsilateral medial rectus subnucleus of cranial nerve III through the MLF. An important side loop connects this pathway to the medullocerebellar neural integrator that all eye movement subsystems use to maintain eccentric gaze.

Damage to one side of the horizontal vestibular pathway creates a unilateral bias, so that the eyes are driven towards the involved side. The brainstem then generates quick phases in the opposite direction, in an attempt to bring the eyes back to the orbital center. This sets up a jerk nystagmus beating away from the side of lesion. If the damage is in the labyrinth or vestibular nerve, the brainstem compensates within days and the nystagmus disappears. No such compensation occurs with unilateral vestibular pathway lesions within the brainstem.

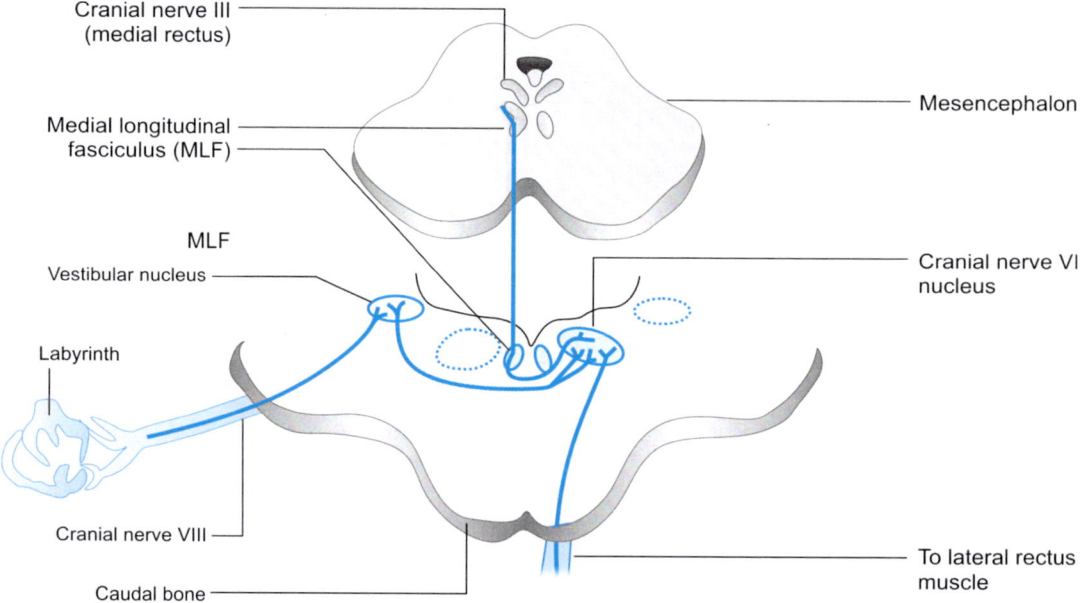

FIG. 4: Control of horizontal vestibulo-ocular movement. This pathway is wholly restricted in the brainstem but does not synapse at PPRF. Vertical vestibulo-ocular pathways travel from vestibular nuclei to midbrain through uncertain pathways.

Equal damage to both labyrinths and vestibular nerves does not create a vestibular tone imbalance, so nystagmus does not occur. However, the VOR is lost, so that quick head or body movements are not compensated by opposing eye movements. As a result even small head or eye movements produce the sensation that viewed objects are moving and blurred (oscillopsia).

Vertical and torsional vestibular eye movements have two separate pathways: (i) Upgaze and contralateral torsion —anterior semicircular canal to superior vestibular nucleus; from there to ipsilateral superior rectus and contralateral inferior oblique subnuclei of cranial nerve III via brachium conjunctivum; and (ii) downgaze and ipsilateral torsion: posterior semicircular canal to medial vestibular nucleus; from there to ipsilateral cranial nerve IV nucleus and contralateral inferior rectus subnucleus of cranial nerve III via uncertain pathways. To maintain the position of the eyes after vestibular stimulation, all vertical vestibulo-ocular signals eventually pass through the INC.

Testing for Vestibular Dysfunction

Vestibular dysfunction is assessed by looking for nystagmus, measuring ocular alignment and testing for deficits in the VOR. The VOR is assessed by the oculocephalic maneuver, the head-shaking test, and the caloric test.

The oculocephalic maneuver is used to assess the VOR in unconscious patients and in awake patients with very reduced excursions of the eyes. In an unconscious patient, eye movements directed opposite to passive head movements indicates that the VOR pathway from medulla to pons or midbrain is intact. In an awake patient who has limited or absent volitional eye movements, the head is turned in the horizontal and vertical planes and the patient is instructed to look straight ahead. The examiner makes notes whether the reflex ocular excursions are greater than the volitional excursions. When the reflex excursions are greater, the lesion causing the gaze disturbance must lie rostral to the midbrain in the diencephalon or cerebral hemispheres bilaterally (supranuclear gaze paresis).

The head-shaking (dynamic) visual acuity test is used to assess the VOR in awake patients who have full-range eye movements. Patients are asked to identify the smallest line possible on the Snellen's near card and then shake head quickly (>1 cycle/s) and read the same line backward. If acuity drops by at least two lines, the VOR is bilaterally deficient. Lesions may lie in the labyrinths, vestibular nerves, or brainstem vestibular pathways.

The caloric test uses thermal convection currents to stimulate the semicircular canals. The supine patient's neck is flexed 30° to place the horizontal canals in the vertical plane. Having ascertained that the tympanic membrane is intact, the right external auditory canal is irrigated with 10–50 mL of ice water. A normal response in an awake patient, occurring within minutes, is an ipsilateral slow conjugate deviation, followed by contralateral quick phases, setting up nystagmus. In a comatose patient, the quick phases are absent, because the PPRF is nonfunctional. Failure of eye deviation suggests disruption of the ipsilateral VOR. The same procedure is repeated on the left side, after a 5 minutes pause to allow dissipation of the caloric effect on the right. To test integrity of downgaze, ice water is instilled in both ears simultaneously; to test upgaze warm water is instilled in both ears.

GAZE DISTURBANCES

Gaze disturbances are usually caused by central nervous system lesions. Less commonly they result from lesions of the peripheral nerves, neuromuscular junction, and extraocular muscles. These conditions usually do not produce binocularly symmetric loss of eye movements and the eyes are misaligned in certain fields of gaze. So the patient may complain of diplopia. In contrast, diplopia is rarely a clinical feature of supranuclear disorders, which affect the movement of both eyes equally.

As already mentioned, two major types of gaze disturbances are: (i) Gaze deviations: Displacement of the eyes into the extremes of the orbit, and (ii) Gaze deficits: Abnormalities in the latency of initiation, speed, amplitude, or accuracy of conjugate eye movements.

In general, gaze deviations are manifestation of acute and often massive brain damage. Gaze deficits are less severe disorders of gaze and are apparent with subacute or chronic lesions and often signify quite discrete involvement of eye movement pathways. The diagnosis of gaze deficits requires systematic examination of saccades and pursuit eye movements.

The approach to gaze deviations and gaze deficits revolves around two questions:

1. **Is the VOR intact?**

If the VOR is intact, the gaze disturbance is called "supranuclear". Focal lesions that cause supranuclear vertical gaze disturbances lie rostral to the midbrain. By contrast, focal lesions responsible for horizontal gaze disturbances lie rostral to the pons. A supranuclear gaze disturbance need not be the result of a focal process. It may be caused by a diffuse or multifocal process that spares the VOR because this pathway is phylogenetically older and more robust than the saccadic and pursuit pathways.

2. **If the VOR is impaired, is the gaze disturbance in the horizontal or the vertical plane?**

Horizontal disturbances with VOR impairment suggest a pontine lesion; vertical disturbances suggest a midbrain lesion. Gaze disturbances limited to one plane with VOR impairment may also be caused by conditions that affect the ocular motor nerves, myoneural junction, and extraocular muscles.

Horizontal Gaze Deviations

If the VOR is preserved, the lesion lies in the cerebrum or diencephalons; if the VOR is not preserved, lesion lies in the pons.

Vestibulo-ocular Reflex Preserved

The important causes are:
- Acute unilateral cerebral hemispheric lesion
- Partial seizure
- Unilateral thalamic lesion.

Conjugate displacement of the eyes to one side is a common manifestation of an acute unilateral cerebral hemispherical lesion. Usually a hemorrhage or an infarct, it lies most commonly in the parietal region, subcortical white matter or internal capsule, more often on the right than on the left. The eyes are deviated towards the side of the lesion, away from the contralateral hemiparesis. The head is typically deviated in the same direction as the eyes. The eyes can usually be driven across the midline with caloric stimuli, but not as consistently with the less potent oculocephalic (doll's eye) maneuver. The larger the lesion, the more persistent is the deviation. However, in most cases the deviation lessens within a week so that the eyes move across the midline with volitional as well as with reflex eye movements.

Episodic horizontal eye deviation can be a sign of a partial seizure, usually originating in the contralateral cerebral cortex. Typically, the patient's head is deviated in the same direction as the eyes, and a jerk nystagmus in the same direction is often present. When the seizure ends, the eyes often briefly deviate toward the opposite side (Ocular Todd's paralysis).

Horizontal conjugate eye deviation may rarely result from a unilateral thalamic lesion, particularly a hemorrhage. The eyes may deviate either toward or away from the side of the lesion. Looking towards the side of the lesion can be explained by interruption of cerebropontine pathways. Looking away from the side of the lesion is difficult to explain and has therefore been called "wrong-way eyes." Thalamic hemorrhages can also produce forced downward deviation of the eyes with convergence and miosis. This usually indicates extension of the hemorrhage in or compressing the midbrain.

Vestibulo-ocular Reflex Not Preserved

Horizontal gaze deviations in the absence of a VOR suggests a unilateral pontine lesion. The eyes always look away from the side of the lesion and toward the hemiparesis. Neither the oculocephalic nor caloric maneuvers move the eyes because the lesion invariably involves either the abducens nucleus or the PPRF, through which the VOR pathways pass without synapsing (fibers of passage).

Gaze deviations caused by pontine lesions are much less common than those caused by cerebral or thalamic lesions. Most pontine lesions cause a horizontal gaze deficit rather than a gaze deviation; that is, the eyes do not move toward the affected side, but they are not conjugately deviated toward the unaffected side.

Vertical Gaze Deviations

Acute vertical gaze deviations usually signify damage to the midbrain and the VOR is rarely intact.

Upgaze deviation is often reported as patients are about to faint and may be a sustained phenomenon after profound central nervous system (CNS) hypoxia or ischemia. The tegmental midbrain is likely a vascular watershed region sensitive to drops in blood pressure. Episodic upgaze is also a feature of oculogyric crisis, usually part of a dystonic reaction to phenothiazines, carbamazepine, or lithium. Tonic upgaze is sometimes a transient event. Finally, it may be a psychogenic manifestation.

Downgaze deviation usually reflects damage to the dorsal midbrain. It is a common sign of acute hydrocephalus (setting sun sign) being the result of compression by a dilated third ventricle, or in a thalamic lesion, usually a hemorrhage or infarction that causes mass effect on the subjacent dorsal midbrain. Chronic downward deviation of the eyes may also be caused by fibrotic contracture secondary to inflammatory extraocular myopathy (especially in Graves' disease). Other signs of orbitopathy are usually present, and the forced duction test is positive (*see* chapters 14 and 15).

Gaze Deficits

Gaze deficits may be classified according to:
- The type of ocular movement affected:
  - Saccadic paresis
  - Smooth pursuit paresis.
- The direction of gaze affected:
  - Both horizontal and vertical gaze (omnidirectional)
  - Primarily horizontal gaze
  - Primarily vertical gaze.

Saccadic Paresis

Paresis of saccades may be evident as delay in despatching them, undershooting the target (hypometria), or slowness of their trajectories.
- *Saccadic delay:* Saccades are dispatched about 200 msec after a visual stimulus. Saccadic delay in all directions can be a sign of cerebral cortical and basal ganglia involvement, in Alzheimer's disease and Parkinson's disease. Reflexive saccades to visual targets are delayed mainly contralateral to parietal lobe lesions. Prolonged saccadic latency is an obvious and fundamental defect in congenital ocular motor apraxia. Patients use head motion to dispatch coincident saccades. Combined motor programs for triggering eye and head movement serve to trigger saccades in ocular motor apraxia. This congenital disorder improves with maturation into adulthood.

  Patients with very delayed onset or very slow saccades also use head motion to shift gaze. Head thrusts are used to initiate saccades. If saccades are extremely slow, head movements are used to activate vestibular eye movements away from the intended gaze direction. Nystagmus fast phases in the direction of head motion aid refixation. If no fast phase occurs, the head thrusts overshoot the target until the eyes achieve fixation; the head then rotates back with fixation maintained until the eyes reach mid-position in the orbit.
- *Hypometric saccades:* Saccadic reflations usually consist of one or two steps. Refixations of three or more low amplitude steps are called multiple step hypometric saccades. They occur in some normal subjects after fatigue or in advanced age. They are conclusively abnormal if they predominate in one direction. Hypometric saccades occur contralateral to cerebral hemispheric damage and ipsilateral to cerebellar cortical lesions. Omnidirectional hypometric saccades accompany bilateral cerebral, basal ganglia, or cerebellar disease.
- *Lateropulsion of saccades:* It is a form of dysmetria that occurs after lateral medullary infarcts. It consists of a triad of: (i) Overshoot of ipsiversive saccades; (ii) Undershoot of contraversive saccades; (iii) Ipsiversive deviation of vertical saccades (vide infra).

  Slow saccades: Damage to excitatory burst neurons or their projections to the ocular motor nuclei, to inhibitory burst neurons, or to pause neurons causes slow saccades. Lesions of the PPRF severely reduce the peak velocities of ipsiversive saccades. Slow saccades are a feature of focal lesions in the pontine tegmentum such as infarcts, tumors, and of degenerations such as progressive supranuclear palsy (PSP), Huntington's disease and variants of spinocerebellar degeneration, multiple sclerosis, lipid storage diseases or infections, e.g., AIDS, Whipple disease, involving the pontine tegmentum (vide infra).

Smooth Pursuit Paresis

When smooth eye movements fail to match the speed of a slowly moving target, catch-up saccades compensate for the low velocity (if smooth tracking, saccadic pursuit is the sign of paresis in smooth pursuit system).

- *Unidirectional pursuit paresis:* Saccadic pursuit occurs (toward the side of posterior parietal and parieto-temporal lobe lesions, particularly involving the angular gyrus and prestriate cortical Brodmann areas 19, 37, and 39 at the temporal–occipital–parietal junction. Frontal lobe lesions may also cause ipsiversive pursuit paresis. The ipsiversive pursuit defects caused by damage to either of two distinct cerebral regions, angular gyrus and dorsolateral frontal lobe, imply parallel routes through which cortical pursuit commands are conveyed to the brainstem.

  Ipsiversive saccadic pursuit also occurs toward the side of lesions that involve the cerebellar flocculus. In contrast to unilateral lesion in the cerebral hemisphere, vestibulocerebellum or rostral pons, unilateral tegmental damage in the caudal pons and vestral medulla impairs contraversive smooth pursuit. Greater paresis of contraversive pursuit after pontomedullary damage may signify disruption of excitatory projections from the vestibular nucleus to the contralateral abducens nucleus, or damage to projections to the cerebellar vermis.

- *Omnidirectional pursuit paresis:* Saccadic pursuit in all directions results from diffuse cerebral, cerebellar or brainstem disease. Multiple sclerosis, Parkinson's disease, Alzheimer's disease and cerebellar degenerations may cause lower smooth pursuit speed, resulting in saccadic tracking of slowly moving targets. Advanced age, sedative drugs, fatigue and inattention also lower smooth pursuit velocities in all directions and thereby cause saccadic tracking.

Horizontal Gaze Deficits

Selective impairment of horizontal gaze usually implies disease of the pons, although a cerebral disorder is sometimes the cause.

The VOR preserved: Important causes are:

- Acute unilateral cerebral lesion
- Congenital ocular motor apraxia.

Acute unilateral cerebral lesions (infarcts, hemorrhages, trauma) in parietal or frontal regions can produce a deficit in contralateral horizontal saccades and pursuit. At outset, an ipsilateral horizontal gaze deviation is often present. Within days, the gaze deviation typically disappears, but voluntary eye movements toward the opposite side remain impaired, pursuit recovers faster than saccades, which may remain hypometric.

The VOR impaired: Important causes are:

- Pontine lesion
- Wernicke's encephalopathy
- Other CNS disorders: Tay–Sachs disease, Maple syrup urine disease, advanced PSP, vitamin E deficiency, Leigh's disease, hepatic encephalopathy, drug overdose (phenytoin, carbamazepine, lithium)
- Mobius syndrome
- Peripheral nervous system disorders.

When voluntary and vestibular eye movements are impaired, the likely CNS cause is a pontine lesion.

Unilateral pontine lesions (infarct, hemorrhage, tumor, demyelination, infection, myelinolysis, and thiamine deficiency) compromise all ipsilateral versional eye movements. In the acute phase, the eyes may be contralaterally deviated. Convergence remains intact, as it is mediated by the midbrain. Because the MLF is so close, an ipsilateral internuclear ophthalmoplegia (INO) often accompanies the gaze palsy. This combination is called a "one-and-a-half syndrome", the "one" referring to the gaze palsy, the "half" to the INO.

Bilateral pontine lesions impair voluntary and reflex horizontal versional eye movements in both directions sparing convergence and vertical eye movements. Considerations include toxic, metabolic and degenerative CNS diseases.

A congenital CNS cause of horizontal gaze deficit is Mobius syndrome, an aplasia of the cranial nerve VI nuclei. Patients often have facial diplegia caused by aplasia of cranial nerve VII, and tongue atrophy with fasciculations caused by aplasia of cranial nerve XII nuclei.

Non-CNS causes of horizontal gaze impairment with loss of VOR include Fisher's syndrome, Botulism, myasthenia gravis, and dystrophic and inflammatory extraocular myopathies.

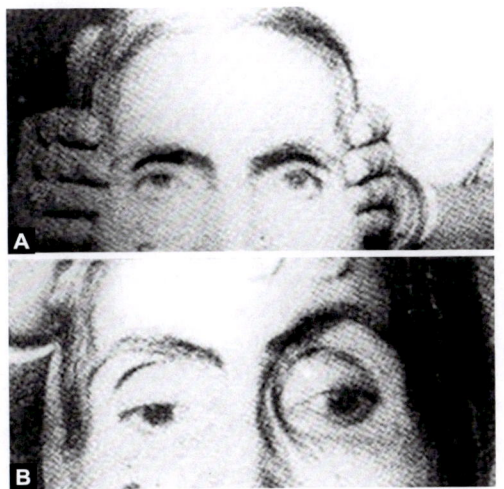

FIG. 5: Illustration showing upgaze **A,** and downgaze; **B,** restriction in a patient with progressive supranuclear palsy.

Vertical Gaze Deficits (Fig. 5)

Selective impairment of vertical gaze implies a lesion of the thalamus, midbrain, or vertically acting extraocular muscles.

The VOR preserved: Important causes are:
- Thalamic lesion
- Progressive supranuclear palsy.

The most common acute cause of supranuclear vertical ophthalmoplegia is a thalamic lesion, typically a medial infarction, occurring as a part of the "top of the basilar" syndrome. Other causes of acute thalamic lesion are hemorrhage, encephalitis, and hydrocephalus.

The most common chronic cause of supranuclear vertical ophthalmoplegia is PSP. Although, downgaze is often more involved than upgaze, the reverse pattern may occur. The nonstructural disorders to consider are Whipple's disease, Creutzfeldt–Jakob disease, Wilson's disease, kernicterus, Niemann–Pick disease type C, and Gaucher's disease.

VOR impaired: Important causes are:
- Midbrain lesion—thalamic lesion
- Pineal lesion—hydrocephalus
- Peripheral nervous system disorders.

Vertical gaze palsy that fails to preserve the VOR is usually attributable to an intrinsic midbrain lesion (stroke, tumor, demyelination). However, external compression by a large thalamic or pineal lesion, or a dilated third ventricle in hydrocephalus must also be considered.

When the lesion damages the dorsal (tectal, posterior commissural, collicular) midbrain, upgaze is often selectively impaired. Often called Parinaud's syndrome, its other neuro-ophthalmologic abnormalities include pupils that fail to constrict to light but do constrict in response to a near target (light-near dissociation), bilateral lid retraction (Collier's sign), convergence-retraction nystagmus, skew deviation, cranial nerve IV palsy, and convergence misalignment. A more ventral midbrain lesion often selectively impairs downgaze; pupils are large and do not constrict in response to light or a near target.

Vertical gaze deficits may also be caused by peripheral disorders, especially myasthenia gravis and inflammatory extraocular myopathy.

Omnidirectional Gaze Deficits

Impairment of conjugate eye movements in all directions may be the result of cerebral or brainstem disorders, but cranial nerve, neuromuscular junction, or extraocular muscle dysfunction can also produce it.

The VOR preserved: Important causes are:
- Bilateral cerebral lesions
- Thalamic lesion
- Progressive supranuclear palsy.

Acute omnidirectional supranuclear gaze deficits follow bilateral cerebral lesions affecting the parieto-occipital and frontal regions, which generate pursuit and saccadic eye movements. The most common cause of such a bilateral cerebral gaze disorder is severe hypotension or hypoxia. Unless the damage has been severe, the deficit usually resolves within weeks. Less common causes are bilateral middle cerebral artery thromboembolic stroke, cerebral venous sinus thrombosis, and infectious, neoplastic, demyelinating, hypertensive, metabolic, and toxic encephalopathies. A second cause for an acute supranuclear omnidirectional ophthalmoplegia is a thalamic lesion, including infarction, hemorrhage, tumor or demyelination.

The most common cause of chronic supranuclear ophthalmoplegia is PSP. Other chronic causes include spinocerebellar ataxia type 7, ataxia-telangiectasia, Whipple's disease, Creutzfeldt–Jakob disease, Niemann–Pick disease type C, and Gaucher's disease types 2 and 3.

The VOR impaired: Important causes are:
- Bilateral midbrain and pontine lesion
- Wernicke's encephalopathy
- Other CNS disorders (as in horizontal gaze deficits)
- Peripheral nervous system disorders.

NONCONJUGATE SUPRANUCLEAR EYE MOVEMENT DISORDERS

As a general principle, supranuclear eye movement disorders affect conjugate eye movements, i.e., movements of both eyes are affected equally, and so diplopia is rare. The exception to this is a small group of nonconjugate supranuclear eye movement disorders in which diplopia is a common symptom. These include:
- Internuclear ophthalmoplegia
- Skew deviation
- One-and-a-half syndrome
- Midbrain convergence with dorsal midbrain syndrome
- Supranuclear paralysis of monocular elevation (Lessell 1975).

Internuclear ophthalmoplegias and one-and-a-half syndrome have been discussed elsewhere in this volume (*see* Chapter 14).

Skew Deviation (Fig. 6)

Skew deviation is a vertical misalignment of the eyes which can be concomitant (hypertropia or higher eye the same in all positions of gaze), or can have varying degrees hypertropia or even crossed hypertropia (e.g., right eye higher on right gaze, left eye higher on left gaze). Skew deviation occurs with a variety of brainstem and cerebellar lesions, most commonly infarction, but also hemorrhage, demyelination or tumor and occasionally raised intracranial pressure due to supratentorial tumors or idiopathic intracranial hypertension. Pontine lesions are the most common site of origin, but medulla, cerebellum, and midbrain lesions are also well described. The supranuclear origin of skew deviation is important to recognize clinically, since it is often misdiagnosed as a peripheral ocular motor nerve or muscle lesion affecting vertical eye movements.

Skew deviation is thought to arise from impairment to or imbalance of otolith inputs, which ascend via the MLF to the ocular motor nuclei. In medullary (Wallenberg's lateral medullary syndrome) or pontine lesions affecting the vestibular nuclei, the lesion is usually on the side of the lower (hypotropic) eye. Unilateral internuclear ophthalmoplegias are also commonly associated with a skew deviation, reflecting concurrent damage to the otolith inputs that are ascending, in the lesioned MLF. With unilateral internuclear ophthalmoplegia, the higher (hypertropic) eye is usually ipsilateral to the lesion. With cerebellar lesions crossed (alternating) skew deviation can occur, with the abducting eye hypertropic. The association of downbeat nystagmus and skew deviation suggests a lesion of the cerebellar flocculus.

Lesions of the midbrain, in or around the region of the INC, commonly cause skew deviation, also with ipsilateral hypertropia, and often accompanied by an ocular tilt reaction. Rarely, periodic alternating skew deviation occurs, usually indicating a midbrain lesion. In general, skew deviation is a relatively transient phenomenon, with acute onset and lasting 4–6 weeks before resolving. Chronic and persistent skew deviation suggests that concomitant cerebellar damage may be present, with impaired compensation for the acquired otolith imbalance.

In neuro-otological practice, a patient with a head tilt along with a skew deviation, the differential would lie between all the central pathologies mentioned above and a simple isolated trochlear palsy in the eye opposite to the head tilt. Such a patient would complain of a vertical diplopia, whereas one with a central cause would feel the environment to be tilted. An alternate cover test would cause reversal of the direction of the skewed eyes. This phenomenon is called ocular counter-roll. The combination of head tilt, skew deviation and ocular counter-roll is called ocular tilt reaction and generally indicates a central lesion affecting central utricular pathway. This is illustrated in Fig. 6.

It would perhaps be appropriate here to mention briefly about the striking eye movement disorders seen in some patients with lateral medullary syndrome (Wallenberg).

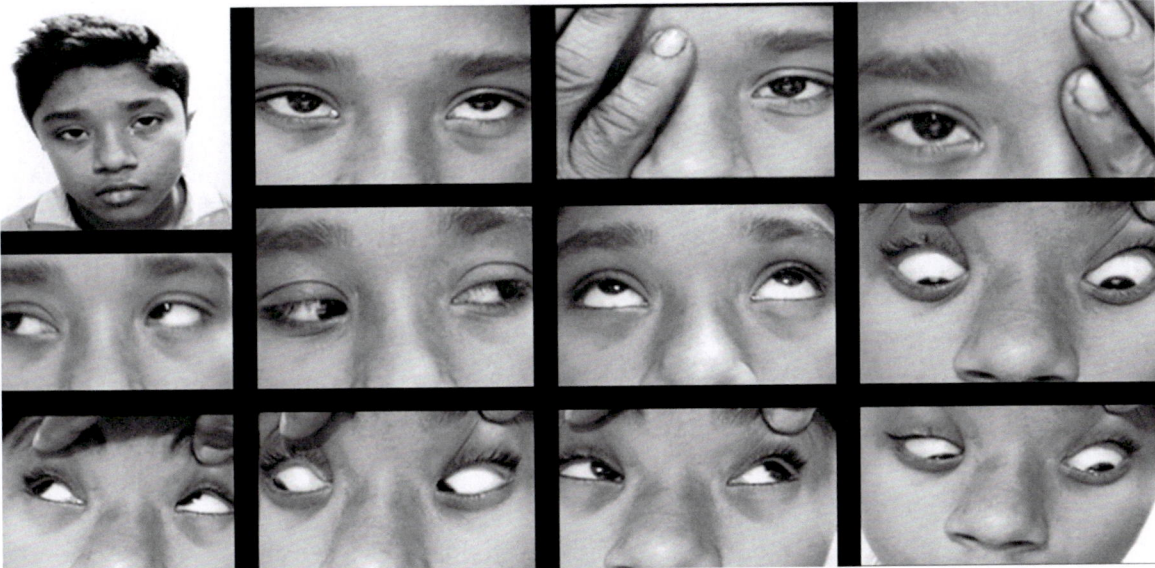

FIG. 6: A 12-year-old boy with head tilt to right for 2 months. He had no double vision. But complained of the surrounding environment to be tilted, to correct it, he adopted the right head tilt. A closer look at him revealed a skew deviation with the right eye at a lower position compared to the left (Ocular tilt). This eye position reversed when his eyes were covered alternately (Ocular counter-roll). Eye movements in all directions were full and there had been no abnormal torsional movement of the left eye on looking down in the adducted position; thus excluding a left trochlear palsy. This combination of head tilt, skew deviation, ocular tilt and ocular counter-roll on alternate cover test is called ocular tilt reaction (OTR). Interestingly, the tilt disappeared on making the boy lie flat on bed. There was no environmental tilt either, confirming the diagnosis of OTR. No cause for this occurrence could be found. *(For color version, see Plate 2)*

Lateropulsion of saccades is a form of dysmetria that occurs after lateral medullary infarcts, a phenomenon we call ipsipulsion in order to specify the direction of saccadic dysmetria relative to the side of the lesion. It consists of a triad of: (i) Overshoot of ipsiversive saccades, (ii) Undershoot of contraversive saccades, and (iii) Ipsiversive deviation of vertical saccades. Lesions of the superior cerebellar peduncle and uncinate fasciculus causes contrapulsion, which is the triad of overshoot of contraversive saccades, undershoot of ipsiversive saccades, and contraversive deviation of vertical saccades. Ipsipulsion may arise from, damage to projections from the inferior olivary nucleus through the inferior cerebellar peduncle to the dorsal vermis; this in turn inhibits the ipsilateral fastigial nucleus, which modulates the accuracy of saccades. Damage to the fastigial nucleus itself might cause ipsipulsion but the typical cause is lateral medullary infarction. Contrapulsion of saccades can be explained by disruption of the uncinate fasciculus as it passes around the superior cerebellar peduncle, conveying projections from the contralateral fastigial nucleus to the PPRE. A medial medullary lesion may also cause contralateral pulsion (contrapulsion) by disrupting olivocerebellar projections before their decussation across the midline.

UTILITY OF VESTIBULO-OCULAR REFLEX TESTING IN VESTIBULAR DISORDERS

One of the major problems in the diagnosis of vestibular disorders is the assessment of patients presenting with an acute vestibular syndrome of which there are two major causes: Acute vestibular neuritis and a posterior circulation stroke presenting with acute onset of isolated vertigo. Neuroimaging may be negative in the early stage. The head impulse test (HIT) is an extremely useful test in such an emergency setting. The test actually checks the integrity of VOR.

The subject is asked to fixate straight ahead. The examiner holds the head with two hands and sharply turns the head to one side. With intact VOR the eyes deviate to the opposite side to the head turn. This is normal and designated as a "negative hit test." The same occurs with a central lesion like a stroke in the posterior circulation. However with a peripheral lesion like vestibular neuritis, the eyes first tend to deviate to side of the head turn and then make a quick corrective saccade and deviate to the opposite side. This is a "positive hit test." This test is claimed to be very sensitive and specific even if imaging is negative. Of course there are pitfalls. A brainstem lesion (central lesion) at the root entry zone of the vestibular nerve like an anterior cerebellar artery infarct or a multiple sclerosis plaque at the same site would reveal a "positive hit." In the former of course, vertigo would be associated with acute hearing loss. In addition vestibular neuritis affecting the inferior division of the nerve (rather uncommon) gives a negative result.

A more sensitive modification of the hit is "video HIT (vHIT)" where the head and eye movements are recorded electrographically simultaneously and the VOR gain is calculated. Normal VOR gain is zero. A value less than 1 indicates a positive hit.

EYE MOVEMENT IN COMA

Comatose patients do not make eye movements that depend on cortical visual or motor processing, and so voluntary saccades and smooth pursuit are absent. Three important aspects of the clinical examination in comatose patients are: (i) The resting position of the eyes, (ii) Spontaneous eye movements, and (iii) Reflexively induced eye movements.

Resting Position of the Eyes

Conjugate horizontal deviation of the eyes is common in coma. For lesions above the brainstem ocular motor decussation, which is between the midbrain and pons (e.g., midbrain, cerebral hemisphere), the eyes are usually directed ipsilesionally (away from the hemiparesis). Vestibular stimuli will usually drive the eyes across the midline. For lesions below the ocular motor decussation (e.g., pons) the eyes are usually directed contralaterally away from the lesion (towards the hemiparesis). Contralesional deviation is typical of pontine lesions, but can also occur with thalamic lesions or rarely with hemispheric lesions (wrong-way deviation).

Intermittent deviation of the eyes and head turning are usually due to seizure activity. At the onset of the seizure, gaze is usually deviated contralateral to the seizure focus, often followed by the eyes drifting back towards the midline and nystagmus quick phases returning them out contralaterally again. Toward the end of the seizure, gaze often drifts to the ipsilesional side and may be paretic.

Tonic downward deviation of the eyes, often accompanied by convergence, occurs typically with thalamic hemorrhages and with lesions of the dorsal midbrain.

Tonic upward deviation of the eyes is uncommon in coma, but may occur following hypoxic–ischemic damage. Downbeating nystagmus may subsequently develop. Tonic upward deviation also occurs with oculogyric crises caused by various drugs, especially neuroleptics. Tonic uninhibited elevation of the eyelids (eyes open coma) may occur in unconscious patients with ponto-mesencephalic damage.

Disconjugate deviations of the visual axes in coma suggest the presence of infranuclear cranial nerve palsies, skew deviation, phoria no longer compensated by visual fusion or restrictive orbital trauma. Clinical evaluation depends on determining the range of eye movements using head rotation (doll's head or oculocephalic maneuver) or caloric stimulation. Impaired abduction suggests sixth nerve lesion. Impaired adduction suggests either third nerve lesion or internuclear ophthalmoplegia. Vertical tropias are usually due to fourth nerve lesions or skew deviation.

Spontaneous Eye Movements

Slow conjugate or disconjugate roving eye movements are similar to those of light sleep (mild loss of consciousness) and imply that the brainstem gaze mechanisms are intact. Ocular bobbing consists of intermittent, usually conjugate rapid downward eye movements, followed by a slower return to primary position. Reflex horizontal eye movements are usually absent. Although ocular bobbing is commonly regarded as a classic sign of an intrinsic pontine lesion (especially hemorrhage), it also occurs with cerebellar lesions and metabolic as well as toxic encephalopathies. Repetitive vertical eye movements that contain convergent-divergent components suggest disease affecting the dorsal midbrain. Other variants of ocular bobbing have less localizing value, although patients with pontine lesions may show several variants of bobbing, suggesting a common underlying pathophysiology. Ping pong gaze consists of slow horizontal conjugate deviations of the eyes alternating every few seconds. It is usually a sign of bilateral hemispheric infarction, but may also occur with posterior fossa hemorrhages. Rapid monocular eye movements with horizontal, vertical, or torsional components can occur with coma and brainstem dysfunction.

Finally, preserved voluntary vertical eye movements and eye opening or closure are critical to recognize as one of the only indicators of the locked-in state. This syndrome typically occurs with pontine infarction and patients are conscious but quadriplegic, with variable loss of some or all horizontal reflex and voluntary eye movements. The presence of eyelid or vertical eye movements may be the only means by which the patient can communicate.

Reflex Eye Movements

In the unconscious patient these are elicited either by head rotation (doll's head maneuver) or by caloric stimulation. Pontine lesions may abolish horizontal reflex eye movements, but spare the vertical responses. Vertical eye movements may be impaired with lesions of the midbrain or with bilateral MLF lesions. If, reflex eye movements are intact in the unconscious patient then the brainstem is likely to be structurally intact. If reflex eye movements are abnormal or absent, the cause may be structural disease, profound metabolic coma, or drug intoxication.

OCULAR MOTOR ABNORMALITIES IN CEREBELLAR DISEASES

This topic merits some detailing especially because of its relevance to some unique Indian studies.

An important function of the cerebellum is to calibrate motor responses to maintain their accuracy in the setting of an ever-changing system and external environment. In the ocular motor system, this means to maintain the accuracy and dynamics of eye movements, to maintain binocular alignment, to maintain gaze stability when the head is still (fixation) and when the head is moving (vestibulo-ocular reflex), to compensate for changes in the visual environment (e.g., spectacles), and to compensate for orbital-position dependencies.

The importance of the cerebellum in the control of eye movements is evident in the variety of ocular motor abnormalities that are observed in patients with cerebellar lesions. In some cases, these eye movement disturbances have profound effects on vision. Patients may have diplopia from impaired ocular alignment. Oscillopsia, an illusion of back-and-forth movement of the visual environment, may occur at rest, due to spontaneous nystagmus, or when the head is moving, due to impairment of the VOR. Saccadic dysmetria may impair functions, such as reading, which require a rapid sequence of accurate scanning eye movements. In addition, abnormalities in eye movements are tied closely to balance and walking. For example, disturbances in the VOR that cause oscillopsia may also affect balance through impairment of the vestibulo-spinal reflexes.

To summarize, the important ocular motor abnormalities in cerebellar diseases include gaze holding—disturbance of which leads to nystagmus which may be of downbeat or gaze-evoked types. These are detailed in the chapter on ocular oscillations (Chapter 17).

Saccadic abnormalities: Both inaccurate (dysmetric) saccades and postsaccadic drift (glissades) occur.

Pursuit abnormalities: Pursuit has a "jerky" appearance, as saccades are substituted to compensate for inadequate smooth tracking. There is a corresponding impairment in the ability to cancel the VOR; nystagmus is seen when a patient attempts to follow a target that is moving with the head.

Disturbances of binocular control with ocular misalignment may also occur. There may be apparent divergence paralysis or an alternating skew deviation.

Structure-function relationship of these various ocular motor disorders to sites of cerebellar lesions have been attempted. These are too complex and often inadequately elucidated. Clearly detailing on these would be beyond the scope of a clinically oriented volume like the present one.

Two interesting ocular motor disorders described in Indian patients with autosomal dominant cerebellar ataxias (ADCA) deserve special mention.

Phenomenon of Slow-saccadic Movement (Fig. 7)

Wadia and Swami first drew attention to this unique ocular motor disorder in some Indian families with ADCA. Subsequent genetic studies established the diagnosis of spinocerebellar ataxias 2 (SCA2) genotype in some such families. The phenomenon has been adequately described by Wadia.

Careful examination revealed a slowing of the horizontal, fast, random, and command eye movements (saccades) without any limitation in their range. A staring look due to the absence of the small fixation saccades was noticed. As the slowing increased, the vertical movements were affected. Finally, the eyes could not be moved voluntarily through their full range, though the doll'seye maneuver and caloric stimulation drove them into the corners. There was no squint, ptosis, diplopia, pupillary abnormality, or nystagmus, optokinetic examination, caloric stimulation, and rotation in a Barany's chair produced an abnormal response. There was merely a conjugate deviation of the eyes or, early in the disease, a slight return oscillation of the eyeballs.

Accompanying the ocular disorder were compensatory head movements and blinking. The patient made an "obligatory" blink or small jerk of the head to initiate a saccade by breaking the heightened ocular fixation reflex. This was an early sign to which attention was sometimes drawn by an alert relative to indicate another affected member, with diminishing velocity a head–eye lag appeared when the patient attempted to look at a target. The head and neck were turned in advance of the eyes, which slowly followed to fixate on the target. Some patients moved the head away from the object of gaze to turn the eyes reflexly toward it.

The same phenomenon had been observed in SCA2 families from Cuba later on.

The phenomenon however is not characteristic of SCA2 genotype alone; this has been observed in patients with other genotypes as well, though the classical head–eye lag had not been encountered in genotypes other than SCA2. The offending lesion probably lies in the burst neurons of the PPRF.

Pursuit Abduction Lag Phenomenon (Fig. 8)

Chakravarty and later Chakravarty and Mukherjee drew attention to an interesting disorder of smooth horizontal tracking (pursuit) in a single asymptomatic member of a genetically proved SCA3 family. Many other affected members of the same family exhibited gross ophthalmoparesis. Although her ocular movements were full and not slowed during horizontal pursuit, a significant "lag" was observed always in the abducting eye. On a closer look at her other family members with gross ophthalmoparesis, the authors were impressed by the finding that the restriction of movement more often affected the abducting eye rather than the adducting eye. It was therefore felt that the "abduction lag" phenomenon is probably an early ocular motility

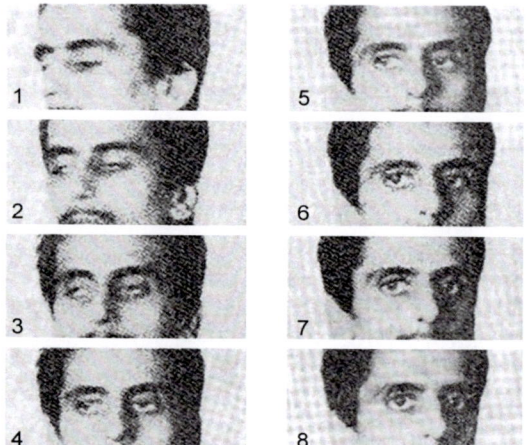

FIG. 7: Illustration of slow saccadic eye movement and head–eye lag in a patient with spinocerebellar degeneration. Patient was asked suddenly to look to the left at an observer. Note that in frames 1–4 he blinks to unfix the eyes. Also note that the face has turned much before the eyes (frames 5 and 6) which are seen to follow the head in the subsequent frames (7 and 8). Ocular movements are full.
Courtesy: Late Professor NH Wadia and Editor Brain

disorder that members of this family with SCA3 suffered from. With progression of the disease, more severe ophthalmoparesis supervened. (Fig. 9)

Again, this phenomenon of "abduction lag" does not appear to be unique to SCA3 families. We have observed this in SCAI genotype and also in some members of SCA families of undetermined genotype. Recently, one such patient has been seen to exhibit both a subtle degree of slow saccadic movement disorder (with obligatory eye blink) and a clear abduction lag phenomenon on horizontal tracking (pursuit).

It is possible that the site of lesion for this phenomenon also lies at or near the PPRF affecting fibers of passage causing either a slow relaxation of the medial rectus or hypofunction of the lateral rectus muscle in the abducting eye.

As mentioned earlier, varying degrees of ophthalmoparesis, progressing over time and culminating in a nearly fixed eyeball, may be seen in many patients with SCA2 and SCA3 genotypes. Judging by the observations of the authors made on Indian (especially, Eastern Indian) patients, they feel that genotype–phenotype correlation in relation to ocular motor abnormalities in patients with dominant ataxias is on the whole inconsistent. This view has been supported by Sinha et al. as well.

In Friedreich ataxia (FA), the prototype of early onset autosomal recessive ataxia, ocular motor abnormalities have been reported to be common. Ocular flutter and square-wave jerks are frequently

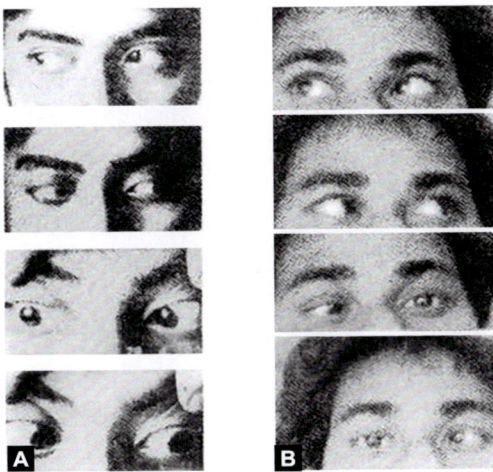

FIG. 8: Illustration of the phenomenon of **A,** abduction lag during slow tracking (pursuit) in an asymptomatic member of an SCA3 family. To note full ocular movement on saccade (upper two). Lag in abduction noted in the abducting eye on slow pursuit to right and left, respectively (lower two). **B,** Abduction lag during pursuit in an SCA1 patient. Full ocular Movements on saccade (upper two) but lag in abduction during slow pursuit in the abducting eye (lower two).

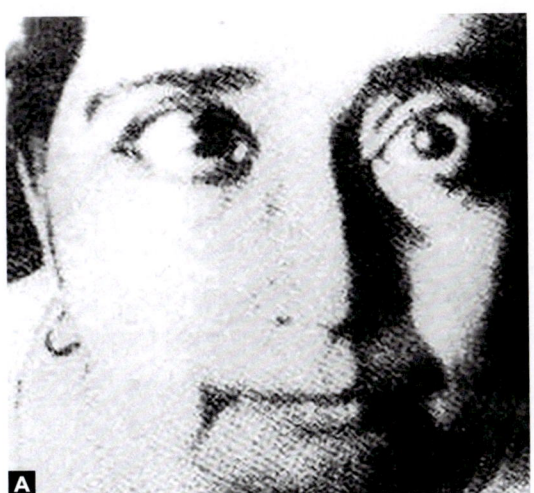
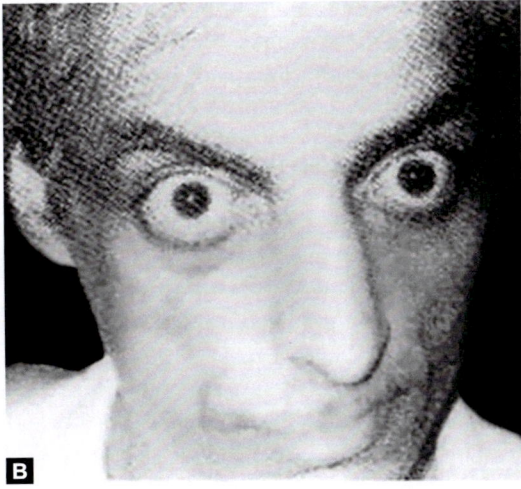

FIG. 9: Two members of an SCA3 family. Note bulging eyes and ophthalmoparesis.

seen, but ophthalmoparesis does not occur. In a relatively small series of Indian patients with early onset, autosomal recessive ataxias, Chakravarty and Mukherjee noted square-wave jerks in two patients and a slow saccadic movement in one case only. There is on the whole a dearth of literature on autosomal recessive ataxia from India.

Occasional cases of ataxia telangiectasia (AT) are encountered by neurologists in this country. Ataxia telangiectasia has nevertheless received great attention because of its association with cancer and DNA repair. It is a recessive disease caused by mutation in the ATM gene. The hallmark oculo-cutaneous-telangiectasia usually do not appear until age 4-6 years though truncal ataxia is noted in infancy. Later, oculomotor dyspraxia and coarse nystagmus become prominent.

Ataxia with oculomotor apraxia (AOA) and hypoalbuminemia. In some respects this autosomal recessive disorder clinically falls between FA and AT. European and Japanese scientists independently discovered the gene defect in AOA in 2001. Only as more cases are uncovered, will the full range of clinical features become clear, though there clearly is some heterogeneity. Nevertheless several generalizations already can be made. First, AOA is the most common recessive ataxia in Japan and likely the third most common recessive ataxia in Europe (after FA and AT). Second, it is characterized by cerebellar ataxia, oculomotor apraxia and in later stages, hypoalbuminemia and hypercholesterolemia. In addition, an axonal motor neuropathy is common and chorea may occur. Immune deficiency status (like in AT) and cerebellar atrophy (like in FA) do not occur. The AOA is caused by mutations in the *APTX* gene. The *APTX* encodes 'aprataxin' a new member of the histidine triad (HIT) protein subfamily and is presumed to be involved in DNA repair.

The present chapter ends with a series of boxes and tables (Boxes 1 to 11, table 1 and 2) to highlight major issues in supranuclear control of eye movements in health and disease discussed in this chapter. For proper understanding on this complex topic it is suggested that the present chapter and the following one (Chapter 17) on ocular oscillations be read together.

Box 1: Cortical control of saccades.

1. *Cortical areas PREPARING saccades*
- Dorsolateral prefrontal cortex
  - Inhibits unwanted saccades (Via superior colliculus)
  - Memorizes saccades sequences (Spatial working memory)
  - Elicits predictive saccades (Through frontal eye field)
- Posterior parietal cortex
  - Visuospatial integration/translation (Accuracy)
  - Visuospatial attention (Latency/neglect)
- Hippocampus/Anterior cingulate
  - Chronological order of sequence
  - Hierarchical prioritization

2. *Cortical areas TRIGGERING saccades*
- Frontal eye field
  - Intentional exploration of visual environment
  - Disengagement of attention
    - Triggering of retinotopic saccades
    - Visually guided
    - Antisaccades
    - Memory guided
    - Predictive
  - Amplitude of predictive retinotopic saccades
  - Not spontaneous saccades in darkness
- Supplementary eye field
  - Prepares motor programs
  - Chronologic aspects of saccade sequence
  - Not retinotopic saccades
- Parietal eye field
  - Reflexive exploration of visual environment
  - Directing visuospatial attention
  - Disengagement from fixation
  - Triggers reflexive visually guided saccades

Box 2: Effects of focal lesions on supranuclear eye movement control

1. *Frontal lesions*
   - Frontal eye field
     - Impaired triggering of different types of intentional saccades
     - Antisaccades: Delayed latency; increased error rate
     - Memory guided: Bilateral increased latency
     - Predictive: Decreased frequency/accuracy, increased latency
     - Decreased accuracy of all retinotopic saccades (Contra lesional >Ipsilesional)
   - Dorsolateral prefrontal cortex
     - Decreased suppression of reflexive saccades (Increased expresses saccades/gap effect)
     - Increased saccades distractibility/fixation losses
       - Saccades intrusions
       - Antisaccade errors/latency
     - Predictive saccades: Decreased frequency
     - Memory-guided saccades: Increased latency, decreased accuracy
   - Supplementary eye field
     - Memory-guided saccades: Impaired chronological sequencing
     - Nonvisual memory-guided saccades: Impaired accuracy

2. *Parietal lesions*
   - Impaired saccadic initiation (Increased latency contra lesional > Ipsilesional)
   - Impaired saccadic accuracy (Contralesional)
   - Impaired optokinetic nystagmus for stimuli towards lesion

3. *Temporo–occipito–parietal junction lesions*
   - "No notion for motion": Impaired ability to estimate speed of moving target within the affected visual field
   - Inaccurate saccades to moving targets in hemifield
   - Impaired initiation of smooth pursuit

4. *Thalamic lesions*
   - Wrong-way deviation (Conjugate away from lesion)
   - Forced downward deviation (± convergence)
   - Downward paralysis
   - Impaired contralateral visually guided saccades (Frequency, latency)

5. *Midbrain lesions*
   - Rostral interstitial nucleus of the medial longitudinal fasciculus
     - Burst neurons for vertical and torsional eye movements
     - Usually infarction in posterior thalamo-subthalamic paramedian artery territory
   - Unilateral
     - Loss of torsional movements
     - Loss of vertical saccades above primary position
     - Slow and limited saccades below primary position
   - Bilateral
     - Impaired downward saccades (?lateral lesion)
     - Loss of all vertical and torsional saccades (?medial lesion)
   - Posterior commissure
     - Loss of upward saccades
     - Dorsal midbrain syndrome (Parinaud's syndrome)
     - Ocular tilt reaction
     - Impaired vertical gaze holding
   - Supranuclear paralysis of monocular elevation
     - Failure of both elevators of one eye (Superior rectus and inferior oblique)
     - Eyes straight in primary position; disconjugate on upgaze
     - Lesion of prenuclear inputs to oculomotor nucleus

6. *Pontine lesions*
   - Horizontal gaze palsy (Ipsilateral)
   - Internuclear ophthalmoplegia
   - One-and-a-half syndrome
   - Slow saccades (Horizontal)

Box 3: Dorsal midbrain syndrome

1. Limitation of upward eye movements (Parinaud's syndrome)
   - Saccades
   - Smooth pursuit
     - Vestibulo-ocular reflex
     - Bell's phenomenon
2. Lid retraction (Collier's sign)
3. Disturbances of downward eye movements
   - Downward gaze preference (Setting-sun sign)
   - Downbeating nystagmus
   - Impaired downward saccades, smooth pursuit (VOR preserved)
4. Disturbances of vergence eye movements
   - Convergence-retraction nystagmus
   - Paralysis of convergence
   - Spasm of convergence
   - Paralysis of divergence
5. Fixation instability (Square-wave jerks)
6. Skew deviation
7. Pupillary abnormalities (Tight-near dissociation)

Box 4: Causes of slow saccades

- Olivopontocerebellar atrophy spinocerebellar degenerations
- Huntington's disease
- Progressive supranuclear palsy
- Whipple's disease
- Lipid storage diseases
- Wilson's disease
- Creutzfeldt–Jakob disease
- Drug intoxications: Anticonvulsants, benzodiazepines
- Tetanus
- Dementias: Alzheimer's disease, AIDS
- Lesions of the paramedian pontine reticular formation
- Internuclear ophthalmoplegia
- Peripheral nerve palsy, disease affecting the neuromuscular junction and extraocular muscle, restrictive ophthalmopathy

Box 5: Supranuclear eye movement abnormalities with acute hemispheric lesions

1. Unilateral lesion
   - Eyes commonly deviate TOWARDS lesion
     - Right > Left hemisphere
     - Parietal > Frontal lobe
   - Resolve within days–1 week
   - Vertical saccades may have oblique component TOWARDS lesion
   - Vestibulo-ocular reflex often intact (Cf. pontine lesion)
   - Bilateral ptosis and upgaze palsy with unilateral right hemispheric lesion.
2. Bilateral lesions (Frontal or parietal)
   - Acquired ocular motor apraxia
     - Loss of voluntary control of horizontal and vertical eye movements with preservation of reflex movements (e.g., VOR)
     - Head thrust/turn often initiates eye movements
     - If parietal, BALINT's syndrome—ocular motor apraxia plus optic ataxia and impaired visual attention/visual field
3. Epileptic seizures
   - Unilateral frontal focus: Eyes move AWAY (Contralesional)
   - Bilateral frontal focus: Eyes may move vertically
   - Parietal–occipito–temporal focus: Eyes move (Contralesional > Ipsilesional)

Box 6: Chronic effects of large unilateral lesions of the cerebral hemisphere

1. Fixation
   - In darkness, eyes drift away (Contralesional)
   - Ophthalmoscopy: Nystagmus quick phases towards lesion
   - Square-wave jerks
2. Saccades
   - Latency: Increased away (Contralesional)
   - Velocity: Decreased bidirectional (Contra lesional > Ipsilesional)
   - Accuracy: Hypometric/hypermetric into blind hemifield
3. Smooth pursuit
   - Reduced gain ipsilesional or bidirectional
4. Optokinetic
   - Reduced gain for stimuli moving ipsilesional
5. Forced eye closure
   - Conjugate deviation away/contralesional (Spasticity of conjugate gaze)

Box 7: Nonconjugate supranuclear eye movement disorders (Central diplopia)

- Internuclear ophthalmoplegia
- Skew deviation
- One-and-a-half syndrome
- Midbrain convergence/dorsal midbrain (Parinaud's) syndrome
- Supranuclear paralysis of monocular elevation.

Box 8: Gaze disturbances—peripheral causes

Acute
- Fisher's syndrome
- Botulism
- Myasthenia gravis

Chronic
- Myasthenia gravis
- Chronic progressive external ophthalmoplegia
- Oculopharyngeal dystrophy
- Myotonic dystrophy
- Inflammatory extraocular myopathy (including Graves disease)

Box 9: Metabolic disorders causing abnormal eye movements

1. Lipid storage diseases
   - Tay–Sachs
   - Adult-onset hexosaminidase A deficiency
   - Niemann–Pick variants
   - Gaucher's disease
2. Aminoacidurias
   - Maple syrup urine disease
   - Hyperglycinemia
3. Wernicke's encephalopathy
4. Leigh's disease
5. Abetalipoproteinemia
6. Wilson's disease
7. Kernicterus

Box 10: Disorders of vertical gaze—causes

1. *Tumor*
   (Especially pineal germinoma/teratoma in adolescent male)
2. *Hydrocephalus*
   (Especially aqueductal stenosis with third ventricle dilation/posterior commissure compression)
3. *Vascular*
   - Midbrain or thalamic hemorrhage/infarction
4. *Metabolic*
   Lipid storage disease (e.g., Niemann–Pick, Gaucher's, Tay–Sachs), maple syrup urine disease, Wilson's disease, kernicterus
5. *Drug-induced*
   E.g. barbiturates, carbamazepine, neuroleptic agents
6. *Degenerative*
   - Progressive supranuclear palsy
7. *Miscellaneous*
   - Multiple sclerosis
   - Whipple's disease
   - Hypoxia
   - Encephalitis
   - Syphilis
   - Basilar aneurysm
   - Trauma
   - Benign transient form of childhood

Box 11: Eye movement abnormalities in progressive neurodegenerative disorders

1. *Parkinson's disease*
   - Hypometric saccades
   - Simple visually guided saccades NORMAL
   - Smooth pursuit impaired (Especially pursuit initiation)
   - Antisaccades increased errors
2. *Progressive supranuclear palsy*
   - Sccades > Pursuit > VOR
   - Saccades
     - Vertical > Horizontal impairment
     - Decreasing velocity, then decreasing amplitude
     - Eventually saccades lost completely
   - Pursuit
     - Vertical > Horizontal impairment
     - Low gain, slow or no catch-up saccades (Tonic deviation)
     - Eventual limitation or loss excursion
   - Fixation
     - Impaired, frequent square-wave jerks
   - Bell's phenomenon absent
   - Apraxia of eyelid opening
   - Frontal lobe dysfunction
     - Increased antisaccade errors/latency
     - Increased express saccades (Gap paradigm)
   - Attentional deficits
     - Vertical plane > Horizontal
3. *Huntington's disease*
   - Voluntary saccade initiation impaired
     - Prolonged latency
     - Blink/head turn
   - Reflexive visual saccade latency normal
   - Saccade velocity slowed
     - Vertical and horzontal
   - Fixation instability
     - Saccadic distractibility
     - Antisaccade errors
4. *Alzheimer's disease*
   - Saccades
     - Increased latency (especially unpredictable targets)
     - Hypometric
     - Increased anticipatory saccades
     - (?) mild slowing of velocity
   - Fixation
     - Large amplitude saccadic intrusions
     - Poor suppression of reflexive saccades
     - Impaired antisaccade task (visual grasp reflex)
   - Smooth pursuit
     - Low gain; catch-up saccades
     - Saccadic intrusions
   - Balint's syndrome if prominent parietal involvement

Table 1: Eye movement characteristics in spinocerebellar ataxias (SCAs)

Abnormality	SCA1	SCA2	SCA3	SCA6	SCA7*	SCA15	SCA17	Friedreich ataxia
Increased square-wave jerks	–	–	+	(+)[‡]	–	ND	–	(+++)
Gaze-evoked nystagmus	+	–	++	(+++)	±	++	±	+
Positional downbeat nystagmus	–	–	–	(+++)	ND	ND	ND	ND
Impaired smooth pursuit	+	±	++	+++	–	++	(++)	++
Decreased saccade velocity	(++)	(+++)	±	–	(+++)	–	–	±
Hypermetric saccades	+	–	±	(++)[§]	–	±	±	+
Hypometric saccades	±	–	++	+	–	±	(++)	±
Supranuclear gaze palsy	±	±	++	–	(++)	ND	++	–
Hypoactive vestibulo-ocular reflex	+	–	++	±	–	(±)	–	(+++)
Hyperactive vestibulo-ocular reflex	–	–	–	+	–	–	(++)	–

Features in brackets are characteristics of the condition.
*With pigmentary retinopathy.
[‡]Square-wave jerks are synchronous with downbeat nystagmus.
[§]Prominent downwards deviation during horizontal saccades.
Abbreviations: –, not present; ±, present in some patients; +, mild; ++, moderate; +++, marked; ND, not determined; SCA, spinocerebellar ataxia.

Table 2: Spontaneous eye movements occurring in unconscious patients

Term	Description	Significance
Ocular bobbing	Rapid downward movement: Slow return to primary position	Structural (especially pons) lesions; metabolic or toxic encephalophathy
Reverse ocular bobbing	Rapid upward movement: Slow return to primary position	Unreliable for localization, e.g., Metabolic disorder
Ocular dipping (Inverse ocular bobbing)	Slow downward movement: Rapid return to primary position	Unreliable for localization, e.g., Hypoxia; ischemia; metabolic disorders
Reverse ocular dipping (Converse bobbing)	Slow upward movement: Rapid return to primary position	Unreliable for localization, e.g., Pontine infarction; AIDS
Vertical myoclonus	Vertical pendular oscillations (2–3 Hz)	Acute brainstem stroke
Ping-pong gaze	Slow, horizontal conjugate deviations of the eyes, alternating every few seconds	Bilateral cerebral hemisphere dysfunction

SUGGESTED READINGS

1. Averbuch-Heller L. Supranuclear control of ocular motility. Ophthalmol Clin N Am. 2001;14:187-204.
2. Barth A, Bogousslavsky J, Caplan LR. Thalamic infarcts and hemorrhages. In: Bogousslavsky J, Caplan LR, editor. Stroke Syndromes. Cambridge: Cambridge University Press; 1995. P. 276-83.
3. Borchert MS. Principles and techniques of the examination of ocular motility and alignment. In: Miller NR, Newman NJ, editor. Walsh & Hoyt's Clinical Neuro-ophthalmology, 5th ed. Vol 1. Baltimore: Williams & Wilkins; 1998. P. 1169-88.
4. Burk K, Fetter M, Abele M, et al. Autosomal dominant cerebellar ataxia type 1: Oculomotor abnormalities

in families with SCA-1, SCA-2, and SCA3. J Neurol. 1999;246:789-97.
5. Caplan IR, Han W. Pontine hemorrhages and infarcts. In: Bogousslavsky J, Caplan LR, editor. Stroke Syndromes. Cambridge: Cambridge University Press. 1995. p. 324-35.
6. Chakravarty A, Mukherjee SC. Autosomal dominant cerebellar ataxias in ethnic Bengalis in West Bengal—an Eastern Indian state. Acta Neurol Scand. 2002;105:202-8.
7. Chakravarty A, Mukherjee SC. Primary degenerative cerebellar ataxias in ethnic Bengalis from West Bengal. Neurol India. 2003;51:227-34.
8. Chakravarty A. Oculomotor abnormalities in a family with Machado Joseph Disease (Abstract) J Neural Sci. 1997;150:196.
9. Corbett JJ. Neuro-ophthalmological complications of hydrocephalus and shunting procedures. Semin Neurol. 1986;6:111-23.
10. Date H, Onodera O, Tanaxa H, et al. Early onset ataxia with ocular motor apraxia and hypoalbuminemia is caused by mutations in a new H9T superfamily gene. Nat Genet. 2001;29:184-8.
11. Fisher CM. Some neuro-ophthalmological observations. J Neurol Neurosurg Psychiatry. 1967;30:383-92.
12. Fletcher WA, Sharpe JA. Saccadic eye movements dysfunction in Alzheimer's disease. Ann Neurol. 1986;20:464-71.
13. Goodwin JA, Kansu T. Vulpian's sign: Conjugate eye deviation in acute cerebral hemisphere lesions. Neurology. 1986;36:711-2.
14. Guitton D, Buchtel HA, Douglas RM. Frontal lobe lesions in man cause difficulties in suppressing reflexive glances and in generating goal-directed saccades. Exp Brain Res. 1985:58:455-72.
15. Hoyt CS, Mousel DK. Transient supranuclear disturbances of gaze in healthy neonates. Am J Ophthalmol. 1980;89:708-13.
16. Keane JR. Sustained upgaze in coma. Ann Neurol. 1981;9:409-12.
17. Kommerell G, Hoyt WF. Lateropulsion of saccadic eye movements. Electro-oculographic studies in a patient with Wallenberg's syndrome. Arch Neurol. 1973;28:313-8.
18. Lasker AG, Zee DA, Hain TC, et al. Saccades in Huntington's disease: Initiation defects and distractibility Neurology. 1987;37:364-70.
19. Leigh R, Newman SA, Folstein SE, et al. Abnormal ocular motor control in Huntington's disease. Neurology. 1983;33:1268-75.
20. Leigh RF, Foley JM, Remler BE, et al. Oculogyric crisis: A syndrome of thought disorder and ocular deviation. Ann Neurol. 1987;22:13-7.
21. Leigh RJ, Zee DS. The Neurology of Eye Movements. 3rd ed. Philadelphia: FA Davis, 1999.
22. Mobius PJ. Ueber angeborone doppelseitige Abducens-FaciaKs-Lahmung. Munch Med Wschr 1888;35:91-4.
23. Moreira Me, Barbot C, Tachi N, et al. The gene mutated in ataxia-ocular apraxia 1 encodes the new H9T/Zn-finger protein aprataxin. Nat Genet. 2001;29:189-93.
24. Morrow MJ, Sharpe JA. Cerebral hemispheric localization of smooth pursuit asymmetry. Neurology. 1990;40:284-92.
25. Morrow MJ, Sharpe JA. Retinotopic and directional deficits of smooth pursuit initiation after posterior cerebral hemispheric lesions. Neurology. 1993;43:595-603.
26. Morrow MJ, Sharpe JA. Smooth Pursuit Eye Movements. In: Sharpe J, Barber HO, editor. The Vestibulo-ocular Reflex and Vertigo. New York: Raven Pressl; 1993. p. 141-62.
27. Orozco Diaz G, Nodarse Fleites A, Cordovez Sagaz R, et al. Autosomal dominant cerebellar ataxia-clinical analysis of 265 patients from a homogeneous population in Holguin. Cuba. Neurology. 1990;40:1369-75.
28. Ouvrier RA, Bill Son F. Benign paroxysmal tonic upgaze of childhood. J Child Neurol. 1988;3:177-88.
29. O'Sullivan EP, Shaunak S, Henderson L, et al. Abnormalities of predictive saccades in Parkinson's disease. Neuroreport. 1997;8(5):1209-13.
30. Pierrot-Deseilligny C, Rivaud S, Gaymard B, et al. Cortical control of saccades. Ann Neurol. 1995;37:557-67.
31. Pierrot-Deseilligny CH, Chain F, Gray F, et al. Parinaud's syndrome: Electro-oculographic and anatomical analyses of six vascular cases with deductions about vertical gaze organization in the premotor structures. Brain. 1982;105:667-96.
32. Sharpe JA, Sylvester TO. Effect of aging on horizontal smooth pursuit. Invest Ophthalmol Vis Sci. 1978;17:465-8.
33. Sharpe JA. Neurol control of ocular motor systems. In: Miller NR, Newman NJ, editor. Walsh & Hoyt's Clinical Neuro-ophthalmology. 5th ed. Vol I. Baltimore: Williams & Wilkins; 1998. P. 1101-68.
34. Shaunak S; O'Sullivan E, Kennard C. Eye movements. Journal of Neurology Neurosurgery and Psychiatry. 1995;59:115-25.
35. Sinha KK, Worth PF, Jha DK, et al. Autosomal dominant spinocerebellar ataxia: SCA2 is the most frequent mutation in Eastern India. Neurol Neurosurg Psychiat. 2004;75:484-52.
36. Sweeney JA, Mintun MA, Kwee S, et al. Positron emission tomography study of voluntary saccadic eye movements and spatial working memory. J Neurophysiol. 1996;75:454-68.
37. Tijseen CC. Contralateral conjugate eye deviation in acute supratentorial lesions. Stroke. l994;25:1516-9.
38. Tijssen CC, Van Gisbergeh JA, Schulte BR. Conjugate eye deviation: Side, site, and size of the hemispheric lesion. Neurology. 1991;41:846-50.
39. Towfighi J, Marks K, Palmer E, et al. Mobius syndrome: Neuropathologic observations. Acta Neuropathol. 1979;48:11-7.

40. Troost B, Weber RB, Daroff RB. Hypometric saccades. Am Ophthalmol. 1914;78:1002-05.
41. Troost BT, Baroff RB. The ocular motor defects in progressive supranuclear palsy. Ann Neurol. 1977;2:397-403.
42. Wadia NH, Peng J, Desai J, et al. A clinico-genetic analysis of six Indian spinocerebellar ataxia 2 (SCA2) pedigrees. The significance of slow saccades in diagnosis. Brain. 1998;21:2341-55.
43. Wadia NH, Swami RK. A mew form of heredofamilial spinocerebellar degeneration with slow eye movements (nine families). Brain. 1971;94:359-74.
44. Wadia NH. A common variety of hereditary ataxia in India. In: Lechitenberg R, editor. Handbook of Cerebellar diseases. New York. Marcel Dekkar Inc. 1993. p. 373-88.
45. Walker MF, Zee DS. Cerebellar control of gaze. In: Sharpe JA, editors. Neurol-ophthalmology at the Beginning of the New Millennium: Proceedings of the International Neuro-ophthalmology Society Meeting. Englewood, NJ. Medimond; 2000. p. 71-81.
46. White OB, Saint-Cyr JA, Tomlinson RD, et al. Ocular motor deficits in Parkinson's disease. II. Control of the Saccadic and Smooth Pursuit Systems. Brain. 1983;106:571-87.
47. Zackon DH, Sharpe JA. Smooth pursuit in senescence: Effects of target velocity and acceleration. Acta Otolaryngol. 1987;104:290-7.
48. Zee DS, Yee RD, Singer HS. Congenital ocular motor apraxia. Brain. 1977;100:581-99.

CHAPTER 17

Ocular Oscillations

Angshuman Mukherjee, Ambar Chakravarty

> "Never write on nystagmus, it will lead you nowhere"
>
> Willbrand, Contemporary Neuro-ophthalmologist (1953)

INTRODUCTION

Ocular oscillations are divided into three types: (i) nystagmus, in which a slow eye movement drift initiates the oscillation; (ii) saccadic disorders, in which a fast eye movement initiates the oscillation; (iii) bobbing and periodic horizontal deviations, in which slow, wide ocular oscillations occur in an unresponsive patient; the nature of the initiating eye movement is uncertain.

The most common type of ocular oscillation encountered in clinical practice is nystagmus.

There are other involuntary ocular oscillations which are not rhythmic and hence do not fit the definition of nystagmus. These include square wave jerks, ocular flutter, opsoclonus, ocular bobbing, ocular flutter and myokymia of superior oblique muscle.

Faced with a patient who has ocular oscillations, the clinician must try to answer three questions:
1. Is this nystagmus or an imitator (saccadic disorder, bobbing, periodic horizontal deviation)?
2. If it is nystagmus, is it physiologic or pathologic?
3. If the oscillation is pathologic, what is causing it?

NYSTAGMUS

Nystagmus is defined as failure of maintenance of ocular posture and characterized by involuntary rhythmic to-and-fro oscillatory movements of the eyes. Nystagmus mainly consists of sinusoidal slow to-and-fro oscillations (pendular nystagmus) or, more commonly, alternating slow drift and corrective quick movements (jerk nystagmus).

Over last over 2 decades research has provided a clearer understanding of pathophysiology and mechanisms of the most forms of nystagmus including other ocular oscillations. These to the clinical neurologist are of much importance for greater accuracy of nystagmus diagnosis and lesion localization.

However, to make proper use of these advances, it is important, therefore, to systematically examine eye movements and interpret the observations in relation to pathophysiology.

PATHOPHYSIOLOGY

Clear vision depends on holding the image steadily on to the central retina at the foveal part. Normally, three mechanisms are involved. Steady, so that our view of the surrounding is clear.

The first mechanism is the vertibulo-ocular reflex, by which the inner ear balancing mechanism (vestibular organ) make eye movements to effectively balance for movements made by the head, which occur during walking and other activities.

The next one is 'visual fixation', which has two divisions. One which detect movement of the image on the retina (drift) and another which make compensatory eye movements, and blocks unwanted eye movements which tend to move the eye away from the target.

The third mechanism working through a network of nerve cells tend to maintain the eyes at a fixed position (like, in lateral gaze).

Disordered function of any of these mechanisms may make the eyes to move away from the object of vision; corrective, fast movements (saccades) may then reposition the central fovea toward the object of visual fixation.

It should be noted that nystagmus is usually referred to by the direction of the quick phase, but it is the slow phase which points to the abnormality. Simply speaking, disordered neural mechanism at various levels may affect visual fixation and would cause a slow drift of the eye to one side (slow phase of nystagmus) but activation of central mechanisms at this stage, trying to restore continued visual fixation on a given target, would work through the elastic recoil of orbital structures to bring the eyes back quickly to the desired position (quick phase of nystagmus). These movements occurring in a repetitive manner would generate the to-and-fro movement called nystagmus. It is important to differentiate pathological nystagmus from physiological nystagmus. During rotation of the head and body in space, both vestibular nystagmus and optokinetic nystagmus act to reduce motion of images of the world on the retina, and so to preserve clear vision. During pathological nystagmus, however, drifts of the eyes away from the target degrade vision.

Nystagmus is best classified by its relationship to the dysfunction of the gaze-holding networks themselves in the brainstem and cerebellum, and their connections which bring informations and can become imbalanced (e.g., in the vestibular system). The principal nuclei for gaze-holding, which act as a neural integrator — are located in the medulla for horizontal gaze (the medial vestibular nuclei and the adjacent nucleus prepositus hypoglossi) and for vertical gaze in the midbrain (the interstitial nucleus of Cajal). The upper part of the vestibular nuclei probably also influence vertical gaze-holding through their connection, via the medial longitudinal fasciculus (MLF), to the interstitial nucleus of Cajal. The midline pons paramedian structures also contain neurons that are important for ocular motor integration. These integrators in the brainstem are connected to the cerebellar flocculus and paraflocculus (tonsils), which are the key cerebellar structures involved in the fine tuning of the integrators in the brainstem for optimum functioning.

APPROACH TO A PATIENT WITH NYSTAGMUS

Certain historical information is helpful in alerting the clinician to the presence and type of nystagmus. One should enquire about how long back the nystagmus was first noticed, whether it interferes with vision or causes oscillopsia (illusory motion of the visual world), and whether it is accompanied by other neurological symptoms like tinnitus, vertigo and nausea. In general, oscillopsia is a feature of acquired, not congenital nystagmus. Oscillopsia which is worse when the patient is in motion implies a vestibular disorder. Time of onset can be very helpful in diagnosis since a nystagmus present from birth or within the first few days of life in an otherwise healthy infant points to the diagnosis of congenital nystagmus. If on the other hand, the eye movement disorder developed weeks to several months after birth, an acquired cause should be sought - most frequently a condition resulting in poor vision.

A careful history should be obtained, including a history of similar ocular movements or visual loss in other family members. Present and past drug usage should be reviewed, including tranquilizers, antibiotics, and antiepileptic medications, as well as alcohol ingestion.

Before starting an evaluation of nystagmus, one should note any abnormality of head posture, examine the visual system (acuity, fields, color, stereopsis), optic nerves, lids, pupils, and look for signs of ocular albinism. Several congenital forms of nystagmus are associated with disorders of the visual system.

The nystagmus itself should be carefully observed in the cardinal eye positions for several minutes and notation made regarding the direction of fast components, the amplitude of movement and the rate. The basic type of nystagmus (pendular or jerk) present in primary position should be recorded. Clinically, pendular nystagmus is characterized by bilateral ocular oscillations that are approximately equal in velocity in both directions. The oscillations may vary in speed and amplitude but are almost always horizontal and often have a jerk component in eccentric gaze with the fast phase in the direction of gaze. Jerk nystagmus is characterized by rhythmic oscillations in which the movement in one direction is recognizably faster than the movement in the other direction. Although the slow movement in this situation is the pathologic movement and the fast movement is corrective, jerk nystagmus is still defined according to the direction of the fast phase or corrective movement. The position in which the intensity of ocular oscillations is minimum is referred to as the null point of the nystagmus and should be noted. The form taken by the nystagmus, that is horizontal, vertical, torsional or mixed in the different fields of gaze should also be recorded. The nystagmus in both the eyes should be compared and should be noted.

If the direction or amplitude of the oscillation differs, or if there is any asynchrony, or if the size of the movements differs in each eye, it is referred to as dissociated nystagmus. If the direction of the movements in each eye differs, it is referred to as disconjugate or disjunctive nystagmus. Each eye needs to be covered in turn to check for latent nystagmus.

Some nystagmus are transitory and require prolonged observation over several minutes. Nystagmus of low amplitude may only be detected during ophthalmoscopy. The effect on nystagmus of removing visual fixation should always be examined. Nystagmus due to peripheral vestibular imbalance may only be apparent when visual fixation is removed. The best way is to observe the nystagmus behind Frenzel glasses or M-glasses (high-positive lenses), which removes visual fixation and also provide the examiner with a magnified, view of the patients' eyes.

All functional classes of eye movements—saccades, smooth pursuit, and vergence should be systematically examined. It is also important to note the effects of each type of eye movement on the nystagmus, as well as effect of head shaking in the horizontal or vertical planes.

Head shaking nystagmus should be examined through Frenzel glasses. Placing the patient into head hanging positions may increase nystagmus due to benign positional vertigo.

It is possible to induce nystagmus in normal subjects with optokinetic stimuli like a moving striped drum or a moving tape measure and this will be discussed later.

To summarize, the points to note in nystagmus evaluation include:
- Direction: 'Right, left, up, down beating, rotatory, torsional
- Amplitude: The width of the swings
- Frequency: The number of oscillations per second
- Intensity: The product of amplitude and frequency
- Symmetry: Whether the waveform and intensity in the two eyes are the same
- Conjugacy: Whether the two eyes are moving in the same direction (conjugate) or opposite directions (disconjugate)
- Position of gaze, whether the nystagmus pattern varies with different ocular gaze positions. The gaze position in which the nystagmus is least obvious is termed the "nullpoint" or "null zone"
- Spontaneity: Whether the nystagmus is present under normal viewing conditions or must be induced by a particular maneuver (Frenzel lenses, head positioning, hyperventilation, tympanic membrane pressure, caloric irrigation, optokinetic drum).

CLINICAL TYPES OF NYSTAGMUS

Physiologic or Endpoint Nystagmus

- The most common physiologic form is the unsustained few beats of nystagmus seen at gaze deviations of 30 degrees or more
- Fatigue nystagmus usually develops after extended maintenance of an extreme gaze position. This variety has been found in up to 60% of normals when horizontal gaze is maximally deviated for a lime exceeding 30 seconds
- Sustained end-point nystagmus begins immediately or within several seconds after reaching an eccentric lateral gaze position and has been found in over 60 percent of normal subjects with horizontal gaze maintenance greater than 40 degrees. This sustained end-point nystagmus may be different in the two eyes, but it is symmetric in both lateral directions. The amplitude is less than 3 degrees.

To summarize, to qualify as physiologic, nystagmus must have the following six features:

- Present only in extremes of horizontal gaze. It appears only when the eyes reach a point where that portion of the sclera located on the side of gaze is no longer visible (30–40° eccentricity)
- Primary trajectory is horizontal and the fast phase beats in the direction of gaze. A torsional component may be present, but pure vertical nystagmus is never physiologic
- Unsustained; it rarely lasts more than three or four beats
- Low amplitude; it is barely visible without magnification (oscillation width <3°)
- Symmetric, both eyes display the same amplitude and waveform
- Unaccompanied by other pathologic neuro-ophthalmic phenomena.

Induced Nystagmus

Drug-induced Nystagmus

This may occur following ingestion of tranquilizers, barbiturates, phenothiazines, anticonvulsants, or alcohol. The nystagmus is usually not present in the primary position but gaze-evoked and horizontal or torsional in direction. Vertical nystagmus is often present in upgaze and only rarely in down gaze.

With severe intoxication, the nystagmus may be dissociated and may be present even in the primary position.

Optokinetic Nystagmus

Optokinetic nystagmus (OKN) is a combination of smooth pursuit and compensatory fast eye movement saccades to pick up fixation on the next target on a rotating OKN drum or a moving OKN tape. Such induced horizontal and vertical OKN is a normal physiologic finding but becomes abnormal when it is asymmetric; that is less OKN demonstrated when targets move in one direction compared to the other. For example, with an infarction of right posterior cerebral cortex that affects secondary visual areas concerned with motion processing, the response will be reduced as the stripes move to the patient's right (ipsilateral impaired smooth pursuit) and less corrective quick phases will be triggered - that is, there will be less nystagmus as the stripes move to the patient's right compared with moving to left. Normal OKNs also provide evidence of at least gross levels of visual function in infants or patients feigning visual loss. In evaluating eye movement disorders this nystagmus can be very helpful when the drum is rotated in the downward direction accentuating convergence–retraction nystagmus with dorsal midbrain lesions. In the clinic OKN may be elicited by moving a measuring tape in front of the eyes and in a subject complaining of loss of vision in both eyes, elicitation of this jerky eye movement is suggestive of psychogenic visual loss.

Caloric Nystagmus

Vestibular nystagmus can be induced by irrigating the external canal with old or warm water or air, which produces a convection current in the endolymph of the labyrinth. In clinical practice, the cold water (30°) caloric test is the most convenient. After checking that the tympanic membrane is intact, the patient's head is elevated 30 degrees to the horizontal plane, to place the lateral semicircular canal in a vertical position.

Ideally, eye movements should be recorded with a nystagmogram or observed with Frenzel glasses. A normal response, consisting of a nystagmus beating away from the stimulated ear, can be elicited with as little as 0.2 mL of cold water. Loss or reduction of caloric response indicates of loss of unilateral vestibular function or dysfunction. A useful mnemonic for remembering the direction of the induced nystagmus is COWS, standing for "cold opposite, warm same", reminding us that irrigation of cold water in the external canal will result in a jerk nystagmus beating away from the irrigated side. Cold irrigation depresses function of the ipsilateral labyrinth and its central connection to the contralateral vestibular nucleus (the same occurs with a destructive labyrinthine pathology). This would result in an unopposed activity of the ipsilateral vestibular nuclear complex which through activation of the closely linked pontine gaze center would deviate the eyes to the side of irrigation (slow phase of nystagmus to same side of cold irrigation). Corrective mechanisms would come into play immediately, quickly moving the eyes to the central point of fixation (i.e., away from the side of irrigation). The last would constitute the fast phase of the nystagmus to the side opposite the side of cold irrigation. This mimics the findings of a destructive labyrinthine process on the irrigative side. An opposite event would occur with nystagmus directed towards the same side with warm water irrigation. The key factor in nystagmus generation in the cold caloric test is the integrity of central corrective mechanism. In an unconscious patient (with intact brainstem mechanism) cold irrigation would only lead to a tonic deviation of eyes to the irrigated side as no corrective mechanism to "re-fixate" the eyes to the central position would be available. With extensive brain, stem damage, even this tonic deviation would not occur (absent vestibulo-ocular reflex).

Voluntary Nystagmus

Voluntary nystagmus consists of bursts of extremely rapid, conjugate, horizontal oscillations that appear pendular but are really back-and-forth saccades. Most subjects cannot sustain this oscillation for longer than 20 or 30 seconds and manifest facial distortions with eyelid closure to rest their eyes. This ability may be hereditary and is said to be present in 5 percent of the population.

Efferent Nystagmus

This is found in association with some limitation of eye movement either due to restriction as in thyroid disease, or an ophthalmoparesis as in the abduction nystagmus of an internuclear ophthalmoplegia. Myasthenia gravis can cause this abduction nystagmus as well, mimicking an internuclear ophthalmoplegia.

Afferent Nystagmus

Afferent nystagmus is usually not present at birth but develops within the first 2-3 months of life and cannot be distinguished by observation alone from true congenital motor nystagmus. Careful examination, however, can usually identify an associated ocular disease, such as ocular albinism, congenital optic atrophy, congenital cataracts, Leber's congenital amaurosis, achromatopsia, or an extremely high refractive error. Children who lose vision before age 2 years will almost always develop nystagmus while those who lose vision after age 6 years usually do not. Those losing vision around age 4 years may or may not develop nystagmus. This sensory or afferent nystagmus is much more common than congenital motor nystagmus in a ratio of 10:1 and, therefore, *any child with "congenital nystagmus" should have a careful ophthalmologic evaluation to rule out an afferent visual problem.*

Specific, Recognizable, Localizing — Types of Nystagmus

These types of nystagmus are either anatomically localizing or recognizable by their constellation of associated findings on clinical examination.

Congenital Nystagmus

This includes all manifest nystagmus noted at birth or within the first few days of life. It may vary from an overt jerk nystagmus to a purely pendular oscillation. On examination, these patients appear to have normal visual sensory systems. Congenital nystagmus usually remains horizontal in all gaze angles and may be suppressed during convergence. Frequently a "null zone" of nystagmus can be identified in which the nystagmus is least marked and the visual acuity is the best. Patients may manifest *a head turn to keep the eyes in this null position.* A characteristic sign of congenital nystagmus is that during testing with a horizontal optokinetic stimulus, the quick phases may be directed in the same direction as drum motion—*optokinetic inversion.*

Latent Nystagmus

Latent nystagmus is a jerk nystagmus induced by monocular occlusion usually of either eye but may be induced by covering one eye only. When one eye is covered, the patient develops a bilateral jerk nystagmus with the jerk component directed away from the covered eye. Movements are bilateral, similar in amplitude and frequency, and symmetric. Latent nystagmus is associated with lack of normal binocular development and childhood strabismus. The importance of latent nystagmus is that it is always congenital in nature and never an acquired phenomenon.

Table 1 summarizes the clinical distinctions between congenital and acquired nystagmus. Both types are pathological.

Spasmus Nutans

Spasmus nutans is a rare, most often benign, triad of head tilt, head nodding and nystagmus,

Table 1: Distinguishing features of congenital and acquired nystagmus

	Congenital nystagmus	Acquired nystagmus
Onset	Within six months of birth	Usually after 6 month
Underlying vision defect	Common	Uncommon
Oscillopsia	Never	Sometimes
Nystagmus trajectory	Usually horizontal; remains horizontal in upgaze	Any direction; often converts to upbeat on upgaze
Nystagmus waveform	Increasing velocity slow phase; foveation periods	Constant or decreasing velocity slow phase; no foveation periods
Null zone	Often eccentric	Centric or absent
Latent component	Common	Never
Optokinetic nystagmus reversal	Common	Never

which usually appears to be monocular on gross inspection. The onset is usually between the ages of 4 and 14 months. It often lasts less than a month but may last several months or years and disappears by age 5 years. The eye movements are frequently pendular, may be horizontal or vertical, of low amplitude, and usually high frequency. On close inspection both eyes are noted to be involved although the involvement is usually asymmetric.

Spasmus nutans is usually a benign condition but rarely, it is associated with developmental nervous system disorders, chiasmal gliomas, third ventricular tumors and degenerative disorders.

Down-beat Nystagmus

Down-beat nystagmus is defined as nystagmus in the primary gaze position, with the fast phase beating in a downward direction. Typically, it is best evoked by looking down and laterally. Downbeat nystagmus is usually encountered with lesions of the vestibulocerebellum, craniocervical anomalies (e.g., Chiari anomaly) and drug intoxications; it is also a feature of the calcium channelopathy episodic ataxia type II.

Upbeat Nystagmus

This consists of nystagmus present in the primary position with the fast phase beating upward upbeat nystagmus have been mainly reported with lesions in the medulla, or close to the superior cerebellar peduncle.

It can also be due to severe drug intoxication. Phenytoin toxicity is a common example.

Pure Torsional Nystagmus

Pure torsional nystagmus with the eye close to the central position is uncommon and is usually seen with medullary lesions, such as syringobulbia and lateral medullary infarction (Wallenberg's). It is often accompanied by ocular tilt reaction or unilateral INO.

Periodic Alternating Nystagmus

Horizontal nystagmus that regularly reverses direction about every 2 minutes is periodic alternating nystagmus (PAN). It is often associated with lesion of cerebellar nodule and with cervicomedullary junction abnormalities.

To identify this conditions, an observation for a few minutes is required, and the periodic alternating head turns should be looked for. A congenital variant of PAN, with no associated cerebellar pathology, usually does not reverse direction at regular intervals.

Convergence Retraction Nystagmus

These jerk convergence retraction movements are due to cocontraction of the extraocular muscles, especially on attempted convergence or upgaze. This usually results from an extrinsic mass in the dorsal rostral mid brain area. Attempted upgaze results in bilateral convergence retraction nystagmus along with bilateral lid retraction. Convergence-retraction nystagmus may be elicited by asking the patient to make an upward saccade, or by using a hand held optokinetic drum or tape, moving the stripes down. Infants with this finding usually have congenital aqueductal stenosis, while a 10 years old has a pinealoma; a 20 years old has these findings due to head trauma; a 30 years old due to a vascular malformation, a 40 years old due to long-standing multiple sclerosis, and a 50 years old due to a basilar artery stroke. Occasional patients with relatively symmetric bilateral thyroid eye disease involving the inferior and medial recti muscles will demonstrate a similar convergence/retraction movement on attempted upgaze. These patients usually have other signs of dysthyroid disease.

See-saw Nystagmus of Maddox

See-saw nystagmus consists of upward movement and intorsion of one eye and synchronous downward movement and extorsion of the other eye in the first half cycle, followed by change in direction during the next half cycle. The see-saw phenomenon is most prominent in primary or downward and lateral gaze. Pendular see-saw nystagmus may occur with disorders that disrupts with crossing axons at the optic chiasma and cause bitemporal hemianopia, such as pituitary Jerk see-saw nystagmus may occur in patients with lesions in the region of the interstitial nucleus of Cajal.

Acquired Pendular Nystagmus

Acquired pendular nystagmus exhibits a quasi-sinusoidal waveform, and often shows directions that are oblique, elliptical, or circular, depending on the size and temporal relation between horizontal and vertical components. Congenital pendular nystagmus is usually horizontal in direction. Acquired pendular nystagmus may be conjugate, dysconjugate or dissociated. It occurs most commonly in association with multiple sclerosis, and after brainstem stroke in the syndrome of oculopalatal tremor.

Oculopalatal Tremor

Palatal tremor consists of brief, rhythmic involuntary movements of the soft palate. Two types are distinguished: essential palatal tremor, which involves the tensor veli palatini, and symptomatic palatal tremor, due to contaction of levator veli palatini. Symptomatic, but not essential palatal tremor, is associated with pseudohypertrophy of the inferior olive. Lesions can be found in these patients affecting the outflow of the cerebellum from the dentate nucleus via the superior cerebellar peduncle, the red nucleus and the central tegmental tract which carries afferents to the inferior olive (Guillain–Mollaret triangle). In oculopalatal tremor, the palatal movement is associated with a vertical pendular nystagmus with a rate of between 100 and 150 oscillations per minute and synchronous with contraction of the soft palate. The nystagmus may have oblique or torsional components.

Convergent–divergent Nystagmus

Pendular oscillations that are about 180° out of phase in the horizontal plane causes a type of convergent, divergent nystagmus, which occurs in some patients with cerebral Whipple's disease, sometimes with associated oscillatory movements of the jaw, face or limbs (oculomasticatory myorhythmia) and vertical gaze palsy. Pendular convergent-divergent nystagmus has also been reported in patients with multiple sclerosis and brainstem stroke.

Vestibular Nystagmus

Nystagmus can occur due to peripheral or central vestibular imbalances. The VOR depends on motion sensors in the inner ear that respond to head movements in different directions. Under normal conditions, the resting discharges from the two vestibular organs are balanced. Sudden cessation of activity from one side would precipitate vertigo and the accompanying nystagmus as maintenance of eye positions is also dependent of balanced discharges from the two vestibular organs. Malfunction of the central integrator of balanced vestibular functions would also cause vertigo and nystagmus in the vertical plane—upbeat or downbeat depending upon the direction of the fast component.

Mixed horizontal-torsional jerk nystagmus that suppresses with fixation is usually attributable to a peripheral vestibular imbalance and is accompanied by vertigo. Peripheral vestibular nystagmus commonly beats away from the side of lesion, and increases when the eyes are turned in the direction of the quick phase (Alexander's law). The direction of nystagmus remains same in all fields of gaze and the movement remains horizontal in vertical gaze. As mentioned earlier, cold water irrigation in the external canal mimics the effects of a destructive lesion of the vestibular end organ while warm water irrigation mimics an irritative lesion. Clinically, of course, most diseases of the end organ cause destructive effects. Thus, cold water in the left ear of a normal subject reproduces the following symptoms of left labyrinthine disease: (i) nystagmus with a fast phase to the right (COWS); (ii) the slow component is to the left; therefore, the environment appears to move to the right; (iii) the subject past points to the left; (iv) Romberg fall is to the left when the head is in the primary position; Romberg fall is backward when the face is turned to the left and Romberg fall is forward when the face is turned to the right. In central vestibular nystagmus, however, the jerk nystagmus may change direction with change in direction of gaze (direction changing nystagmus or more clearly speaking a gaze evoked nystagmus). Tinnitus, deafness, and vertigo are usually less prominent symptoms, and the Romberg direction of fall does not vary with change in the position of the head. Visual fixation has a dampening effect on the peripheral vestibular nystagmus (and it is best observed through a Frenzel glass) but not on central vestibular nystagmus.

Positional Nystagmus

Nystagmus that is present only when induced by positional testing (Dix Halpike or Nylan Barany maneuver) is a feature of benign paroxysmal positional vertigo. The nystagmus has a latency, is torsional, upbeat (in posterior canal vertigo but downbeat in anterior canal vertigo) and shows fatigue on repeated testing and is associated with severe vertigo. In contrast, a central or malignant form of positional nystagmus, starts immediately, is purely vertical, usually downbeat, does not show fatigue and is associated with mild systemic symptoms.

Gaze-evoked Nystagmus

This is a common form of nystagmus encountered in clinical practice and occurs only when the eyes are moved into eccentric gaze, especially in lateral and upgaze. This gaze-evoked nystagmus has quick phases that are directed away from the central position. Holding the eyes in such eccentric positions requires a tonic contraction of the extraocular muscles, which is achieved by a sustained discharge of motoneurons. The gaze holding neural network includes the nucleus prepositus hypoglossi and medial vestibular nucleus for horizontal gaze, the interstitial nucleus of Cajal for vertical gaze, and the vestibulocerebellum, which optimizes gaze holding.

Gaze–evoked nystagmus is caused by cerebellar and brainstem disorders as well as in a number of intoxications, including sedatives, anticonvulsants and alcohol. When patients with gaze-evoked nystagmus attempt to hold eccentric gaze for a number of seconds, and then return their eyes to the central position, a transient *"rebound nystagmus,"* with quick phases opposite to the direction of the prior eccentric gaze, may occur. Such rebound nystagmus is prominent in patients with disease affecting the vestibular cerebellum.

Brun's Nystagmus

Acoustic neuromas grow so slowly that adaptive mechanisms often obscure the clinical vestibular manifestations. A vestibular nystagmus beating away from the side of the lesion may be present, particularly if fixation is eliminated. As the tumor expands to compress the brainstem, a slow gaze evoked nystagmus is often added. Therefore, a combination of a small amplitude, rapid primary position jerk nystagmus beating away from the side of lesion and a slower, larger-amplitude, gaze-evoked nystagmus towards the side of the lesion occurs with this tumor and other extra-axial masses compressing the brainstem, including certain cerebellar tumors.

Nystagmus of Lateral Medullary Syndrome

Patients with Wallenberg's lateral medullary syndrome have a distinct constellation of findings, including ipsilateral loss of pain and temperature sensation in the face and contralateral loss in the trunk and limbs, dysarthria and dysphagia; ipsilateral Horner's syndrome, ataxia of the ipsilateral limbs, vertigo and a distinctive type of nystagmus. When the eyes are open there is a horizontal jerk nystagmus beating away from the side of the lesion. With a disruption of fixation or closing of the eyes, nystagmus either stops or reverses. Additionally, these patients may demonstrate ocular lateropulsion, or a tendency for the eyes to deviate toward the side of the lesion.

Epileptic Nystagmus

Ocular oscillations often occur during partial seizures. The initial eye movement is contraversive (rarely ipsiversive) conjugate head and eye deviation. A few seconds later, as the head and eyes remain deviated, jerk nystagmus begins in the same direction. During the oscillation, the patient may maintain some level of interaction with the surroundings, but focal clonic movements of the contralateral face, arm and leg or automatisms are often present. Thereafter, the seizure may generalize and render the patient unconscious. In the postictal state, the eyes may be deviated toward the side of the seizure focus (ocular Todd's paralysis). A seizure may also induce a sustained horizontal (or vertical) deviation of the eyes without causing an oscillation (saccadic deviation).

Other Ocular Oscillations

These are involuntary eye movements that do not fit the definition of nystagmus.

Square wave jerks: These can occur in healthy subjects, but are a prominent finding in progressive supranuclear palsy and some spinocerebellar atrophies (especially Friedreich's ataxia). They are small, conjugate saccades, ranging from 0.5 to 5.0 degree in size, which take the eye away from the fixation position and then return it there after a period of about 200 ms. They may be most evident during smooth pursuit.

The fast initial movement and the pause at its end are clues that this is not nystagmus. Square wave jerks may, however, be confused with unintentional eye movements that carry the eyes away from fixation (saccades of distraction). Saccades of distraction differ from square wave jerks in being of extremely wide and varying amplitudes.

Macrosaccadic oscillation: These usually consist of horizontal saccades that occur in bursts, building up and then decreasing in amplitude, with intersaccadic intervals of about 200 ms. These oscillations are usually induced by a gaze shift. They are a sign of midline cerebellar disease (affecting the fastigial nucleus), including spinocerebellar degenerations, but have also been reported with pontine lesions.

Ocular dysmetria: Ocular dysmetria is an oscillation that occurs at the termination of a refixational eye movement, akin to an extremity intention tremor. It is more apparent when saccades move from the lateral gaze position to the primary position than when they travel in the opposite direction. The eyes, overshoot the target, and repetitive saccades of decreasing amplitude bracket the target until the eyes settle on it. In some cases, ocular dysmetria looks like a quiver movement of the eyes that seems to interrupt fixation. In fact, the eyes are making tiny but inaccurate – oscillatory refixational movements (microsaccades).

Ocular dysmetria nearly always signifies cerebellar system disease. It occurs in the very same cerebellar system disorders that cause intention tremor of the extremities, ataxic speech, and midline (truncal and gait) ataxia. Like square wave jerks, ocular dysmetria causes no visual symptoms.

Ocular flutter: This consists of bursts (6-12 Hz) of horizontal saccadic oscillations (2-5° amplitude) without intersaccadic interval. These horizontal back to back saccades typically occurs in bursts of several cycles. Unlike ocular dysmetria, ocular flutter is not triggered by a refixational movement, it interrupts fixation.

Opsoclonus: This consists of saccadic oscillations with horizontal, vertical and torsional components. The frequency of oscillation is typically 10-15 cycles per second, being higher with smaller size movements. It is frequently associated with axial myoclonus (Kinsbourne opsoclonus – myoclonus syndrome).

Flutter and opsoclonus in childhood may reveal a neuroblastoma in half the cases. In adults they may appear after several infectious diseases, during brainstem encephalitis or with malignant pathology (paraneoplastic syndrome). They may be induced by drugs (lithium, haloperidol) or by fluid imbalance and electrolyte abnormalities.

Management strategies of opsoclonus may be summarized as follows:
1. In children, rule out neuroblastoma and in adults, rule out lung, breast, ovarian, or other primary cancers. If negative, rule out meningoencephalitis, hydrocephalus, focal or multifocal brain disorders, and medication or toxin exposure.

2. If neuroblastoma is found, treat that. Opsoclonus often improves as tumor is eliminated. Use of intravenous corticosteroids is optional.
3. If cancer is found in an adult, therapy for the tumor and for opsoclonus is probably not helpful. Death will occur within 3–6 months regardless of therapy.

If opsoclonus appears to be post-infectious rather than paraneoplastic, use of intravenous corticosteroids or immunoglobulin is optional.

Ocular Bobbing

This peculiar movement consists of an initial rapid downward movement of the eyeballs and then after a few seconds a slow upward movement to the original position. This cycle would continue to be repeated. Cerebellar or pontine lesions produce such movements. The opposite type of movement is termed inverse bobbing or dipping: slow downward shift and fast corrective upward movement. If initial movement is upward, then reverse bobbing occurs. All these movements, seen in unconscious patients, generally suggest widespread cerebral damage.

Ping-pong gaze refers to alternating high amplitude horizontal eye movements and suggests diencephalic dysfunction.

Superior oblique myokymia: This is a monocular rotatory fast eye movement. Abnormal eye movement restricted to one eye should raise this possibility caused by spontaneous firing of superior oblique muscle fibers. The patients complain of episodic oscillopsia or diplopia. The etiology of the condition is unknown but the clinical course is usually benign with spontaneous remission. Superior oblique myokymia is discussed in some detail in the Chapter on Nuclear and Infranuclear Ophthalmoplegias (Chapter 14).

Ocular neuromyotonia: This is characterized by episodes of diplopia that are usually precipitated by holding the eyes in eccentric gaze, often sustained adduction. These episodes are caused by involuntary, sometimes painful, contraction of one or more muscles innervated by one oculomotor nerve. Most reported patients have undergone previous radiation treatment to the parasellar region. The mechanism responsible for ocular neuromyotonia is unknown, but ephaptic neural transmission has been suggested. Carbamazepine may prove an effective treatment.

A diagnostic approach of ocular oscillations is shown in Flowchart 1.

Drug Treatment for Ocular Oscillations

Drug treatments are now available for some forms of acquired nystagmus and other ocular oscillations that disrupt clear vision (Table 2).

Table 2: Summary of current drug treatments for nystagmus

Vestibular forms of nystagmus	
A) Peripheral imbalance	Diphenhydramine, promethazine, prochlorperazine, ondansetron for relief of attendant vertigo and nausea; resume activity as soon as able
B) Central imbalance	
• Downbeat nystagmus	Clonazepam, baclofen, trihexyphenidyl; acetazolamide (for nystagmus associated with episodic ataxia type II); 4-aminopyridine;
• Upbeat nystagmus	Baclofen ; ? 4-aminopyridine
C) Central instability	
• Periodic alternating nystagmus	Baclofen
Nystagmus associated with visual system disorder	
• Seesaw nystagmus	Baclofen, clonazepam, alcohol, gabapentin
Nystagmus from disorders of the gaze holding mechanism	
• Acquired pendular nystagmus	*In association with disease of central myelin:* gabapentin, mementine, clonazepam, trihexyphenidyl, scopolamine; cannabis, alcohol. *As part of the syndrome of oculopalatal tremor ("Myocloniaus"):* gabapentin, valproate; trihexyphenidyl.

Continued

Continued

Saccadic intrusions and oscillations	
• Square wave jerks	Methylphenidate
• Opsoclonus and ocular flutter	Clonazepam, popranolol, gabapentin, corticosteroids, intravenous immunoglobulin, plasma exchange.
Miscellaneous abnormal movements	
• Superior oblique myokymia	Gabapentin, carbamazepine, propranolol
• Ocular neuromyotonia	Carbamazepine

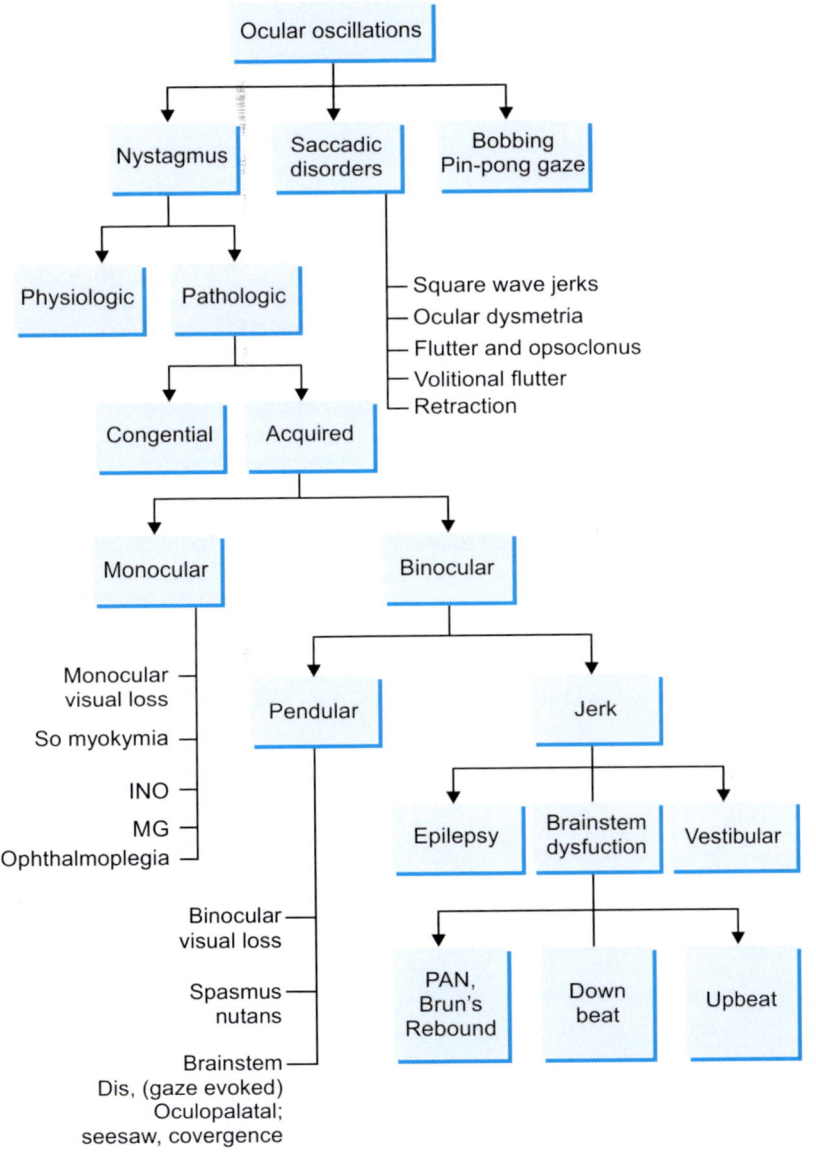

FLOWCHART 1: Pathways in diagnosis of ocular oscillations

SUGGESTED READINGS

1. Abel LA, Parker L, Daroff RB, et al. End point nystagmus. Invest Ophthalmol Vis Sci. 1978;17:539.
2. Anderson JR. Latent nystagmus and alternating hyperphoria. Br J Ophthalmol. 1954;38:217.
3. Arnold DB, Robinson DA. The oculomotor integrator: Testing of a neural network model. Exp Brain Res. 1997;113:57-74.
4. Averbuch-Heller L, Leigh RJ. Nystagmus and related ocular motility disorders. In: Miller NR, Newman N, editors. Walsh and Hoyt's clinical neuro-ophthalmology. 5th ed. Vol. 1. Baltimore: Williams and Wilkins; 1998. pp. 1461-500.
5. Averbuch-Heller L, Zivotofsky AJ, Remla BP, et al. Convergent-divergent pendular nystagmus: Possible role of the vergine system. Neurology. 1995;45:509-15.
6. Averbuch-Heller L, Zivotofsky AZ, Das VE, et al. Investigations of the pathogenesis of acquired pendular nystagmus. Brain. 1995;188:369-78.
7. Baloh RW, Jen JC. Genetics of familial episodic vertigo and ataxia. In: Kaminski HJ, Leigh RJ, editors. The neurobiology of eye movements, from molecules to behavior. Ann NY Acad Sci. 2002;956:338-45.
8. Baloh RW, Konrad HR, Dirks D, et al. Cerebellar-pontine angle tumors: Results of quantitative vestibulo-ocular testing. Arch Neurol. 1976;33:507.
9. Bataller L, Graus P, Saiz A, et al. Clinical outcome in adult onset idiopathic or paraneoplastic opsoclonus - myoclonus. Brain. 2000;124:437-43.
10. Bonder RL, Sharpe JA, Lewis AJ. Rebound nystagmus in olivocerebellar atrophy: A clinico pathological correlation. Ann Neurol. 1984;15:474-7.
11. Cogan DG. Ocular dysmetria: Flutter-like oscillations of the eyes, and opsoclonus. Arch Ophthalmol. 1954;451:316-35.
12. Dell' Osso LF, Daroff RB. Nystagmus and saccadic intrusions and oscillations. In: Glaser JS, editor. Neuro-ophthalmology. 3rd ed. Philadelphia: Lippincott, Williams and Wilkins; 1999. pp. 369-401.
13. Glaser JS. Myasthenic pseudo-internuclear ophthalmoplegia. Arch Ophthalmal. 1966;75:363.
14. Halmagyi GM, Aw ST, De Haene I, et al. Jerk-waveform see-saw nystagmus due to unilateral meso-diencephalic lesion. Brain. 1994;117:775-88.
15. Hoyt WF, Keane JR. Superior oblique myokymia: Report and discussion on five cases of benign intermittent uniocular microtremor. Arch Ophthalmol. 1970;84:461.
16. Kaminski HJ, Leigh RJ. The neurobiology of eye movements: From molecules to behavior. Ann NY Acad Sci. 2002;956:1-615.
17. Minigar A, Sheremata WA, Tusa RJ. Perverted head shaking nystagmus: A possible mechanism. Neurology. 2001;57:887-9.
18. Morrow MJ, Sharpe JA. Torsional nystagmus in lateral medullary syndrome. Ann Neurol. 1998;24:390-8.
19. Mukherjee A, Chakravarty A. Vertigo, dizziness and epilepsy. In: Chakravarty A. Borderlands of epilepsy. J Assoc Neurosci Eastern India. Kolkata. 2003. pp. 253-72.
20. Mukherjee A, Chatterjee SK, Chakravaty A. Vertigo and dizziness—a clinical approach. J Ass Phys Ind. 2003;51:1095-101.
21. Nakoda T, Kwee IL. Oculopalatal myoclonus. Brain. 1986;109:431-41.
22. Norton EW, Cogan DG. Spasmus nutans: A clinical study of twenty cases followed two years or more since onset. Arch Ophthalmol. 1954;52:442.
23. Schon F, Hodgson TL, Most Di, et al. Ocular flutter associated with a localised lesion in the paramedian pontine reticular formation. Ann Neurol. 2001;50:413-6.
24. Schwartz MA, Selhorst JB, Ochs AL, et al. Oculomasticatory myorhythmia: A unique movement disorder occurring in Whipple's disease. Ann Neurol. 1986;20:677-83.
25. Shults WT, Stark L, Hoyt WF, et al. Normal saccadic structure and voluntary nystagmus. Arch Neurol. 1977;95:1399.
26. Smith JL, Zieper I, Gay AJ. Nystagmus retractions. Arch Ophthalmol. 1954;62:864.

18. Ptosis and Blepharospasm

Ravindranath M Chowdhury, Sanjib Sinha

PTOSIS

Ptosis, also referred to as blepharoptosis, is defined as an abnormal low-lying upper eyelid margin with the eye in primary gaze. The word 'ptosis' is derived from the Greek 'πτωσις', which means 'to fall'. The official definition of ptosis is an upper marginal reflex distance below 2 mm or an asymmetry of more than 2 mm between the eyes. The normal adult upper lid lies 1.5 mm below the superior corneal limbus and is highest just nasal to the pupil. Ptosis, which is a droopy upper eyelid, is the result of dysfunction of one or both upper eyelid elevator muscles. These muscles are the levator palpebrae superioris (LPS) and its aponeurosis and Müller's muscle. Ptosis may occur secondary to pathology of muscle or connective tissue, neuromuscular junction, oculomotor nerve or its nuclei and supranuclear causes. The causes of ptosis can range from benign to life threatening emergency conditions, hence careful clinical assessment can prevent inappropriate expensive investigations and sometimes it can be life saving.

Clinical Anatomy and Physiology

Levator palpebrae superioris (40 cm long), is a voluntary muscle, and supplied by the upper division of the oculomotor nerve, arises from the lesser wing of the sphenoid bone. Passing forward to the Whitnall ligament, it turns inferiorly as an aponeurosis which gets inserted into the anterior aspect of the tarsal plate (Fig. 1). Sending attachments to the skin and forming the upper eyelid crease. This is the major elevator of the upper lid. A smooth muscle named Müller's muscle, is supplied by the sympathetic, originates from the undersurface of the levator palpebrae muscle, and is a weak elevator, raising the upper lid by only about 2 mm. The way that the LPS attaches to the tarsal plate is modified by the underlying Müller's muscle. Two other muscles affecting the final position of the eyelid are the frontalis muscle and the orbicularis oculi, both supplied by the facial nerve. Frontalis contraction helps to elevate the lid by acting indirectly on the surrounding soft tissues, while orbicularis oculi contraction depresses the eyelid.

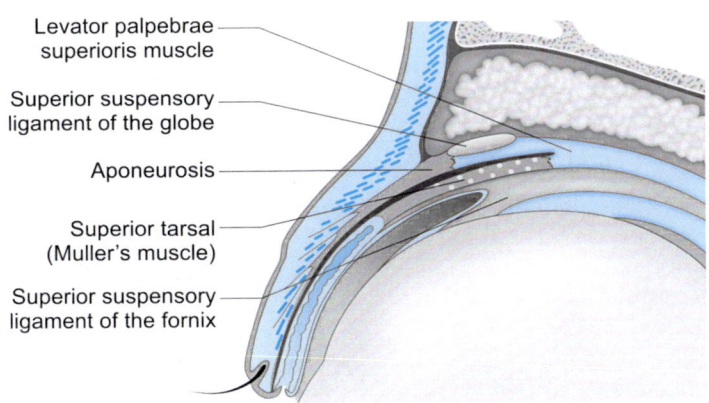

FIG. 1: Shows the anatomy of eyelid muscles and their attachments

Clinical Features

Most often ptosis is noticed accidentally or when it causes cosmetic problems. However, when drooping of eyelids cover the pupil, it may impair vision. In chronic and congenital cases it may result into amblyopia. Even without visual axis obstruction, the drooped lid may induce refractive errors, especially astigmatism resulting in amblyopia or constriction of the superior visual fields. The patients may complain of blurred vision, increased tearing and difficulty with activities of daily living, such as driving, reading, and climbing stairs, affecting the patient's quality of life. Patients may complain that they tire easily when reading and experience frontal headaches as they lift their eyebrows in an effort to keep the eyelids open. They may have associated symptoms depending on cause of ptosis, e.g., myasthenia gravis (MG) patients may have associated diplopia and bulbar symptoms.

Evaluation of Ptosis

History

- Onset, duration, variability, progression, and severity of ptosis
- Has there been any history of trauma to head, eye or neck, eye surgery, contact lens use?
- Has there been diplopia, blurring of vision?
- Any proptosis?
- History of associated lid abnormality
- Any symptoms of MG or other neuromuscular dysfunction?
- History of systemic diseases—thyroid or cardiac illness
- Family history of muscle disease or mitochondrial cytopathies
- Review of old photographs!

Physical Examination

- General physical examination
- Complete neurologic examination.

Ocular Examination

- Note the eye brow position
- Visual acuity (VA)
- Examine the pupil
- Examine the extraocular movements
- Look for Horner's syndrome
- Slit lamp examination
- Posterior chamber examination.

In addition to documenting the VA, the patient's ocular motility and pupillary function should be evaluated.

Horner's syndrome should be investigated fully. Degree of ptosis, should be assessed by various eyelid measurements taken with frontalis muscle relaxed. If needed frontalis contraction should be nullified by holding the brows in their relaxed position. The brows may be lifted to observe the lid level for measurement which would include:

- The Palpebral fissure height (PFH) which is the distance between the upper and lower eyelid margins at the vertical axis of the pupil (normal 9–12 mm) (Fig. 2C)
- Marginal reflex distance (MRD), distance between the central corneal light reflex and upper eyelid margin with eyes in primary position should be taken (normal 4–5 mm). The MRD gives a better assessment of the severity of ptosis than PFH (Fig. 2B)
- Levator function is evaluated by asking the patient to look downward as a measuring device is positioned with a mark adjacent to the upper lid margin. Next with the examiner's hand eliminating any brow movement by the patient, the patient looks upward as far as possible without any change in his/her head position. The amount of lid elevation is measured in millimeters (mm). This is called eye lid excursion is recorded in millimeters (mm) of levator function (Figure 2 left-side image).

Classification of Levator Function

Levator function should be evaluated in all cases. The patient looks downward as a measuring device is positioned with a mark adjacent to the upper lid margin. With the examiner's hand eliminating any brow action by the patient, the patient looks upward as far as possible without changing his/her head position. The amount of lid elevation also called eyelid excursion is recorded in millimeters (mm) of levator function (Fig. 2A).

Levator function is graded as poor: 0–5 mm elevation; fair: 6–11 mm elevation; good: >12 mm elevation. The position of the drooped eyelid in down-gaze should be assessed, as it helps in

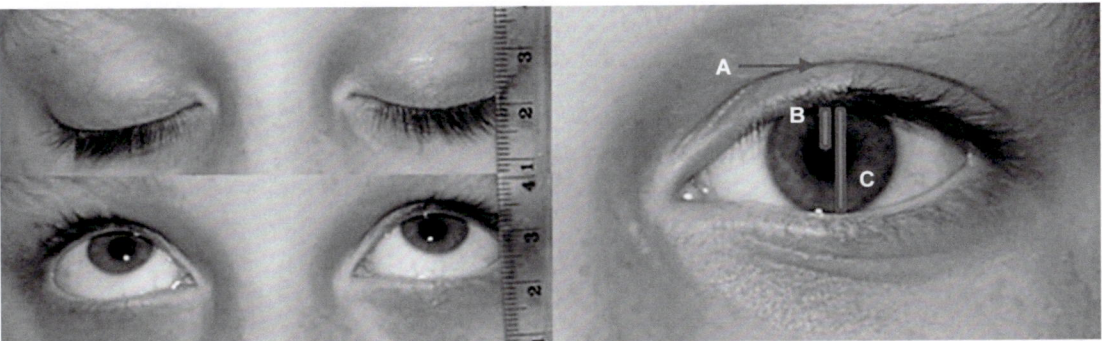

Fig. 2: Measurement of eyelid excursion. The top left image shows the margin of the closed eyelid at a level of 20 mm. When the eyelids are fully elevated (bottom left), this increases to 33 mm, giving a normal eyelid excursion of 13 mm. The right-sided image shows a normal eyelid crease (A), upper marginal reflex distance (B) and palpebral fissure (C).

differentiating congenital from acquired ptosis. Congenitally drooped eyelid remains higher in down-gaze due to lid lag.

Causes of Ptosis (Box 1 and Fig. 1)

Contralateral Lid Retraction (Pseudoptosis)

Subtle lid retraction of one upper lid may make the other lid appear ptotic, even though it is in normal position. A visibility of sclera above the superior limbus indicates upper lid retraction on opposite side and suggests that the suspected "ptotic" lid is in normal position.

Apraxia of Lid Opening

This is the inability to initiate lid opening voluntarily in presence of normal sphincter and lid elevator and first described by Schilder in 1927. Most patients have extrapyramidal disease, but unilateral and bilateral hemispheric disease has been implicated in causing lid apraxia. Patients may lift the lids manually or at times use head thrusting movements.

Hysterical Ptosis

Two types are described: pseudoparalytic and flaccid. It may pose diagnostic and therapeutic problems when present.

Supranuclear Causes

Ptosis from a cerebral hemisphere lesion is a rare sign. It may be apparent on the side opposite to the cerebral lesion. This was described in the pre CT/MRI era and the cause is said to be because of

Box 1: Causes of ptosis

A. Congenital
- Congenital ptosis
- Congenital myopathies
- Neonatal myasthenia
- Congenital myasthenia
- Birth injuries
- Jaw-winking phenomenon

B. Acquired
- Aponeurotic
  - Senescence or involutional
  - Chronic inflammation of lids or its apparatus
  - Long-term contact lens use
- Neurogenic
  - Horner's syndrome
  - Third cranial nerve palsy (supranuclear, nuclear/infranuclear)
  - Synkinetic neurogenic ptosis (Marcus Gunn jaw-winking)
  - Hemispheric ptosis
  - Brainstem ptosis
- Muscle and myoneural junction
  - Myasthenia gravis
  - Chronic progressive external ophthalmoplegia
  - Mitochondrial cytopathy
  - Oculopharyngeal muscular dystrophy
  - Myotonic dystrophy

transtentorial herniation of temporal lobe. Ptosis caused by cerebral hemisphere dysfunction could be uni- or bilateral. Lepore et al. found bilateral ptosis in 13 patients with right hemisphere stroke.

Congenital Ptosis

It may be isolated or may be associated with difficulty in elevating the ipsilateral eye due to under action of LPS and superior rectus muscle. The superior division of third cranial nerve supplies both of these muscles. Ptosis may be part of more complex syndrome of multiple congenital abnormalities like Turner syndrome, Smith–Lemli-Opitz syndrome.

Congenital Myopathies

Ptosis at birth or early in life may be part of congenital myopathic disorder such as myotubular, congenital fiber type disproportion or centro nuclear myopathies and congenital myotonias.

Neonatal Myasthenia

Children born of MG mothers may show evidence of ptosis or other signs of MG beginning within 24 hours. This may last for few weeks and may require supportive treatment with anticholinesterase agents. Transplacental transfer of antibodies causes this.

Congenital Myasthenia

These are due to variety of pathophysiological mechanisms, but symptoms typically begins in neonatal period or early childhood. It is not anti-acetylcholine receptor antibody mediated.

Marcus-Gunn Jaw-winking Phenomenon

Infants may manifest intermittent retraction of a ptotic lid while chewing or otherwise moving the jaw or sucking. This movement results from a presumed miswiring between the oculomotor and trigeminal nerve motor division. Spontaneous improvement with age occurs.

Brainstem Ptosis

Lesions of brainstem may produce bilateral ptosis by involving the LPS sub nucleus of third cranial nerve. Bilateral ptosis along with down-gaze paresis is attributed to destruction of brainstem inputs to levator subnucleus. In this case while the eyes do not descend below midline, the lids do depress as if the eyes were in down gaze.

Lesions of Oculomotor Nuclei

A lesion in the levator portion of the third nerve nucleus produces bilateral ptosis, which may be severe and symmetric. Usually the lesion is caudally placed. There may be associated medial rectus palsy and exotropia. Paralysis of upward gaze and pupillary functions occur when whole of nuclei is involved.

Lesions of Third Nerve

This is commonly unilateral or rarely bilateral, commonly associated with other extraocular muscle weakness and with or without pupillary involvement. Nuclear and infranuclear lesions can cause it. Associated neurological signs can differentiate these and can suggest site of lesion. Diabetes and vasculitis are common causes of isolated partial third nerve palsy.

Pupillary Abnormality with Ptosis

The presence of a dilated and poorly reactive pupil ipsilateral to ptotic lid suggests third cranial nerve palsy. The association of ptosis and ipsilateral miosis suggests an oculosympathetic paresis or Horner syndrome. Rarely Miller Fisher variant of Guillain–Barré syndrome (GBS) and botulism may present with ptosis early in the course of disease.

Myasthenia Gravis

Myasthenia gravis is characterized by impaired transmission of impulses across the neuromuscular junction, due to antibodies to acetylcholine receptors. These antibodies may cause blocking and accelerated receptor degradation. Ocular signs, particularly ptosis may be the initial manifestation of MG in up to 75% of patients. The symptoms may remain restricted to ocular muscles or may become generalized. Fatigability is the hallmark of MG. When ptosis is asymmetrical, the patients may use the frontalis muscle to elevate both lids, producing lid retraction on one side. If the examiner manually lifts the more ptotic lid, the previously retracted lid will fall and this has been termed enhanced ptosis. Cogan et al. has described the lid-twitch sign as being characteristic of myasthenic ptosis. The patient looks down for 10–15 seconds and is then asked to make a rapid refixation to primary position. A positive lid-twitch sign consists of an upward overshoot of the lid, which then will slowly droop to its previous ptotic position. The diagnosis of MG can be established based on clinical features, edrophonium test, electrophysiological studies (repetitive nerve stimulation test and single fiber EMG) and serum anti\acetylcholine receptor antibody testing (Figs. 3 and 4). Ocular myasthenia is further discussed in chapter 13.

Muscular Dystrophy

Myotonic dystrophy is characterized by prominent myotonia, ptosis, distal weakness, and typical facial features (long face, frontal baldness, hollowed masseter, and temporalis). It usually begins in second or third decade. Patients usually have associated cardiac abnormalities.

Oculopharyngeal muscular dystrophy usually presents in fifth and sixth decade. Initially patients present with extraocular muscle weakness and ptosis. Ptosis may be asymmetrical in onset. Later on patients develop pharyngeal weakness. Histologically it is characterized by presence of small intranuclear tubulofilaments.

Mitochondrial Cytopathies

Several types of mutation or deletion in respiratory chain enzyme genes cause mitochondrial cytopathies. Ocular involvement is an important feature of this group of diseases. Kearns-Sayre syndrome (see Chapter 13) presents in childhood or early adulthood. It presents as slowly progressive and symmetrical external ophthalmoplegia and ptosis. It can lead to total immobility of eyes. Retinitis pigmentosa can be associated with it. Usually it is associated with cardiac conduction disorder and this can lead to sudden death. Rarely, Leigh disease may also be associated with ophthalmoplegia.

Idiopathic (Senile) Ptosis

An isolated ptosis in nonmyasthenic older patients may be classified as senile ptosis. This is believed to be due to disinsertion or dehiscence of the LPS aponeurosis.

Key Points in Evaluation of Ptosis

- Ptosis with proptosis, with or without chemosis—cavernous sinus thrombosis, caroticocavernous fistula or orbital lesion
- Ptosis with ipsilateral miosis and anhidrosis—Horner's syndrome
- Ptosis with slowly progressive bilateral symmetrical ophthalmoplegia—mitochondrial cytopathy or muscular dystrophy
- Unilateral ptosis with dilated pupil and restricted extraocular movements—third nerve palsy
- Acute onset ptosis with ophthalmoplegia and with or without areflexia—Miller Fisher variant of GBS, toxic
- Ptosis with diplopia and fluctuating weakness of ocular and other muscles—MG.

Management

If any correctable cause is found on evaluation like MG, it should be treated accordingly. If

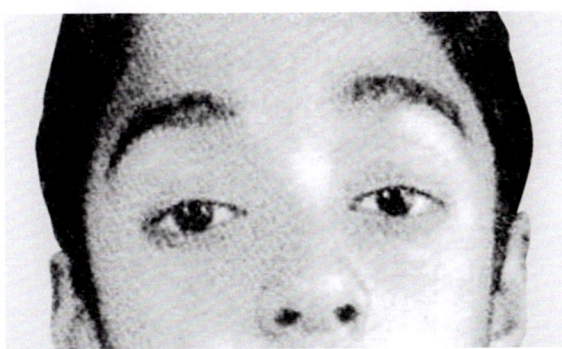

FIG. 3: Illustration of childhood ocular myasthenia. Note bilateral ptosis and fixed eyeballs. Neostigmine test was positive.

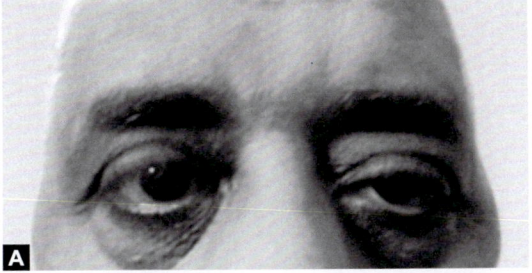
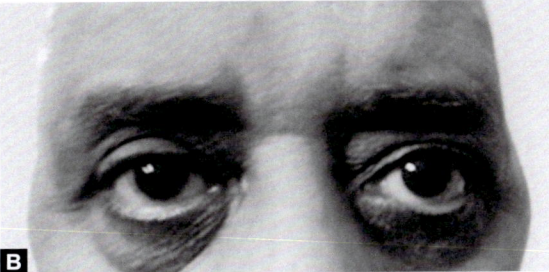

FIG. 4: A, Baseline—moderate ptosis on left-side. Palpebral fissure width (left more than right); **B,** At 45 minutes after neostigmine injection, left-sided ptosis had improved fully.

no correctable cause is found ptosis is treated symptomatically (Flowchart 1).

If condition is slight and not causing much visual or cosmetic problem, it is best left alone. Some relief may be obtained by using special spectacle frames. This is indicated in temporary ptosis and in those who are not good candidates for surgery. Surgery is the treatment of choice for both visual and cosmetic problems.

Various surgical procedures used are listed below:
- Müllerectomy
- Fasanella-Servat procedure
- Levator palpebrae superioris aponeurosis repair
- Frontalis suspension
- Whitnall sling operation.

BLEPHAROSPASM

Blepharospasm is persistent or repetitive involuntary contraction of orbicularis oculi muscle. Blepharo means "eyelid" and "spasm" means "uncontrolled muscle contraction". The term blepharospasm can be applied to any abnormal blinking or eyelid tic or twitch resulting from any cause, ranging from dry eyes to Tourette's syndrome to tardive dyskinesia. People with blepharospasm have normal vision. Visual disturbance is due solely to the forced closure

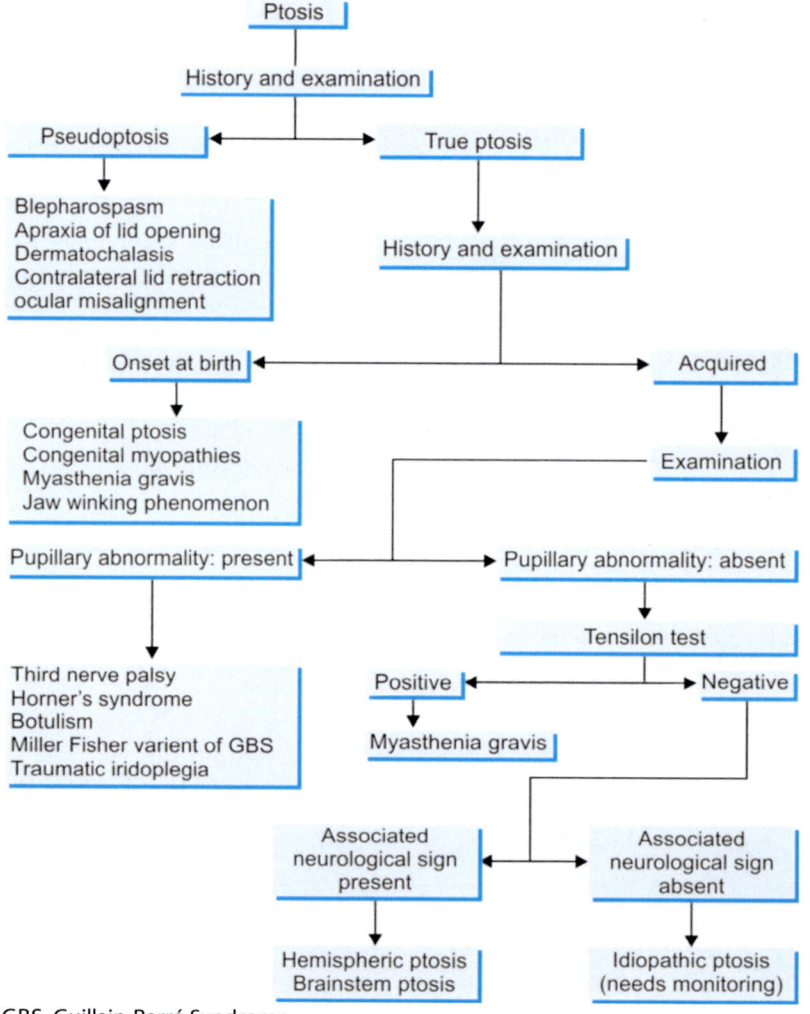

GBS, Guillain-Barré Syndrome.

FLOWCHART 1: Flowchart for evaluation of ptosis (modified from reference 2).

of the eyelids. The prevalence of blepharospasm in the general population is approximately 5 in 100,000. Blepharospasm has a female-to-male preponderance of 1.8:1. The mean age of onset of blepharospasm is 56 years, and two thirds of patients are age 60 years or older.

Clinical Features

Blepharospasm affects the eye muscles and usually begins gradually with excessive blinking and/or eye irritation. The early symptoms of blepharospasm include increased blink rate (77%), eyelid spasms (66%), eye irritation (55%), midfacial or lower facial spasm (59%), eyebrow spasm (24%), and eyelid tic (22%). Early blepharospasm may only occur with specific precipitating factors, like bright lights, fatigue, and emotional tension. It is always present in both eyes. As the condition progresses, it occurs more frequently. The spasms disappear in sleep, and some people find that after a good night's sleep, spasms do not appear for several hours after waking.

Blepharospasm can occur with dystonia affecting the mouth and/ or jaw (oromandibular dystonia, Meige's syndrome). If blepharospasm causes any type of impairment, it is because muscle contractions interfere with normal function. On the whole, the therapeutic response is unsatisfactory and prognosis is difficult to predict.

Pathophysiology

Normally when we blink, eyelid closure results from coinhibition of two groups of muscles, the eye closing muscles (i.e., orbicularis oculi, corrugator superciliaris, and procerus muscles) and the elevators of the eyelids (i.e., LPS, frontalis muscles). During the normal blink, these two groups of muscle function only at separate times. In patients with blepharospasm, this inhibition between the two groups is lost.

Essential blepharospasm may be considered a form of segmental dystonia and believed to be due to abnormal functioning of the basal ganglia, which are deep brain structures involved with the control of movement. The basal ganglia assist in initiating and regulating movement. Exact mechanism in the basal ganglia is still unknown. An imbalance of dopamine, a neurotransmitter in the basal ganglia, may underlie several different forms of dystonia, but much more research needs to be done for a better understanding of the brain mechanisms involved with dystonia. Blepharospasm currently considered as a network defect in dynamic circuit activity, rather than a defect at a specific locus. Fayers et al. have found a decrease in corneal sensitivity in patients with blepharospasm, implying an impairment in cortical processing of sensory input, with a resultant loss of blink reflex inhibition.

Though a history of eye trauma may be obtained in some patients, the relationship between trauma and blepharospasm has not been established. In most people it develops spontaneously with no known precipitating factor. Cases of inherited blepharospasm have been reported, usually in conjunction with early-onset generalized dystonia, which is associated with the *DYT1* gene. Blepharospasm may also be secondary or symptomatic, occurring in association with other disorders such as tardive dystonia, parkinsonian syndromes etc. (Table 1).

Diagnosis

Diagnosis of blepharospasm is based on information from the affected individual and the physical and neurological examination. At this time, there is no test to confirm diagnosis of

TABLE 1: Causes of secondary blepharospasm

- Ocular
  - Allergic conjunctivitis
  - Anterior nongranulomatous uveitis
  - Conjunctival and corneal irritation, iritis, uveitis
  - Dacryocystitis
  - Eyelid myokymia
  - Keratoconjunctivitis sicca
- Neurological
  - Bell's palsy
  - Vascular loop
  - Huntington's disease
  - Wilson's disease
  - Hemifacial spasm
  - Gilles de la Tourette syndrome
  - Meningitis
  - Drugs— antipsychotic, antiemetics, levodopa, anorectics, etc.
- Parkinsonism
  - Meige's syndrome Cruetzfeldt–Jakob disease
  - Postencephalitic syndrome
  - Subarachnoid hemorrhage
  - Habit spasms
  - Tardive dyskinesia

blepharospasm, and, in most cases, laboratory tests are normal.

Blepharospasm should be differentiated from the following:
- Ptosis—drooping of the eyelids caused by weakness or paralysis of levator muscles of the upper eyelid. In blepharospasm the eyebrow is lower than normal but in ptosis it is elevated. The lower lid margin is higher in blepharospasm and normal in ptosis and apraxia of eyelid opening
- Blepharitis—an inflammatory condition of the lids due to infection or allergies. This can be identified by careful local examination
- Hemifacial spasm—a nondystonic condition involving various muscles on one side of the face, often including the eyelid, and caused by irritation of the facial nerve. The muscle contractions are more rapid and transient than those of blepharospasm, and the condition is always confined to one side, while blepharospasm is usually bilateral
- Facial nerve injury with aberrant regeneration—this condition causes symptoms like hemifacial spasm after recovering from previous lower motor neuron facial weakness
- Benign eyelid twitch (also called eyelid myokymia): This is a fine fasciculation (tiny muscle contractions) generally affecting one eyelid (more often a lower eyelid, but upper eyelids as well). Twitching is episodic, lasting seconds-to-hours over minutes-to-months, but always eventually resolves on its own. Associated with stress, fatigue, and caffeine use.

Treatment

Treatment for blepharospasm is designed to lessen the symptoms of spasms, pain, and functions. Most therapies are symptomatic, attempting to cover up or release the spasms. No single strategy is appropriate for every case. The goal of any treatment is to achieve the greatest benefits while incurring the fewest risks. The approach for treatment of blepharospasm is usually three-tiered: oral medications, botulinum toxin injections, and surgery. These therapies may be used alone or in combination. Complementary care, such as physical therapy and speech therapy, may also have a role in the management depending on the form of dystonia. For many people, supportive therapy provides an important adjunct to medical treatment.

Although there is currently no known cure for dystonia, we are gaining a better understanding of dystonia through research and are developing new approaches to treatments.

Medications

The fact that a multitude of drugs has been enlisted in its management, prove that none is effective. Drug therapy for blepharospasm and facial dystonias usually are based upon the following three unproven pharmacologic hypotheses: (i) cholinergic excess, (ii) GABA hypofunction, and (iii) dopamine excess. Some patients gets some mild benefit when treated with such medications as clonazepam, trihexyphenidyl, baclofen, etc. but usually at the expense of side effects. Clozapine is particularly effective in blepharospasm due to neuroleptic drug use.

Botulinum Toxin

This is the treatment of choice. Injection sites are variable depending upon the choice of the doctor concerned. Usual sites include corners of each eyelid, under the lids, to the side of the eye, and in the brow. A total of 25–50 units is generally given. Benefit may start early but may not last more than 3 months. Most do well during this period. Minor transient side effects including diplopia may occur.

Other than high cost of treatment, the injections need to be repeated every 4–6 months with a chance of antibody production, thereby causing decreased response.

Surgery

Before surgery is recommended, people are advised to try nonsurgical therapies such as medication or botulinum toxin injections. At present, protractor myectomy (removal of some or all of the muscles responsible for eyelid closure) has proven to be the most effective surgical treatment for blepharospasm. Deep brain stimulation of the globus pallidus internus and pallidotomy have been described for Meige syndrome.

Complementary Therapy

Dark glasses is a common aid for people with blepharospasm. The glasses fulfill two functions by reducing the intensity of sunlight that bothers many people with blepharospasm, and they hide the person's eyes from curious onlookers. The use of sensory tricks may also be effective in dealing with blepharospasm. Some of the most common "tricks" are pulling on the upper eyelid, pinching the neck, talking, humming, yawning, singing, sleeping, reading, looking down, or concentrating. Different sensory tricks work for different people, and if a person finds a sensory trick that works, it usually continues to work.

SUGGESTED READINGS

1. Arunabh, Jain S, Maheshwari MC. Blepharospasm hemi facial spasm and tremors possibly due to isolated caudate nucleus lesions. JAPI. 1992;40:687-9.
2. Ben Simon GJ, McCann JD. Benign essential blepharospasm. Int Ophthalmol Clin. 2005;45(3):49-75.
3. Berlin Al, Vestal KP. Levator aponeurosis surgery. Ophthalmology. 1989;96:1033-7.
4. Bever CT Jr, Aquino AV, Penn AS, et al. Prognosis of ocular myasthenia. Ann Neurol. 1983;14:516-9.
5. Boghen D. Apraxia of lid opening: A review. Neurology. 1997;48:1491-503.
6. Boghen DR, Lesser RL. Blepharospasm and hemi facial spasm. Curr Treat Options Neurol. 2000;2(5):393-400.
7. Burde RM, Savino PJ, Trobe JD. Blepharospasm. In: Clinical decision in neuro ophthalmology. 2nd ed. London: Mosby Co.; 1992. pp. 365-78.
8. Burde RM, Savino PJ, Trobe JD. Eyelid disturbances. In: Clinical Decisions in Neuro Ophthalmology. 3rd ed. London: Mosby Co.; 2002. pp. 272-96.
9. Buttner-Ennever JA, Acheson JF, et al. Ptosis and supra nuclear downgaze paralysis. Neurology. 1989;39:385-9.
10. Calace P, Cortese G, Piscopo R. Treatment of blepharospasm with botulinum neurotoxin type A: Long-term results. Eurj Ophthalmol. 2003;13(4):331-6.
11. Chiba A, Kusonoki S, Obata H, et al. Serum anti-GQlb IgG antibody is associated with ophthalmoplegia in Miller-Fisher syndrome and Guillain Barre syndrome: clinical and immunological studies. Neurology. 1993;43:1911-7.
12. Cogan DG. Myasthenia gravis: A review of the disease and description of lid twitch as a characteristic sign. Arch Ophthalmol. 1965;74:217-21.
13. Crawford IS. Repair of ptosis using frontalis muscle and fascia lata: A 20-year review. Ophthalmic Surg. 1971;8:31-40.
14. Defazio G, Brancati F, Valente EM, et al. Familial blepharospasm is inherited as an autosomal dominant trait and relates to a novel unassigned gene. Mop Disord. 2003;18(2):207-12.
15. Digre K, Corbett JJ. Hemi facial spasm: Differential diagnosis, mechanism and treatment. Adv Neurol. 1988;49:151-76.
16. Dortzbach RK, Sutula FC. Involutional blepharoptosis: A histopathological study. Arch Ophthalmol. 1980;98:2045-9.
17. Drachman DB. Myasthenia gravis (first part). N Engl J Med. 1978;298:136-42.
18. Evinger C, Bao JB, Powers AS, et al. Dry eye, blinking, and blepharospasm. Mop Disord. 2002;17(Suppl 2):s75-8.
19. Fayers T, Shaw SR, Hau SC, et al. Changes in corneal aesthesiometry and the sub-basal nerve plexus in benign essential blepharospasm. Br J Ophthalmol. 2015;99(11):1509-13.
20. Gorelick PB, Rosenberg M, Pagano RJ. Enhancedptosis in myasthenia gravis. Arch Neurol. 1981;38:531.
21. Grandas F, Elston J, Quinn N, et al. Blepharospasm: A review of 264 patients. Neurol Neurosurg Psychiatry. 1988;51:767-72.
22. Hallett M. Blepharospasm: Recent advances. Neurology. 2002;59:1306-12.
23. Jankovic J, Ford J. Blepharospasm and orofacial-cervical dystonia: Clinical and pharmacological findings in 100 patients. Ann Neurol. 1983;13:402-11.
24. Jankovic J, Orman J. Blepharospasm: Demographic and clinical survey of 250 patients. Ann Ophthalmol. 1984;16(4):371-6.
25. Jankovic J, Patel SC. Blepharospasm associated with brainstem lesions. Neurology. 1983;33:1237-40.
26. Jankovic J. Dystonia: medical therapy and botulinum toxin. Adv Neurol. 2004;94:275-86.
27. Jankovic J. Etiology and differential diagnosis of blepharospasm and oromandibular dystonia. Adv Neurol. 1988;49:103-16.
28. Johnson JC, Rosenbaum DM, Picone CM, et al. Apraxia of eyelid opening secondary to right hemisphere infarction. Ann Neurol. 1989;25:622-4.
29. Lepore FE. Bilateral cerebral ptosis. Neurology. 1987;37:1043-6.
30. Levin H, Reddy R. Clozapine in the treatment of neuroleptic-induced blepharospasm: A report of 4 cases. J Clin Psychiatry. 2000;61(2):140-3.
31. Misbahuddin A, Placzek MR, Chaudhuri KR, et al. A polymorphism in the dopamine receptor DRD5 is associated with blepharospasm. Neurology. 2002;58:124-6.
32. Misulis KE, Fenichel GM. Genetic forms of myasthenia gravis. Paedir Neurol. 1989;5:205-10.
33. Nutt JG. Lid abnormalities secondary to cerebral hemisphere lesion. Ann Neurol. 1977;1:149-51.
34. Sibony PA, Evinger C. Anatomy and physiology of normal and abnormal eyelid position and movement. In: NR Muller, NJ Newman, editors. Walsh and Hoyt's Clinical Neuro-Ophthalmology. 5th ed. Vol. 1. Baltimore: Williams & Wilkins; 1998. pp. 1509-92.
35. Silverman IE, Lui GT, Galetta SL. The crossed paralyses. The original brainstem syndromes of Miller-Gubler, Foville, Weber and Raymond-Ceston. Arch Neurol. 1995;52:635-8.
36. Wang A, Jankovic J. Hemi facial spasm: Clinical findings and treatment. Muscle Nerve. 1998;12:1740-7.

19 Proptosis

Ajitesh Das, Sudip Chatterjee

INTRODUCTION

Proptosis is the pathological forward displacement of one or both eyes. The normal range of ocular protrusion, as measured by exophthalmometry, is 14–21 mm in adults. Although, a 2-mm difference between fellow eyes is generally considered normal, any disparity between the eyes in a patient being evaluated for orbital disease must be regarded as suspicious. As exophthalmometry is not always available in a general neurology or medical clinic, close visual inspection has to be relied upon quite often. It is best to visualize the eyes either from the sides or from the top of the head to assess the degree as protrusion beyond the orbital bony margin and to note any disparity between the two sides. When viewed from the side, visibility of the white sclera between the upper border of the lower lid and the lower border of the cornea, usually suggests a protruded globe. It is also often helpful to compare the appearance of the eyes at the time of examination from those recorded earlier in old photographs.

Once proptosis is confirmed, certain measures need to be performed to make an etiological diagnosis:
- Looking for upper lid retraction: This strongly suggests thyroid-associated ophthalmopathy (TAO) or Graves' ophthalmopathy (GO) and usually excludes other causes of proptosis
- Balloting the eyes for increased resistance to retropulsion, which suggests a mass or orbital congestion
- Palpating for anterior masses
- Listening for bruits over the eyes and orbit, which may be heard with cavernous sinus fistulas or arteriovenous malformations (AVMs)
- Having the patient perform a Valsalva maneuver. A marked increase in proptosis suggests an orbital venous anomaly, which might not be detected on routine imaging
- Looking for contralateral enophthalmos, which can masquerade as proptosis of the normal eye
- Ocular movements must be tested and if restricted, attempt should be made to assess whether due to mechanical hindrance in the orbit or due to actual muscle paralysis (difficult to decide at times). At times, patients with unilateral multiple external ocular muscle palsies have a proptotic looking eye due to laxity of the holding muscles.

The patient who has apparent proptosis without increased resistance to retropulsion probably does not harbor an orbital lesion. Increased resistance to retropulsion, however, does not necessarily indicate a mass lesion. TAO, other orbital inflammations, and increased orbital bone formation, often increase the resistance to retropulsion. On the other hand, the absence of increased resistance to retropulsion must make one wonder whether the condition is truly proptosis. Patients with unilateral high myopia may appear proptotic, since the myopic eye has a much greater axial length.

PROPTOSIS WITH LID RETRACTION

On most occasions, the diagnosis here is TAO/GO. In the absence of primary position of ocular misalignment, the upper lid covers the superior limbus by 1–2 mm. If sclera is visible between the superior limbus and the upper lid, the upper lid is retracted. The upper lid may be tardy in following the eyes as they move into downward gaze. This momentary "hung up" of the upper lid

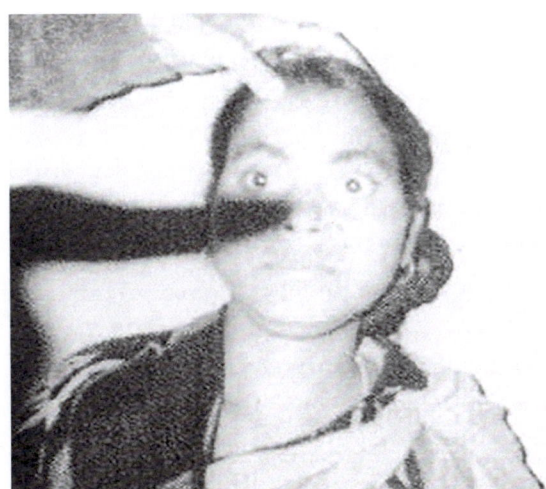

FIG. 1: Illustration of exophthalmos, lid retraction, and lid lag (specially left eye) in a patient of hyperthyroidism.

is termed "lid lag" (Fig. 1). The cause of dysthyroid lid retraction remains unknown. It is believed that retraction is innervational at first but it is cicatricial later. Lid retraction is not related to the state of thyroid function.

Thyroid-associated Ophthalmopathy (Graves' Ophthalmopathy)

Thyroid-associated ophthalmopathy is an immunological disorder where there is increase in orbital volume due to accumulation of glycosaminoglycans and enlargement of the extraocular muscles. Both are due to infiltration of $CD4^+$ T lymphocytes, macrophages, and B-cells and their secretory products and increase in fibroblasts. It has long been known that this is due to sharing of antigens between orbital tissue and thyroid. Other autoantigens [e.g., insulin-like growth factor-1 (IGF-1) receptor, thyroglobulin] have been implicated in the pathogenesis of Graves' orbitopathy. In 90% cases, the disorder is associated with hyperthyroidism but in 10% cases, TAO is associated with hypothyroidism with no previous hyperthyroidism or with the euthyroid state. The disease may be unilateral in 15% of cases. When bilateral, the affection is often asymmetric.

Severe TAO occurs in 3–5% of cases of Graves' disease but mild forms detected by increased intraocular pressure on upgaze has been recorded in 61% cases while orbital computed tomography (CT) can detect it in 70–100% of cases. After an initial report in 1987 that TAO is worsened by smoking, numerous workers have confirmed this phenomenon.

Clinical Assessment

Clinically TAO is evaluated by the "NO SPECS" classification (though not commonly used now) developed by the American Thyroid Association as follows:
- No physical signs or symptoms
- Only signs, no symptoms (upper lid retraction, stare, lid lag, and proptosis to 22 mm)
- Soft tissue involvement (symptoms and signs)
- Proptosis over 22 mm
- Extraocular muscle involvement
- Corneal involvement
- Sight loss.

Objective assessment should also include:
- Documentation of eye fissure width
- Assessment of exposure keratitis with Rose Bengal or fluorescein
- Quantitation of extraocular muscle function with the use of the Hess chart or Maddox rod test
- Measurement of visual acuity, visual fields, and color vision
- Measurement of intraocular pressure on forward and if necessary, upgaze.

Many patients of TAO have mild clinical disease. For example, in the study cohort studied, by Perros et al., 59 out of 101 patients attending a thyroid eye clinic were judged not to require any treatment. After a 5 years follow-up, 15% of these patients deteriorated while 67% improved.

With the passage of time, the active inflammatory process subsides, leaving behind fibrous tissue both in the orbit and within the extraocular muscles. A duration of 18–24 months is most often cited for the inflammatory process though longer duration of disease is often seen.

Management decisions are made on the basis of disease activity and severity. This active phase is best described by the clinical activity score (CAS). The elements are painful feeling behind the globe over last 4 weeks, pain with eye movement during last 4 weeks, redness of the eyelids, redness of the conjunctiva, swelling of the eyelids, chemosis, swollen caruncle, increase in proptosis more than or equal to 2 mm, decreased eye movements more than or equal to 5° in any direction, and decreased visual acuity more than or equal to one line on Snellen chart. The score ranges from 0 to 10 and predicts response to anti-inflammatory therapies. A 7-point scale, lacking the last three elements, is used when no previous assessment is available. GO is considered active in patients with a CAS 3 or more.

As per consensus statement by the European Group on Graves' Orbitopathy, the main gradations of disease severity are mild, moderate-to-severe, and sight threatening. In mild category, immunosuppressive or surgical treatment is usually not needed. In moderate-to-severe, group immunosuppression (if active) or surgical intervention (if inactive) is justifiable. In case of sight-threatening TAO (dysthyroid optic neuropathy and/or corneal breakdown), immediate intervention is necessary.

Orbital scanning with gallium-67 citrate has been used to determine disease activity with more precision and also radiolabeled octreotide (octreoscan) and magnetic resonance imaging (MRI), but these are not practical for routine clinical use. Clinical scoring systems have been devised, but in the final analysis, the assessment of disease activity remains largely confined to the clinical parameters alluded to earlier.

Disease severity is not synonymous with disease activity. For example, a patient may have severe TAO with an inactive disease. Again, there are no set guidelines but most clinicians will consider the following to reach a decision on disease severity:
- Evidence of optic neuropathy
- Evidence of exposure keratitis
- Disabling diplopia especially on downgaze or reading.

Patients are most often concerned with periorbital soft tissue swelling. This is more related to disease activity and vascular congestion than to disease severity.

Management

Simple management measures include elevation of the head end of the bed, wearing tinted glasses and methylcellulose eye drops, and cessation of smoking.

Diuretics are probably not useful and neither are eye drops containing beta-blockers. For mild active disease, recently the European Thyroid Association recommends a 6-month course of selenium (100 mcg twice daily).

In the management of moderate-to-severe active disease, glucocorticoids are the most well-established treatment. These can be used orally, intravenously, or locally either subconjunctival or retrobulbar. Steroids exert the most benefit on optic neuropathy and soft tissue swelling and less so on proptosis and ocular movements. Initial doses are in the range of 40–80 mg per day of prednisolone. After 3 months or so, the dose is generally tapered down and held at the lowest dose, which suppresses disease activity and then stopped. The problem of relapse on stopping steroids is well known. Apart from the usual steroid-associated side effects, early cataract formation is a troublesome sequel.

Methylprednisolone pulses with a cumulative dose of 1–21 g in different studies have been of the most benefit in the patients with greatest disease activity and severity. However, very high intravenous (IV) doses (cumulative doses greater than 8 g) have been seen to induce liver failure and must be avoided. There are various dose regimen of IV methylprednisolone exist like 500 mg for weeks 1–6, then 250 mg for weeks 7–12.

For more severe or progressive cases, initial IV therapy is appropriate. Several recent studies suggest that it is more efficacious and associated with fewer side effects than oral therapy.

Retrobulbar steroids have been tried to reduce the systemic side effects of steroids. In a recent study, 44 patients received orbital cobalt irradiation with retrobulbar methylprednisolone in a dose of 40 mg every 20–30 days for 14 injections. Only 25% had a favorable response compared to 60% in those receiving oral steroids.

Orbital radiotherapy requires a specialized center with high-energy machines. Linear accelerators delivering 4–6 mV are used. Bilateral field settings delivering 20 Gy per eye given in 2 Gy doses over 2 weeks are usually administered. There may be a transient worsening of the ophthalmopathy. The benefits are similar to the benefits of steroids and in fact radiation is steroid sparing. Concerns exist with regard to cataract formation, radiation retinopathy, and future carcinogenic potential. This form of therapy has hardly been used in India.

Orbital decompression surgery aims at increasing the space within the bony orbit by removal of one or more walls of the orbit. Most current data are on the transantral approach, which leaves no external scar and very effectively decompresses the apex of the orbit (which is the site of optic nerve compression). Garrity from Mayo Clinic published data on 453 eyes, where 89% improved their visual acuity, 91% improved their visual fields, 94% improved papilledema, and 92% improved exposure keratitis. Complications were sinusitis (4%), lower lid entropion (9%), numb lip (5%), cerebrospinal fluid (CSF) leakage (3.5%), and frontal lobe hematoma in one patient. The major problem is new onset of diplopia after the procedure, which can affect up to two-thirds of patients and has medicolegal consequences. Once fibrosis of the extraocular muscles sets in, further, surgery can of course be done to correct diplopia.

Other treatment modalities have been tried. Particularly, if high-dose glucocorticoid therapy is contraindicated or ineffective, options include rituximab, mycophenolate mofetil, etc. Rituximab, an anti-B-cell monoclonal antibody, has been reported to be as effective as glucocorticoids.

Rituximab induces a fall in thyrotropin receptor antibody (TRAb) levels and depletion of B-cells in the retro-orbital tissues. Current regimen of two infusions of 1 g each may be effective in TAO and allow immunosuppression to be avoided.

Other trials are ongoing to assess the efficacy of future treatment like tocilizumab (an interleukin-6 antibody), and teprotumumab (an IGF-1 receptor antibody).

Most are uncontrolled studies on small numbers of patients. Two randomized controlled studies have been done with cyclosporine and both showed a good response. There is a small study on the use of intravenous immunoglobulins (IVIGs) where 34 patients were randomized with 76% responding to IVIG and 66% responding to steroids. A list of the other treatments studied so far is given here. There is no data to suggest that any of these treatments are superior to the standard treatments available. The list includes:
- Plasmapheresis
- Azathioprine
- Colchicine
- Octreotide and lanreotide
- Bromocriptine
- Acupuncture.

Treatment of associated hyperthyroidism is an important part of the treatment for eye disease. In general, the greater the hyperthyroidism, the worse is the eye disease.

Treatment with methimazole (carbimazole, more commonly used in India, is a precursor) does not seem to affect progression of eye disease, but it may decrease eyelid retraction and stare. Also, if hypothyroidism develop during the course of therapy, it may have an adverse effect on the orbitopathy. Therefore, during and after treatment of hyperthyroidism, patients require strict monitoring. On the other hand, ablation of the thyroid with I is associated with a worsening of the eye disease in 15% cases. This, however, is temporary and can be tide over by the use of steroids. Surgery of the thyroid also does not seem to affect progression of eye disease, although some studies have demonstrated a benefit of total (as opposed to subtotal) thyroidectomy.

There is a well-known association between GO and myasthenia gravis. Treatment of the former has been known to relieve symptoms of the latter in two-thirds of the patients. In some cases, thymectomy can favorably affect both the diseases. Ocular myasthenia can coexist with thyroid ophthalmopathy in the same patient.

LID RETRACTION NOT PRESENT

Proptosis in the absence of lid retraction is unlikely to be caused by GO. Orbital imaging is the appropriate next step. CT and MRI of orbits are complimentary technologies, each having advantages. When detail of bony structures of orbit is needed, CT is certainly preferable. Contrast studies are often required. The imaging study would reveal whether an orbital mass lesion is present or not causing the proptosis.

Orbital Mass Lesions Causing Proptosis

Cavernous hemangioma, among the most common of orbital tumors, may occur anywhere in the orbit but has an affinity for the intraconal space. Cavernous hemangiomas are found mainly in adults and enlarge slowly over a period of many years. A well-encapsulated mass that enhances markedly after IV contrast injection on MRI is characteristic of these lesions. Hemangiomas usually produce an MRI picture of a well-circumscribed mass that is isointense to muscle on T1-weighted images. Regions of high intensity on T2-weighted images probably represent thrombosis. While proptosis is usually the only sign, at times optic nerve compression with visual loss can result if the mass is expanding or compressing the optic nerve. Complete surgical excision of hemangiomas within their capsule is the treatment of choice in these circumstances. Other well-circumscribed lesions indistinguishable from cavernous hemangiomas on imaging include schwannomas, fibrous histiocytomas, neurofibromas, and hemangiopericytomas.

Venous anomalies (varices, lymphangiomas) can also cause proptosis. Some patients experience increased proptosis during the Valsalva maneuver or when bending forward. Bleeding from orbital varices and lymphangiomas may produce painful proptosis, sometimes associated with subconjunctival hemorrhage. On imaging, venous anomalies are usually distinctive enough to establish the diagnosis because of the specific imaging characteristics of blood. The imaging pattern varies with flowing blood or thrombosis. Should bleeding occur, the imaging pattern varies with the age of thrombus. Surgical removal of a venous anomaly is seldom necessary (and usually not possible).

Optic nerve sheath meningiomas produce proptosis and progressive visual loss over a period of months to years. In a review of 22 patients with optic nerve meningiomas, 17 patients (77%) had visual loss. Transient visual obscurations were noted in five patients (23%), but other ophthalmic symptoms, including proptosis, were infrequent. The optic disk appearance included disk elevation in 13 patients (59%) and atrophy in nine patients (41%). Optociliary shunt vessels were detected in five patients (23%).

Enlargement of the optic nerve with increased density peripherally and decreased density centrally (tram-track sign) is the characteristic CT finding of an optic nerve sheath meningioma. But diffuse enlargement of the optic nerve signal, at times with angulation, is also found. The meningioma may involve the entire intraorbital optic nerve or any portion thereof. Two advantages of MRI over CT are the ability to visualize the tumor's extent through the optic canal, and the ability to detect the tumor with gadolinium diethylenetriaminepentaacetic acid.

The management principles of optic nerve sheath meningiomas can be summarized as follows:
- If the patient has adequate vision or if progressive visual loss has been documented, consider three-dimensional conformal radiation of the lesion
- If patient elects no treatment, follow-up imaging (MR) studies to be done at 6 months interval
- If expansion of an intracranial component is documented, consider surgical debulking or radiation.

Enlargement of an optic nerve on CT in a child is more likely to be caused by a glioma than a meningioma. Other stigmata of neurofibromatosis should be sought. Treatment of optic nerve gliomas continues to be a subject of much controversy. Some who consider these tumors to be benign hamartomas have suggested observation alone. Others, who view these lesions as potentially more aggressive, suggest complete surgical removal to prevent extension to the optic chiasm. Primary radiation after age 5 years and chemotherapy in children of all ages are viable treatment options. Observation in lieu of treatment is acceptable as long as the visual loss is not severe or progressive. No treatment has ever been properly tested in a randomized trial. Optic pathway gliomas are also discussed in Chapter 11 : Chiasmal Disorders

Metastatic tumor causing proptosis may be the first sign of cancer. Histologic verification that the lesion is producing proptosis is advisable before treatment is begun, since other causes of proptosis are possible. In certain patients, fine-needle aspiration biopsy of orbital tumors is an alternative to biopsy through an orbitotomy.

The most common orbital metastases derive from breast (42%), lung (11%), or prostate (8.3%). Enophthalmos (and not proptosis) may be produced when scirrhous breast carcinoma metastasizes to the orbit.

In children, metastatic neuroblastoma in the orbit may produce rapidly progressive proptosis.

Both orbits are involved in as many as 50% of patients, and frequently, radiographic evidence of metastasis to the bones of the skull is found. Only 5% of neuroblastoma patients initially present with orbital signs, however.

Orbital Mass Lesions Not Detected

When imaging of the patient with proptosis fails to disclose an orbital mass, the examiner must consider a variety of nontumorous causes. The most common is idiopathic orbital inflammation (orbital pseudotumor). Others include, nonidiopathic orbital inflammations due to sarcoidosis, Wegener's granulomatosis, syphilis, tuberculosis, and collagen vascular diseases. Other causes of proptosis include lymphoproliferative disorders, orbital cellulitis, carotid-cavernous fistula, orbital trauma, spontaneous orbital hemorrhage, and orbital dysplasia.

Orbital Pseudotumor

Orbital pseudotumor or idiopathic orbital inflammation may involve any orbital structure—sclera (posterior scleritis), lacrimal gland (dacryoadenitis), and classically extraocular muscle (myositis). Some authorities would include Tolosa–Hunt syndrome in this category on the ground that this may be due to an inflammatory disorder of the superior orbital fissure or cavernous sinus.

Distinguishing between orbital pseudotumor and orbital lymphoproliferative disorders (including lymphoma) may be difficult. Orbital pseudotumor presents with relatively acute periocular pain, whereas lymphoproliferative disorders are typically painless and their development more indolent. Histopathologically, orbital pseudotumor consists of a mixed cellular infiltrate including lymphocytes, neutrophils, and eosinophils. Monotonous sheets of lymphocytes are more typical of the lymphoproliferative disorders.

The imaging pattern of orbital pseudotumor varies with the orbital region that is preferentially affected. In one study, the CT characteristics of 21 patients with the clinical diagnosis of orbital pseudotumor included contrast enhancement (prevalence 95%), retrobulbar fatty infiltration (76%), proptosis (71%), extraocular muscle enlargement (57%), apical fat edema (48%), muscle tendon sheath involvement (43%), optic nerve thickening (38%), and uveoscleral thickening (33%). While extraocular muscle enlargement may resemble that of GO, myositis generally involves the area of the tendinous insertion to the globe, and Graves' myopathy usually spares this region. Orbital pseudotumor is also more likely to be unilateral. The paranasal sinuses are rarely abnormal in patients who have orbital pseudotumor.

Magnetic resonance imaging may be useful to further distinguish orbital pseudotumor from more invasive lesions. Using surface coil MRI in patients with orbital pseudotumor, the lesions were found to be hypointense to fat and isointense to muscle on T1-weighted images. On T2-weighted images, the lesions were isointense or only minimally hyperintense to fat. Orbital metastases instead appeared markedly hyperintense relative to fat on T2-weighted images.

The investigation of the patient with signs of noninfectious orbital inflammation includes ruling out underlying systemic disease. A complete blood count (CBC) and erythrocyte sedimentation rate (ESR), Venereal Disease Research Laboratory (VDRL)-rapid plasma reagin (RPR), urinalysis, SMA-12, cytoplasmic antineutrophil cytoplasmic antibody (c-ANCA), angiotensin-converting enzyme level, and chest plain films should be performed.

Patients with pseudotumor, who do not have any evidence of an underlying systemic disease, should receive a course of oral prednisolone (60–80 mg/day). The response is often striking; the prednisolone may be continued for few days and then gradually tapered, and the patient maintained on a suitably tolerated dose. A lesion that does not resolve dramatically is probably not a pseudotumor and orbital biopsy should be considered.

Orbital Cellulitis

Proptosis, periorbital swelling, and ophthalmoplegia in a febrile patient suggest orbital cellulitis. The presence of ophthalmoplegia implies postseptal orbital involvement by the infection, whereas periocular edema alone suggests that the infection likely is limited to the preseptal area.

Most patients have contiguous sinus disease, with the ethmoid sinus involved most often, especially in young patients. The maxillary and frontal sinuses are less often affected, although pansinusitis is not unusual.

Any diabetic or immunocompromised patient who develops signs of orbital inflammation should be considered to have orbital mucormycosis until another cause is identified. Diabetic patients need not to be in ketoacidosis. The nonseptate hyphae of mucormycosis cause obliterative arteritis with necrotic lesions in the orbit and nasal cavity. Paranasal sinus involvement is universal but initially may present only as subtle mucosal thickening on imaging. If mucormycosis is suspected, a complete nasal examination should be performed to detect the typical black eschars. Their absence, however, does not exclude mucormycosis, since the eschars appear later in the course of the disease. Reports link the appearance of mucormycosis with deferoxamine, a drug used to treat iron or aluminum excess. Although, most of these patients have developed systemic (not orbital) mucormycosis, any patient under deferoxamine treatment who develops orbital signs should be investigated for orbital mucormycosis.

Management principles include: early diagnosis with biopsy, correction of underlying metabolic disorder, aggressive local treatment with excision and debridement of devitalized oral, nasal, sinus, and orbital tissue, and administration of systemic amphotericin B (or its lyophilized form) in adequate doses.

Carotid-cavernous Fistula

Proptosis associated with chronic conjunctival injection and an audible bruit is highly suggestive of carotid-cavernous fistula. Review of three studies shows the relative frequency of these and other signs and symptoms of carotid fistula.

Arterialization of conjunctival veins, which appear as corkscrew vessels that go to the limbus, is the response to sustained arterial blood flow directly into venous channels. The intraocular pressure may be elevated as a result of the increased episcleral venous pressure. "Machine-like" bruits, synchronous with the pulse, may be detected with a stethoscope placed over the patient's eye or temporal area.

Risk of visual loss is variable. Six potential causes of visual loss with carotid-cavernous fistulas have been reported:
1. Glaucoma due either to increased episcleral venous pressure or rarely to iris neovascularization
2. Anterior segment ischemia
3. Corneal decompensation from exposure
4. Maculopathy: Cystoid macular edema, hemorrhage in the macula, or macular ischemia
5. Retinal artery occlusion
6. Optic nerve ischemia.

Refinements in cerebral angiography have resulted in the reclassification of fistulas according to the velocity of blood flow through the shunt (low-flow and high-flow) and the anatomic origin of the arteries supplying the fistula. Fistulas may be spontaneous or traumatic: type A is usually traumatic; types B, C, and D are actually AVMs that develop spontaneously into fistulas. Ocular signs are usually ipsilateral to the fistula, but because of ample venous communication between the two cavernous sinuses, bilateral signs may appear with unilateral fistula, and rarely, the ocular manifestations may be contralateral to the fistula.

Spontaneous resolution of these fistulas may occur. Low-flow fistulas resolve spontaneously in some 30–50% of patients, whereas high-flow carotid-cavernous fistulas resolve spontaneously in fewer than 5%. Imaging may assist in correctly identifying a fistula as the cause of patient's signs or symptoms. The most consistent sign is enlargement of the superior ophthalmic vein. However, this sign can also be associated with orbital pseudotumor, cavernous meningioma, and GO. Color Doppler ultrasonography of the orbit may assist in identifying a fistula as the cause of an enlarged superior ophthalmic vein. Blood flow characteristic of arterial instead of venous circulation in the enlarged superior ophthalmic vein is compelling evidence of a fistula. Enlargement of the extraocular muscles similar to that of GO also may be found, owing to venous congestion of the extraocular muscles. The definitive diagnosis of carotid-cavernous fistula is made by selective arteriography. Intra-arterial angiography with selective catheterization is needed to detect all fistulous communications before treatment may be attempted.

Several sophisticated methods are available for closing a carotid-cavernous fistula while preserving carotid patency. For direct (type A) fistulas, detachable balloons may be introduced endoarterially through the internal carotid artery or endovenously through the inferior petrosal sinus or the superior ophthalmic vein. Successful occlusion of the fistula with retention of internal carotid artery patency is the goal of treatment. Injection of isobutyl cyanoacrylate (glue) or particles of polyvinyl alcohol foam, or the insertion of steel coils is the treatment for slow-flow dural (types B–D) fistulas. Thrombogenic needles or wires also may be introduced into the cavernous sinus through a temporal craniotomy. Direct surgical repair of a fistula is technically difficult and fraught with complications. Cerebral and ocular ischemia can result from any of these treatment attempts.

SUGGESTED READINGS

1. Atlas SW, Grossman RI, Savino PJ, et al. Surface-coil MR of orbital pseudotumor. AJR Am J Roentgenol. 1987;148:803-8.
2. Atlas SW. Magnetic resonance imaging of the orbit: Current status. Magn Reson. 1989;5:39-96.
3. Auerbach DB, Bilyk JR, Miller NR, et al. Lung cancer, proptosis, and decreased vision. Sun Ophthalmol. 1999;43:405-12.
4. Barrow DL, Spector RH, Braun IF, et al. Classification and treatment of spontaneous carotid-cavernous sinus fistulas. J Neurosurg. 1985;62:248-56.
5. Bartalena L, Baldeschi L, Boboridis K, et al. The 2016 European Thyroid Association/European Group on Graves' Orbitopathy Guidelines for the Management of Graves' Orbitopathy. Eur Thyroid J. 2016;5:9-26.
6. Bartalena L, Baldeschi L, Dickinson AJ, et al. Consensus statement of the European group on Graves' orbitopathy (EUGOGO) on management of Graves' orbitopathy. Thyroid. 2008;18:333-46.
7. Bartalena L, Maococci C, Bogazzi F, et al. Relation between therapy for hyperthyroidism and the course of Graves' ophthalmopathy. N Engl J Med. 1998;338:73-8.
8. Bartalena L, Pinchera A, Marcocci C. Management of Graves' ophthalmopathy: reality and perspectives. Endocr Rev. 2000;21:168-99.
9. Baschieri L, Antonelli A, Nardi S, et al. Intravenous immunoglobulin vs. corticosteroid in treatment of Graves' ophthalmopathy. Thyroid. 1997;7:579-85.
10. Boelaert JR, Fenves AZ, Coburn JW. Mucormycosis among patients on dialysis. N Engl J Med. 1989;321:190-1.
11. Burch HB, Wartofsky L. Graves' ophthalmopathy: current concepts regarding pathogenesis and management. Endocr Rev. 1995;14:747-93.
12. Char DH. Thyroid eye disease. Br J Ophthalmol. 1996;80:922-6.
13. Chavis RM, Garner A, Wright JE. Inflammatory orbital pseudotumor: A clinicopathologic study. Arch Ophthalmol. 1978;96:1817-22.
14. Costa VP, Molnar LJ, Cerri GG. Diagnosing and monitoring carotid cavernous fistulas with color Doppler imaging. J Clin Ultrasound. 1997;25:448-52.
15. Daly AL, Velazquez LA, Bradley SF, et al. Mucormycosis: Association with deferoxamine therapy. Am J Med. 1989;87:468-71.
16. Debrun GM, Vinuel F, Fox AJ, et al. Indications for treatment and classification of 132 carotid-cavernous fistulas. Neurosurgery. 1988;22:285-9.
17. Derang J, Huang Y, Long Y, et al. Treatment of carotid-cavernous sinus fistulas retrograde via the superior ophthalmic vein (SOV). Surg Neurol. 1999;52:286-93.
18. Dolene V. Direct microsurgical repair of intracavernous vascular lesions. J Neurosurg. 1983;58:824-31.
19. Eshaghian J, Anderson RL. Sinus involvement in inflammatory orbital pseudotumor. Arch Ophthalmol. 1981;99:627-30.
20. Fladers AE, Mafee MF, Rao VM, et al. CT characteristics of orbital pseudotumors and other orbital inflammatory processes. Comput Assist Tomogr. 1989;13:40-7.
21. Flaharty PM, Lieb WE, Sergott RC, et al. Color Doppler imaging: A new noninvasive technique to diagnose and monitor carotid cavernous fistulas. Arch Ophthalmol. 1991;9:522-6.
22. Forbes G, Gorman CA, Brenan MD, et al. Ophthalmopathy of Graves' disease: computerized volume measurements of the orbital fat and muscle. Am J Neuroradiol. 1986;7:651-6.
23. Gamba JL, Woodruff WW, Djang WT, et al. Craniofacial mucormycosis: Assessment with CT. Radiology. 1986;160:207-12.
24. Gamblin GT, Harper DG, Galantine P, et al. Graves' disease: evidence of frequent subclinical ophthalmopathy. N Engl J Med. 1983;308:420-24.
25. Garrity JA. Fatourechi V, Bergtralh EJ, et al. Results of transantral orbital decompression in 428 patients with severe Graves' ophthalmopathy. Am J Ophthalmol. 1993;116:533-47.
26. Goldberg RA, Rootman J. Clinical characteristics of metastatic orbital tumors. Ophthalmology. 1990;97:620-4.
27. Hagg E, Aspland K. Is endocrine ophthalmopathy made worse by smoking? Brit Med J. 1987;295:634-5.
28. Heufelder AE. Pathogenesis of Graves' ophthalmopathy: recent controversies and progress. Eur J Endocrinol. 1995;132:532-41.
29. Hoyt WF, Baghdassarian SA. Optic glioma of childhood: Natural history and rationale for consecutive management. Br J Ophthalmol. 1969;53:793-8.
30. Kahaly G, Diaz M, Hahn K, et al. Indium 111-pentreotide scintigraphy in Graves' ophthalmopathy. J Nucl Med. 1995;36:550-4.

31. Kahaly G, Schrezenmeir J, Krause U, et al. Ciclosporin and prednisone v. prednisone in treatment of Graves' ophthalmopathy: a controlled, randomized and prospective study. Eur J Clin Invest. 1986;16:415-22.
32. Kohn R, Hepler R. Management of limited rhino-orbital mucormycosis without exenteration. Ophthalmology. 1985;92:1440-4.
33. Konuk O, Atasever T, Unal M, et al. Orbital gallium 67 scintigraphy in Graves' ophthalmopathy. Thyroid. 2002;12:603-8.
34. Krieger CC, Neumann S, Place RF, et al. Bidirectional TSH and IGF-1 receptor crosstalk mediates stimulation of hyaluronan secretion by Graves' disease immunoglobins. J Clin Endocrinol Metab. 2015;100:1071-7.
35. Kupersmith MJ, Berenstein A, Flamn E, et al. Neuro-ophthalmologic abnormalities and intravascular therapy of traumatic carotid cavernous fistulas. Ophthalmology. 1986;93:906-12.
36. Marcocci C, Bartalena L, Bogazzi F, et al. Orbital radiotherapy combined with high dose systemic glucocorticoids for Graves' ophthalmopathy is more effective than orbital radiotherapy alone: results of a prospective study. J Endocrinol Invest. 1991;14:853-60.
37. Marcucci C, Bartalena L, Panicucci M, et al. Orbital cobalt irradiation combined with retrobulbar or systemic corticosteroids in Graves' ophthalmopathy: a comparative study. Clin Endocrinol (Oxf). 1987;27:33-42.
38. Marino M, Ricciardi R, Pinches A. Mild clinical expression of myasthenia gravis associated with autoimmune thyroid disease. J Clin Endocrinol Metab. 1997;82:438-43.
39. Mori S, Yoshikawa N, Horimoto M, et al. Thyroid stimulating antibody in sera of Graves' ophthalmopathy patients as a possible marker for predicting the efficacy of methylprednisolone pulse therapy. Endocr J. 1995;42:442-8.
40. Mossein LH, Debrun GM, Miller NR, et al. Treatment of carotid-cavernous fistulas via the superior ophthalmic vein. Am J Neuroradiol. 1991;12:435-9.
41. Mottow-Lippa L, Jakobiec FA, Smith M. Idiopathic inflammatory orbital pseudotumor in childhood. II. Results of diagnostic test and biopsies. Ophthalmology. 1981;88:565-74.
42. Mourits MP, Koornneef L, Wiersinga WM, et al. Clinical criteria for the assessment of disease activity in Graves' ophthalmopathy: a novel approach. Br J Ophthalmol. 1989;73:639-44.
43. Mourits MP, Prummel MF, Wiersinga WM, et al. Clinical activity score as a guide in the management of patients with Graves' ophthalmopathy. Clin Endocrinol (Oxf). 1997;47:9-14.
44. Mullan S. Treatment of carotid-cavernous fistulas by cavernous sinus occlusion. J Neurosurg. 1979;50:131-44.
45. Packer RJ, Lange B, Ater J, et al. Carboplatin and vincristine for progressive low-grade gliomas of childhood. J Clin Oncol. 1992;11:850-7.
46. Packer RJ, Lange B, Ater J, et al. Carboplatin and Vincristine for progressive low-grade gliomas of childhood. J Clin Oncol' 1992;11:850-857
47. Packer RJ, Savino PJ, Bilaniuk LT, et al. Chiasmatic gliomas of childhood: A reappraisal of natural history and effectiveness of cranial irradiation. Childs Brain. 1983;10:393-402.
48. Palestine AG, Younger BR, Piepgras DG. Visual prognosis in carotid-cavernous fistula. Arch Ophthalmol. 1981;99:1600-3.
49. Parkinson D, Downs AR, Whytehead LL, et al. Carotid cavernous fistula: direct repair with preservation of carotid. Surgery. 1974;76:882-9.
50. Perros P, Crombie AL, Kendall-Taylor P. Natural history of thyroid-associated ophthalmopathy. Clin Endocrinol (Oxf). 1995;42:45-50.
51. Perros P, Crombie AL, Matthews JN, et al. Age and gender influence the severity of thyroid-associated ophthalmopathy: a study of 101 patients attending a combined thyroid-eye clinic. Clin Endocrinol (Oxf). 1993;38:367-72.
52. Peyster RG, Savino PI, Hoover ED, et al. Differential diagnosis of the enlarged superior ophthalmic vein. J Comput Assist Tomogr. 1984;8:103-7.
53. Phelps CD, Thompson HS, Ossoinlg KO. The diagnosis and prognosis of atypical carotid-cavernous fistula (red-eyed shunt syndrome). Am J Ophthalmol. 1982;23:423-36.
54. Prummel MF, Wiersinga WM, Mourits MP, et al. Effect of abnormal thyroid function test on the severity of Graves' ophthalmopathy. Arch Intern Med. 1990;2:171-8.
55. Salvi M, Vannucchi G, Campi I, et al. Efficacy of rituximab treatment for thyroid-associated ophthalmopathy as a result of intraorbital B-cell depletion in one patient unresponsive to steroid immunosuppression. Eur J Endocrinol. 2006;154:511-7.
56. Sanders MD, Hoyt WF. Hypoxic ocular sequelae of carotid-cavernous fistulas. Study of the causes of visual failure before and after neurosurgical treatment in a series of 25 cases. Br J Ophthalmol. 1969;53:82-97.
57. Sibony PA, Krauss HR, Kennerdell JS, et al. Optic nerve sheath meningiomas: Clinical manifestations. Ophthalmology. 1984;91:1313-26.
58. Sridama V, DeGroot LJ. Treatment of Graves' disease and the course of ophthalmopathy. Am J Med. 1989;87:70-3.
59. Stiebel-Kalish H, Robenshtok E, Hasanreisoglu M, et al. Treatment modalities for Graves' ophthalmopathy: systematic review and meta-analysis. J Clin Endocrinol Metab. 2009;94:2708-16.
60. Teng MM, Guo WY, Huang CL, et al. Occlusion of arteriovenous malformations of the cavernous sinus via the superior ophthalmic vein. Am J Neuroradiol. 1988;9:539-46.
61. Trokel SL, Jakobiec FA. Correlation of CT scanning and pathologic features of ophthalmic Graves' disease. Ophthalmology. 1981;88:553-64.

62. Van Johnson E, Kline LB, Julian BA, et al. Bilateral cavernous sinus thrombosis due to mucormycosis. Arch Ophthalmol. 1988;106:1089-92.
63. Wartofsky L. Classification of eye changes of Graves' disease. Thyroid. 1992;3:235-6.
64. Wiersinga WM, Prummel MF. Retrobulbar irradiation in Graves' ophthalmopathy. Clin Endocrinol Metab. 1995;80:345-7.
65. Wiersinga WM. Advances in treatment of active, moderate-to-severe Graves' ophthalmopathy. Lancet Diabetes Endocrinol. 2017;5:134-42.
66. Wiersinga WS. Immunosuppressive treatment of Graves' ophthalmopathy. Trends Endocrinol Metab. 1990;1:377-81.
67. Wright JE, Sullivan TJ, Garner A, et al. Orbital venous anomalies. Ophthalmology. 1997;104:905-13.
68. Yaman A, Yaman H. Ocular myasthenia gravis coincident with thyroid ophthalmopathy. Neurol India. 2003;51:100-1.
69. Yokoyama N, Nagataki S, Uetani M, et al. Role of magnetic resonance imaging in the assessment of thyroid-associated ophthalmopathy. Thyroid. 2002;12:223-7.
70. Zimmerman CF, Shatz NJ, Glaser JS. Magnetic resonance imaging of optic nerve meningiomas: Enhancement with gadolinium-DTPA. Ophthalmology. 1990;97:585-91.

20 Psychogenic Neuro-Ophthalmologic Disorders

Ambar Chakravarty

INTRODUCTION

Nearly every symptom and sign described in this book has one time or other been a contrivance, a creation of psychogenic illness. Somatic manifestations of psychogenic origin are however prevalent in all fields of medicine. In contrast to these, visual loss is an apt expression of a psychogenic disorder because it shields disturbing persons from view, evokes sympathy and precludes the performance of unpleasant duties. At the same time, it is less debilitating than many other disturbances (e.g., psychogenic seizures, paralysis, etc.) and is difficult for the physician to expose.

Psychogenic disturbances are caused by psychiatric or behavioral disorders rather than structural or biochemical abnormalities. These are different from psychosomatic disturbances and should not be termed "functional" because it may suggest that something is functioning. Both hysterical and malingered defects may be encountered and the distinction need to be made and underlying psychopathology delineated.

The principal ophthalmic manifestations of psychogenic origin are persistent visual acuity loss (VAL)[7] and visual field loss (VFL). Others include transient visual loss, visual illusions and hallucinations, and hypersensitivity or aversion to light, geometric patterns, bright colors, or moving objects.

Principal nonvisual manifestations of psychogenic origin include spasm of the near reflex, gaze deviations, paralysis of eye movements, convergence insufficiency, voluntary nystagmus, pseudoptosis due to blepharospasm, pharmacologically dilated pupils, and pain syndromes of the periocular region.

This chapter would principally concentrate on evaluation of VA and field loss of psychogenic origin.

PERSISTENT VISUAL ACUITY LOSS

Persistent psychogenic VAL takes three different forms: (i) monocular acuity loss, (ii) mild binocular acuity loss, and (iii) severe binocular acuity loss verging on total blindness. Three strategies are available for dealing with such patients.

Strategy 1: Getting the Patient to Report Normal Visual Acuity without Realizing

This strategy is satisfying because it provides direct evidence of feigned visual loss. It works best in cases of monocular VAL. The patient must be suggestible and naive enough to believe that the acuity in the "good eye" is being tested.

Strategy 2: Demonstrating Inconsistency between Subjective Test Results

The examiner must show that performance on nonacuity tests is incompatible with depressed VA. Unlike strategy 1, this strategy provides only indirect evidence, but it is superior in that the patient does not appreciate the relationship between VA and these other tests.

Strategy 3: Using Objective Tests to Invalidate Subjective Responses

The swinging-light pupil test, electroretinography (ERG), and visual evoked potentials (VEPs) are used to refute evidence gained from subjective tests. Unfortunately, each objective test has limitations. The swinging-light pupil test is useful only when monocular or asymmetric visual loss is in question. Standard ERG is insensitive to disease confined to the fovea. The VEP can be deformed by deliberate "defocusing."

These three strategies are deployed according to the pattern of visual loss.

SUBNORMAL VISUAL ACUITY IN ONE EYE

Fogging

While acuity testing with both eyes viewing the chart, covertly place before the "normal" eye a high convex or astigmatic lens, which blurs the image for that eye. The patient will continue to read with the 'blind' eye. This does not work if the patient closes only one eye at a time.

Duochrome Test

Place a red spectacle over one eye, a green spectacle over the other, and instruct the patient to view a special screen designed to make some letters invisible to the right eye and other invisible to the left eye.

Pupil-Splitting Prism Test

Use a finger to block the vision in the eye with the alleged poor vision. Place a 5-diopter prism base down so that it splits the pupil of the normal eye. Ask whether the patient sees two Snellen charts with the "good eye" (the pupil-splitting prism should create monocular diplopia). Tell the patient to begin reading the letters from the bottom chart. Once the patient has begun reading, simultaneously slide the prism down so that its midportion is centered on the pupil; then remove your finger from in front of the "bad" eye. The patient should be concentrating on reading the letters, and will not notice that the bottom chart is now being viewed only by the "bad" eye.

Pupillary Reactions

Asymmetric optic neuropathy can readily be excluded by finding normal pupillary reactions with the swinging-light pupil test. Subtle afferent pupil defects; however, can easily be overlooked if technique is faulty, and bilateral optic neuropathy with asymmetric VAL can lead to false-negative conclusions. Moreover, normal pupillary reactions do not exclude either a foveal cause of monocular visual loss or amblyopia.

Ophthalmoscopy

Examine the foveal region and optic disc for structural abnormalities to rule out many causes of subnormal acuity, bearing in mind that some rare conditions produce little or no structural alteration. Fluorescein angiography and ERG may be useful in the diagnosis of these cases, but should be reserved for instances when skilled, high-magnification ophthalmoscopy has failed to disclose a diagnostic structural abnormality.

Base-out Prism Test

Instruct the patient to fixate the 20/20 distant Snellen letter, and introduce a 5-diopter base-out prism over the "bad" eye. Observe for inward deviation of that eye, a response to be expected if that eye is foveating. Then remove the prism and observe for the expected outward refixational movement of that same eye. When these refixation movements occur, a substantial central scotoma in the "bad" eye is ruled out; VA must be at least 20/50.

Subnormal Visual Acuity in Both Eyes

For patients who claim severe vision loss, a combination of strategy 2 and strategy 3 must be used. Among the cruder techniques in strategy 2 are the following:

Threat

Briskly wave your hand towards the patient's eyes, as if to strike them, being sure to avoid creating an air current on the cornea. An appropriately timed blink suggests at least some vision, though it may be rudimentary.

Mirror Movement

A mirror large enough to fill the patient's central field is held at a distance of about 6 inches from the eyes and rotated side-to-side. Seeing the reflected image of the eyes provokes an irresistible urge to move the eyes.

Optokinetic Stimulus

Rotate an optokinetic drum or black and white measuring tape at a distance of 6 inches from the patient's eyes and observe for nystagmus. Again, only rudimentary vision is necessary to mount this reflex response.

Ambulation

Patients with severe organic VAL and preserved peripheral vision do not bump into door frames, furniture, or other obstacles. If they have lost both acuity and field, they have learned to lead with their hands, take short steps, and walk cautiously. Patients with psychogenic VAL lurch forward and go out of their way to collide with obstacles, miraculously avoiding serious harm to themselves. This phenomenon can be demonstrated in an obstacle course of the examiner's devising.

Proprioceptively Mediated Tasks

If proprioception is intact, organically blind patients should be able to bring their outstretched fingers toward one another and have them touch. They should also be able to sign their names legibly.

When strategy 2 maneuvers do not work, turn to the objective tests of strategy 3:
1. Swinging-light Pupil Test: With proper technique, this test is extraordinarily sensitive to asymmetric optic nerve disease, but does not detect symmetric optic neuropathies, most retinopathies, and retrogeniculate disorders
2. Visual evoked potentials: If the VEPs are normal, yet the patient claims very poor acuity, the test has worked. However, there are pitfalls. Despite attempts at monitoring fixation, fakers manage to defocus or look away from the target enough to degrade the signal. VEPs have often been perfectly intact in blind patients despite anatomic evidence of destruction of extrastriate visual cortex. These tests evidently sample only a part of the pathway needed for seeing
3. Electroretinography: It is a valuable tool for detecting widespread retinopathies that do not produce ophthalmoscopic abnormalities, such as paraneoplastic retinopathy. However, the standard ERG is insensitive to inner retinal and focal outer retinal disorders. The multifocal ERG may offer greater sensitivity to the diagnosis of the latter.

PERSISTENT VISUAL FIELD LOSS

A determined subject can fake any visual field defect under any testing method, but some defects are easier to fake than others. Central scotoma is a challenge, but hemianopia, quadrant anopia, and altitudinal defects are relatively easy to fake, particularly on the most commonly used automated instrument, the Humphrey Field Analyzer (HFA).

Faking field loss on the HFA is easy. Its testing strategy is based on the patient's threshold visual sensitivity to targets displayed in each field quadrant at the beginning of the test. Thus, if the initial bright stimulus is not detected in a given quadrant, all subsequent stimuli displayed in that quadrant will be bright, allowing the patient to differentiate them from stimuli displayed in other quadrants, where initial sensitivity may have been higher. Do not be surprised if the "reliability indices" look perfectly normal.

Can kinetic perimetry, performed with skill, "smoke-out" deceptions produced on automated perimeters? Not reliably; when six subjects were instructed to fake on Humphrey and Goldmann perimeters, even the most practiced kinetic perimetrists mapped counterfeit defects. In fact, the more experienced perimetrists unwittingly gave the subjects cues that aided in the deceptions.

The techniques used to identify psychogenic VFL are deployed in accordance with the pattern of the VFL, as follows:

Visual Field Constriction

The most common pattern of psychogenic VFL is one whose peripheral borders are so contracted that only a peephole is left in the center. The two common organic causes of this pattern of VFL- diffuse outer retinal disorders and optic neuropathies should produce structural changes apparent on ophthalmoscopy. There is a third organic cause that does not produce ophthalmoscopic changes—bilateral visual cortex disorders with macular sparing. Given the absence of ophthalmoscopic abnormalities, making this diagnosis may be difficult. However, the psychogenic nature of constricted fields usually becomes apparent with skilled use of one or more of the following techniques:

Testing at two distances

By finger confrontation, establish the limits of the visual field at l/3 m and at 1 or 2 m distances from the patient. If the field constriction is organic, the borders will markedly expand (funnel field). If the defect is psychogenic, the field borders wall not expand (tunnel field).

Persuading the Patient hat This is Not a Visual Field Test

Tell the patient that the finger confrontation test is a measure of response latency, that is, "the speed of your reflexes". Start displaying fingers well within the central peephole. Once the patient is lulled into responding, begin displaying fingers further and further from center. Psychogenic field constriction gradually widens to normal.

Demonstrating That the Retained Field Perimeter is Not Stable

Display two vertically oriented fingers, one within the previously acknowledged border, the other outside it. If the patient identifies only one finger, display the two fingers in the horizontal plane with fingertips inside the acknowledged border. A faker will steadfastly report seeing only one finger.

Using Distracting Verbal Cues

Tell the patient that you will cue each presentation by asking "Do you see it now?" and that he or she is to respond by saying "yes" or "no". Begin by presenting fingers well within the central peephole. At first the responses will be cautious, but because the fingers lie well within acknowledged borders, a routine of "yes" responses soon develops. Once the routine is established, introduce a finger outside the acknowledged border without cueing the patient. The lulled patient will utter either a "yes" or a "no"!

Using "Magical" Remedies

Play on the patient's suggestibility by explaining that the constricted field comes from having pupils that are too small to admit all the light. Instill a "special dilating eyedrop" (in reality a standard mydriatic), exhorting the patient to experience a "miraculous expansion" of the visual field. If it works, prescribe the topical nostrum for temporary instillation at home.

Be aware that many of the narrow fields produced on formal kinetic or static automated perimetry are the result of procedural artifacts. Patients may be poorly positioned or incorrectly refracted. Others are tired, inattentive, confused, or mistakenly withholding a response until the target is clearly seen. In kinetic perimetry, patients must be told to signal on first sighting a moving stimulus. With static perimetry, they must be reminded to pay attention and to press the buzzer even if they are not certain they have seen a white dot.

Monocular Temporal Hemianopia

Complete temporal hemianopia is a common accompaniment of psychogenic VAL in the ipsilateral eye. A two-step process is used to disclose the nonorganic nature of this defect.

Confrontation Fields with One Eye Occluded

This establishes that the hemianopia is limited to one eye. Now go to the second step:

Confrontation Fields with Both Eyes Open

The intact nasal field in the contralateral "good" eye should reduce an organic monocular temporal hemianopia to a tiny peripheral crescent. A faking patient describes complete temporal hemianopia. Even if this maneuver yields equivocal results, be aware that no case of organic monocular temporal hemianopia has ever been described without an ipsilateral afferent pupil defect. A pseudo-hemianopic defect could, of course, arise from retinal disease (detachment, retinoschisis, and inflammation).

Postfixational Blindness

Tell the patient to fixate on a small target at 1/3 m from the eyes. Now display a finger 1/3 m behind the fixated target. If the defect is organic, the finger will be invisible within the absent temporal field–organic field cut "funnels" out (vide supra). If field cut is psychogenic, the finger will be visible.

Binocular Perimetry

If perimetry is performed with both eyes open, the intact nasal fields should overlap all, but the outermost crescents of the organic temporal defects found on monocular perimetry and erase those portions. In psychogenic bitemporal hemianopia, the defects will not change in size.

Binasal Hemianopia

The methods used to uncover this psychogenic defect are similar to those used to uncover psychogenic bitemporal hemianopia.

Prefixational Blindness

Tell the patient to fixate on a target positioned at 1 m from the eyes. Then place a second target in front of the first one. If the binasal defect is organic, the closer target will be hidden within the absent nasal field.

Binocular perimetry

With binocular perimetry, the intact temporal fields should entirely overlap organic nasal defects found on monocular perimetry and erase them completely. Binasal hemianopia with visual field defects aligned to the vertical meridian is never caused by organic disease. One might imagine that bilateral compression of the optic chiasm would selectively damage the "noncrossing" axons emanating from temporal retina, but this does not happen. Binasal nerve fiber bundle defects are however very common in ischemic, compressive, inflammatory, and postpapilledemic optic neuropathy, whereas their borders may appear to "respect the vertical meridian," closer inspection reveals that these defects "spill over" into the temporal fields.

Homonymous Hemianopia

Psychogenic homonymous hemianopia is difficult to expose. Fortunately, it is a rare manifestation of nonorganic VFL. It may be limited to a single quadrant.

VISUAL ELECTROPHYSIOLOGY

The International Society for Clinical Electrophysiology of Vision stresses the need for doing in all patients with unexplained visual loss standardized electroretinography, pattern electroretinography, and pattern appearance visually evoked cortical potentials (VECPs). On the other hand, other forms of electrophysiological tests such as electrooculography, bright electroretinography and flash VECPs are noncontributory in such cases and are therefore unnecessary. Visually Evoked Cortical Potentials VECPs originating from the occipital cortex, are recorded to investigate the integrity of the retinogeniculo striate pathway. However, in the context of unexplained visual symptoms the VECP has several limitations. First, normal or near-normal cortical potentials in response to sinusoidal and checkerboard gratings have been reported in many patients of cortical visual loss indicating that recordable electrical signals can be generated in the absence of sufficient viable striate cortex. Second, some subjects, especially those with malingering, can voluntarily influence the pattern VECP. Purposeful defocusing of the test stimulus causing retinal blur may result in decreased amplitude and prolonged latency of the cortical response. Some subjects can even completely obliterate their VECP response on instruction, and others can reduce its amplitude through volitional suppression. Volantary de-fixation can also result in abnormal VECP responses. Careful monitoring of patients therefore is of utmost importance during testing. Hence, electrophysiological demonstration of a normal pathway between the retina and primary cortex is neither necessary nor sufficient to establish a diagnosis in many cases as co-existing pathology of the visual system is relatively common in patients with nonorganic visual loss. Despite all these limitations, VECP is a measure of pathway integrity and therefore remains a vital tool in the assessment of unexplained visual loss when used judiciously in the context of clinical findings. Pattern Electroretinography: The pattern electroretinogram is a retinal response to viewing a temporally modulated pattern stimulus of constant total luminicense (grating or checkerboard) and depends on the functional integrity of the retina and the optic pathway. Its utility is two-fold. It will not only detect photoreceptor dysfunction syndromes with subtle fundoscopic signs but also would indicate that the image on the retina is well focussed and that fixation by the patient was adequate. Consequently, the simultaneous recording of ERG and the VECP appears complimentary and to be particularly useful in cases of psychogenic and feigned visual symptoms

MANAGEMENT

The management of patients suspected of having psychogenic disturbances is often characterized by several missteps.

Ordering Expensive, Misleading, or Low-Yield Test

Retinal fluorescein angiography, VEPs, ERG, and brain imaging are often ordered "defensively" even when the examiner has ample evidence that the manifestations are psychogenic. These tests consume expensive resources, often turn up noncontributory abnormalities that compel further inappropriate tests, and fortify the patient's sense that there is a somatic disorder.

Failure to Document Unequivocally that the Cause is Psychogenic

Evasive and noncommittal gestures on the part of the physician fortify the misimpression of organic illness, invite therapies of dubious value, and create a paper trail to support wasteful litigation.

Failure to Differentiate Between Underlying Psychiatric and Behavioral Disturbances

Most physicians are so angry at being manipulated that they fail to distinguish between conscious and unconscious duplicity. However, some fakers are not malingering; they are convinced that they are ill. Guiding them to the appropriate therapist leads to a more effective resolution of the underlying problems. Effective disposition of these difficult patients require an understanding of the psychosocial conditions that underlie their behavior. At one end of the spectrum is faking with conscious motivation and full awareness—that is maligning. At the other end is faking with unconscious motivation and poor insight—somatoform disorder. Between these respective conditions lies faking with conscious motivation and poor insight—factitious disorder. It is essential to differentiate between these disorders, and psychiatrists' help is often needed. Except for the "hard core deceivers" most patients with somatoform disorders improve with a sympathetic approach to their problems. Formal psychotherapy is generally not needed.

SUGGESTED READINGS

1. Aldrich MS, Alessi AG, Beck RV, et al. Cortical blindness: Etiology, diagnosis and prognosis. Ann Neurol. 1987;21:149-58.
2. American Psychiatric Association. Diagnostic and Statistical Manual of Mental Disorders. 4th ed. Washington, DC: American Psychiatric Association, 1994.
3. Bodis I, Atkin A, Raab E, et al. Visual association cortex and vision in man: Pattern evoked occipital potentials in a blind boy. Science. 1977;198:629-31.
4. Bumgartner J, Epstein CM. Voluntary alteration of visual evoked potentials. Ann Neurol. 1982;12:475-8.
5. Celesia GG, Bushnel D, Cone-Toleikis S, et al. Cortical blindness and residual vision: Is the second usual system in humans capable of more than rudimentary visual perception ? Neurology. 1991;41:862-9.
6. Celosia GG, Archer GR, Kurosiwa Y, et al. Visual function of the extra genieulocalcarine system in man: Relationship to cortical blindness. Arch Neurol. 1980;37:704-6.
7. Donzis PB, Rappazzo A, Burde RM, et al. Effect of binocular variations of Snellen's visual acuity on titmus stereoacuity. Arch Ophthalmol. 1983;101:930-2.
8. Eisendrath SJ. Current overview of factitious disorders. In: Feldman MD. Eisendrath SJ (eds). The Spectrum of Factitious Disorders. Washington DC: American Psychiatric Press: 1996. P. 3-49.
9. Gittinger JW. Functional monocular temporal hemianopsia. Am J Ophthalmol. 1986;101:226-31.
10. Glovinsky Y, Quigley HA, Bisset RA, et al. Artificially produced quadrantanopsia in computed visual field testing. Arm Ophthalmol. 1990;110:90-1.
11. Hess CW, Meienberg O, Ludin HP. Visual evoked potentials in acute occipital blindness: Diagnostic and prognostic value. Neurol .1982;227:193-200.
12. Kaplan HI, Sadock BJ. Concise Textbook of Clinical Psychiatry. Baltimore: Williams Wilkins: 1996. P. 219-29.
13. Kathol RG, Cox TA, Corbett JJ, et al. Functional visual loss: I. A true psychiatric disorder. Psychol Med. 1983;13:307-14.
14. Keane R. Hysterical hemianopia: The "missing half" field defect. Arch Ophthalmol. 1979;97:865-6.
15. Keane R. Neuro-ophthalmic signs and symptoms of hysteria. Neurology. 1982;32:757-62.
16. Keltner JL, May WN, Johnson CA, et al. The California syndrome. Functional visual complaints with potential economic impact. Ophthalmology. 1985;92:427-35.
17. Kramer KK, LaPiana FG, Appleton B. Ocular malingering and hysteria: Diagnosis and management. Surv Ophthalmol. 1979;24:89-96.
18. Levi L, Feldman RM. Use of the potential acuity meter in suspected functional visual loss. Am J Ophthalmol. 1987;114:502-3.
19. Levy NS, Click EB. Stereoscopic perception and Snellen visual acuity. Am J Ophthalmol. 1974;78:722-4.
20. Miller BW. A review of practical tests for ocular malingering and hysteria. Surv Ophthalmol. 1973;17:241-6.
21. Miller NR, Keane R. Neuro-ophthalmologic manifestations of nonorganic disease. In Miller NR, Newman NJ (eds). Walsh & Hoyt's Clinical Neuro-Ophthalmology, 5th ed. Baltimore: II Williams & Wilkins: 1998. P. 1765-86.

22. Minkowski JS, Palese M, Guyton DL. Potential acuity meter using a minute aerial pinhole aperture. Ophthalmol. 1983;90:1360.
23. Morgan RK, Nugent B, Harrison JM, et al. Voluntary alteration of pattern visual evoked responses. Ophthalmology. 1985;92:1356-63.
24. Perley MJ, Guze SB. Hysteria - the stability and usefulness of clinical criteria. N Engl J Med. 1962;266:421-6.
25. Pilley SF, Thompson HS. Binasal field loss and prefixation blindness. In: Glaser JS, Smith JI, (eds). Neuro-Ophthalmology. Vol. 8. St Louis: G.V. Mosby: 1975. P. 277-284.
26. Smith CH, Beck RW, Mills RP. Functional disease in neuro-ophthalmology. Neurol Clin. 1983;1(4):955-71.
27. Smith TJ, Baker RS. Perimetric findings in functional disorders using automated techniques. Ophthalmology. 1987;94:1562-66.
28. Spehlmann R, Gross RA, Ho SU, et al. Visual evoked potentials and postmortem findings in a case of cortical blindness. Ann Neurol. 1977;2:531-4.
29. Tan CT, Murray NMF, Sawyers D, et al. Deliberate alteration of the visual evoked potential. Neurol Neurosurg Psychiatry. 1984;47:518-23.
30. Thompson HS. Functional visual loss. Am Ophthalmol. 1985;100:209-13.
31. Thompson JC, Kosmorsky GS, Ellis BD. Fields of dreamers and dreamed-up fields. Ophthalmology. 1996;103:117-25.
32. Weller M, Wiedemann P. Hysterical symptoms in ophthalmology. Doc Ophthalmol. 1989;73:1-33.

CHAPTER 21: Idiopathic Intracranial Hypertension

Barun K Sen, Arabinda Mukherjee

INTRODUCTION

Idiopathic intracranial hypertension (IIH), also known as pseudotumor cerebri or benign intracranial hypertension is well known as a disorder that predominantly affects overweight and obese women in the child-bearing age. The incidence in women in age group between 15 and 44 years has been 19–24 per 100,000. The incidence may be lower in countries where there is less obesity. While rare in children, it occurs in them with equal sex incidence. The clinical presentation consists of headache, papilledema, visual disturbances, etc. due to raised intracranial pressure. It causes significant long term disability including permanent visual loss and disabling headache.

NOMENCLATURE

The appropriate nomenclature to describe this condition has evolved over time and is debatable. Historically, multiple terms were used to describe the condition like meningitis serosa, otitic hydrocephalus, hypertensive meningeal hydrops, pseudotumor cerebri, benign intracranial hypertension, IIH, and pseudotumor cerebri syndrome. German physician, Heinrich Quincke reported the first case as "serous meningitis" probably in 1890. Nonne in 1904 renamed it pseudotumor cerebri. Foley coined the term benign intracranial hypertension. The term IIH was introduced by Buchheit et al. in 1969. The term was preferable to pseudotumor cerebri as the term tumor carries a lasting impression on the patient. Also, the term benign intracranial hypertension is a misnomer as 10% of all cases of IIH develop serious visual problem. As there is no entirely satisfactory terminology, the term IIH can be used to describe the condition.

EPIDEMIOLOGY

Though, IIH is mostly seen in young obese women (<45-year-old), it can occur in children and less frequently in males, especially after the onset of puberty. The incidence and prevalence of the disorder is highly variable in different nations worldwide, mostly because of diversity in overweight and obesity. The overall annual incidence in the general population worldwide is in between 1 and 3 per 100,000, but when stratified in young women suffering from obesity, the incidence of IIH rises to be 12–28 per 1 million. The incidence and prevalence is likely to rise further considering the increasing trends in obesity worldwide.

RISK FACTORS FOR IDIOPATHIC INTRACRANIAL HYPERTENSION

There are multiple risk factors of IIH, most important of which is overweight/obesity. Rapid weight gain over the preceding few months is also a significant risk factor. Systemic diseases associated with obesity like polycystic ovary syndrome and obstructive sleep apnea also are risk factors for development of IIH (Box 1).

PATHOGENESIS

The exact pathogenesis of IIH is uncertain. Raised intracranial pressure (ICP) is a uniform feature, but the exact mechanism of raised ICP in IIH is not clear. Most theories focus on cerebrospinal fluid (CSF) outflow resistance or intracranial

Box 1: Secondary causes associated with increased intracranial pressure

Pharmacological Causes
- Tetracyclines including tetracycline, minocycline and doxycycline, nalidixic acid, sulfa drugs, vitamin A and related products, antiarrhythmics like amiodarone, nitrofurantoin
- Lithium, hormonal products like levonorgestrel, growth hormone, thyroxine, and steroid withdrawal

Systemic and Medical Causes
- Head trauma, subarachnoid hemorrhage, decreased CSF absorption
- Prior intracranial infection or hemorrhage, cerebral venous thrombosis
- Bilateral jugular vein thrombosis or surgical ligation
- Increased right heart pressure resulting from arteriovenous fistulas, superior vena cava syndrome
- Hypercoagulable states, renal failure, liver failure
- Sleep apnea
- Systemic Lupus erythematosus, sarcoidosis, endocrinopathies like hypoparathyroidism, Addison's disease, Behçet's disease, middle ear or mastoid infection, hypercapnia, Pickwickian syndrome, anemia
- Turner syndrome, Down syndrome, infections like bacterial and viral meningitis,
- Lyme disease, human immunodeficiency virus infection, poliomyelitis, Coxsackie B virus infection
- Viral encephalitis, Guillain-Barré syndrome, infectious mononucleosis
- Syphilis and malaria

CSF, cerebrospinal fluid.

venous hypertension. Excess CSF production is not confirmed in patients with IIH.

There are few proposed theories:
- Increased venous sinus pressure
- Obesity hypothesis
- Abnormal vitamin A metabolism.

Increased Venous Sinus Pressure

Over last few years, increased venous sinus pressure has been hypothesized as the principal causative factors of IIH. Increased venous sinus pressure may occur due to intracranial venous hypertension or venous sinus microthrombi.

There is another hypothesis that presence of venous sinus microthrombi particularly in patients with thrombophilia may affect CSF absorption. It blocks arachnoid granulations and decrease CSF absorption.

Mostly accepted hypothesis is that instead of thrombus obstructing venous blood flow, venous hypertension is thought to result from transverse sinus stenosis in the distal part. Magnetic resonance (MR) venography and conventional angiography have identified the presence of venous sinus stenoses in a large majority (>90%) of patients with IIH compared to few in body mass index (BMI)-matched controls. Whether such sinus stenosis truly cause venous hypertension or merely serve as radiological surrogates of raised ICP is unclear. However, angiography and symptom improvement following endovascular transverse sinus stenting support this hypothesis. On the other hand, stenosis may occur without any evidence of raised ICP and persistence of stenosis in IIH patient after medical treatment and normalization of ICP making the significance of stenoses in the pathogenesis of IIH and the role of stenting as treatment of such patients remains controversial.

There is another theory of "self-sustained venous collapse". Prolonged venous hypertension interfere with CSF absorption via the arachnoid granulations, which results in increased ICP and further venous sinus compression. The cyclical mechanism which links these physiological processes is described below:

Self-sustained Venous Collapse

Raised ICP → venous collapse → transverse sinus stenosis → venous outflow obstruction venous hypertension → reduced absorption of CSF → raised ICP

Obesity Hypothesis

Obesity is one of the most important risk factors for the development of IIH. The fact that the majority of patients with IIH are young obese females and there might be some relationship. Correlations between BMI and risk of IIH have been demonstrated. There is also association between weight gains with disease recurrence and weight loss with improvement of vision.

Despite the association between IIH and obesity, the pathological mechanisms are unclear. IIH is a rare disorder, while obesity is very common. The pattern of obesity, distribution of adiposity determines the ICP. Initially, it was thought that centrally distributed adiposity transmits pressure, generating raised ICP, but studies of waist: hip ratios in IIH patients shows adiposity is predominantly in the lower body by contrast with central adiposity of typical obesity. Elevated level of adipokines and cytokines in CSF was thought to be associated with IIH, but a number of studies evaluating cytokine and adipokines profiles in the serum and CSF of patients with IIH shows inconsistent result. In one study, leptin, an adipokine which regulates satiety at the hypothalamus, was elevated in the serum and in CSF in IIH patients compared with controls matched for BMI, age, and gender. However, dysregulation of adipokines and cytokines are pathogenic in dysregulating ICP, or merely reflect a consequence of the disease has to be established.

Abnormal Vitamin A Metabolism

There is some association between vitamin A level and IIH. Retinol binding protein and retinol elevated in some patients with IIH and when they are elevated in serum they are also transported into the CSF. Elevated CSF retinol is toxic to the arachnoid granulation affecting CSF reabsorption mechanisms. In one study, 24% of 21 patients with IIH demonstrated high (>25 nm) vitamin A levels compared to 0% of 19 patients with elevated ICP due to other causes and 2.5% of 40 patients with normal ICP. Overall 83% of six patients with elevated CSF vitamin A had IIH and indicated a strong association. It is unclear whether elevated CSF retinol is a simply marker of excess CSF production by the choroid plexus or toxic to the CSF absorption mechanism.

Some Possible Mechanisms

Sodium and water retention: Abnormalities in sodium and water homeostasis in brain was thought as possible mechanism of IIH for many years, but there was no histological evidence of brain edema in patients with IIH postmortem.

Sleep apnea: Carbon dioxide retention in sleep apnea patient causes cerebral vasodilation and subsequent raised ICP. Sleep apnea is common among obese males and may exacerbate rather than cause IIH.

CLINICAL FEATURES

A typical presentation of IIH is a young obese female patient presenting with headache with transient visual obscuration with papilledema on fundoscopy.

In a case series of Idiopathic Intracranial Hypertension Treatment Trial (IIHTT), common symptoms of IIH were as follows:
- Headache (84–92%)
- Transient visual obscurations (68–72%)
- Intracranial noises (pulsatile tinnitus) (52–60%)
- Photopsia (48–54%)
- Back pain (53%)
- Retrobulbar pain (44%)
- Diplopia (18–38%)
- Sustained visual loss (26–32%).

Headache (Box 2)

Headache is the most common presenting symptom and is attributed to high CSF pressure. However, there may be several other factors which are responsible for headache in IIH.

Headaches in IIH:
- Due to high CSF pressure (most common)
- Post-lumbar peritoneal shunt (low flow)— Low-pressure syndromes
- Post-lumbar puncture
- Post-lumbar peritoneal shunt leak
- Valve problem (high flow)
  - Cerebrospinal fluid rhinorrhea
  - Transcribriform plate
  - Transphenoidal (empty sella).
- Analgesic-rebound headaches (IIH masquerading as chronic daily headache).

Headache characters are variable, may be holocranial, bifrontal, unilateral, or occipitonuchal, may be like any primary headache including migraine or tension type headache. Localization of headache is seldom helpful in diagnosis.

Headache of IIH may be intermittent or constant and more severe than previous headaches. Some patients describe headache exacerbation with changes in posture and characteristically, headache is relieved by spinal tap. The relief may be permanent or headache may return after days. Further, over medication of analgesics may lead to analgesic rebound headache. Hence, persistence

> **Box 2: Characteristics of idiopathic intracranial hypertension (IIH) headaches according to International Classification of Headaches Disorder (ICHD-3) (criteria A-D must be fulfilled)**
>
> A. Any headache fulfilling criterion C
> B. IIH has been diagnosed, with CSF pressure >250 mm H$_2$O (measured by lumbar puncture performed in the lateral decubitus position, without sedative medications, or by epidural or intraventricular monitoring)
> C. Evidence of causation demonstrated by at least two of the following:
>   1. Headache has developed in temporal relation to IIH, or led to its discovery
>   2. Headache is relieved by reducing intracranial hypertension
>   3. Headache is aggravated in temporal relation to increase in intracranial pressure
> D. Not better accounted for by another ICHD-3 diagnosis
>
> CSF, cerebrospinal fluid.

of headache does not always mean elevated CSF pressure and an indication for lumbar puncture. Among younger children, headache is a less universal finding.

Transient Visual Obscuration

Transient visual obscuration (TVO) is a common symptom of patients with swollen optic disc. It occurs in about two-thirds of patients with IIH. These visual loss episodes are brief (lasting for seconds) attacks of graying, whitening, or blackening of vision affecting one or both eyes. The attacks are often precipitated by change of posture (usually standing, but sometimes lying down or bending over) or valsalva procedures. The attacks may occur only rarely or there may be hundreds of attacks in one day. In contrast to transient visual loss of transient ischemic attack (TIA), the visual loss in TVO is gradual. The symptoms of TVO are almost certainly due to intermittent ischemia of the optic disc but it is not a symptom confined to patients with papilledema. It has also been reported in cases of anomalous elevation of optic disc, disc anomalies and glaucoma. Transient visual obscuration is essentially a benign symptom and has not been reported to cause sudden catastrophic visual loss. Transient visual obscuration alone is not an indication for surgical intervention. Transient visual obscuration tends to improve after lumbar puncture and less responsive to medical treatment. Transient visual obscuration frequency and occurrence does not correlate with the severity of raised ICP or degree of papilledema or is not predictive of future visual loss or optic atrophy.

Other than TVO, photopsias, brief sparkles or flashes of light are also seen in patients with IIH. Few patients with IIH having more rapid or fulminant course with rapid progression of visual loss within few weeks of onset.

Diplopia

Diplopia is an uncommon symptom. Patients with IIH complain of intermittent or continuous horizontal diplopia and this is typically due to a unilateral or bilateral sixth cranial nerve palsy or divergence restriction due to increased ICP. The commonest nerve affected is the sixth cranial nerve. Third nerve affection is rare.

Occasionally patients develop lateral rectus palsy after lumbar puncture because of intracranial shift.

Intracranial Noises or Tinnitus

Pulsatile tinnitus is common in patients with IIH, sometimes is disturbing and encourages the patient to consult otolaryngologist. Headache with pulsatile tinnitus is very suggestive of IIH. Patients complain of intermittent or constant hearing rushing water or wind and the noise disappears after CSF removal. This suggestive of vascular pulsations transmitted by CSF under high pressure to the venous sinuses.

Other Nonspecific Symptoms

Low back pain and paresthesias in all extremities are often seen in IIH patients. These are due to dilation of nerve root sleeves secondary to increased ICP. Some patients complain of aching legs that may be due to extra pressure on lumbar roots at the level of the dural sleeve.

Arthralgia in large joints particularly shoulders, knees, and hips is seen in some patients with IIH as a minor complaint.

Round and Keane reported that momentary ataxia occurred in some patients due to brief hypoperfusion of the brain stem.

EXAMINATION

The most common signs in IIH are:
- Papilledema
- Visual field loss
- Sixth nerve palsy.

Papilledema

Papilledema is the single most important finding. It is the hallmark sign of IIH. Papilledema is the physical sign which may lead to visual loss in IIH. Papilledema is usually bilateral, but may be unilateral. In the IIH Treatment Trial (IIHTT), asymmetric papilledema was noted in 7%. Papilledema can be graded in severity according to the Frisén scale. Higher grades of papilledema have been associated with more severe visual loss.

Patients with headache without papilledema, but on lumbar puncture elevated opening pressure to meet the diagnosis of IIH have been described but are rare.

Risk of visual loss is significantly lower in patients without papilledema compared to typical patients with IIH with papilledema. Commonest error occurs when a patient of headache is diagnosed as IIH in presence of pseudopapilledema without measuring the CSF pressure. Such patients may unnecessarily be subjected to prolonged medical treatment or surgical intervention. Ophthalmologic evaluation is advised to confirm the presence of papilledema and to evaluate those patients with questionable or subtle papilledema and it is therefore mandatory for the physician to establish the diagnosis of IIH by unequivocal demonstration of elevated CSF pressure (>250 mm) before subjecting the patient to prolonged medical therapy or surgical interventions.

Other ophthalmoscopic findings are as follows:
- Macular exudates
- Macular edema
- Choroidal folds across the macula
- Choroidal neovascularization
- Serous retinal elevation around the nerve head.

Visual Acuity and Visual Field Loss

Visual acuity and visual field loss is a major problem to the treating clinician. Visual loss may not be apparent until weeks or months after detection of papilledema. Loss of visual acuity may result from collapse of the entire visual field or more commonly due to macular affection. Subretinal hemorrhage or anterior ischemic optic neuropathy are two other important causes of visual loss. Sudden drop of blood pressure due to over energetic use of antihypertensives or diuretics can cause ischemic changes in the optic disc which has a compromised blood supply due to papilledema. Changes in visual acuity is often detected late. Up to 30% of patients, on presentation, show visual acuity to be less than 20/20. Tests for central vision should include distant and near vision testing, contrast sensitivity testing, Amsler grid, color vision, and fluroscein angiogram in selected cases.

Visual field is almost universally affected depending on the type of visual field examination done (Fig. 1). With standard Humphrey perimetry, field defect can be found in about 90% cases of IIH. The universal defect associated with papilledema is enlargement of the blind spot. However, this is not a useful sign to follow the progress of the disease because enlarged blind spot may persist long after the papilledema has subsided. The next most common field defect to appear is inferior nasal quadrantic defect. Like nasal step seen in glaucoma, it indicates the first sign of nerve fiber layer damage at the optic disc. As the visual field constricts it merges with the enlarging blind spot giving rise to centrocecal scotoma. When this is bilateral it may be mistaken as a bitemporal field defect of chiasmal lesion. Visual evoked potential, contrary to earlier expectations, does not play an important role in prediction of visual loss. Since, VEP is an indicator of central vision which is affected late in the course of the disease it has no predictive value in the management of the disease.

Cranial Nerve Deficits

Cranial nerve deficits mostly seen in patients with IIH is unilateral or bilateral sixth cranial nerve (abducens) because of long intracranial course before exiting the skull. This reflects false localizing sign of raised ICP. Some others cranial nerve

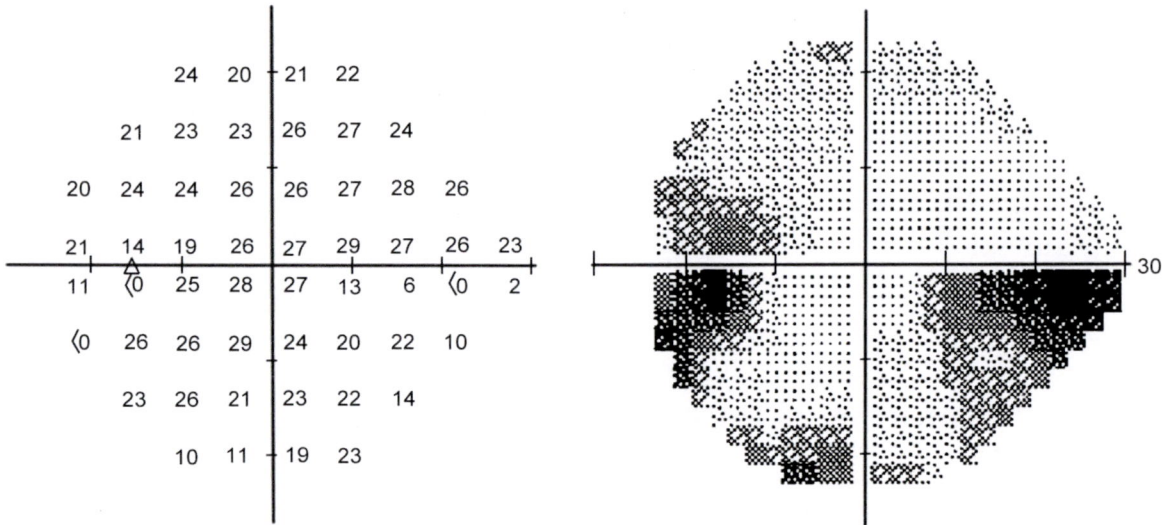

FIG 1: Visual field loss in the left eye of a patient with idiopathic intracranial hypertension who presented late.

involvement may be seen in patients with IIH particularly in children as follows:
- Olfactory
- Oculomotor
- Trochlear nerve
- Trigeminal nerve
- Facial nerve
- Auditory nerve.

DIAGNOSIS

A diagnosis of IIH can be suspected on the basis of clinical history and ophthalmological examination alone prior to neuroradiological exclusion of other causes of raised ICP and confirmatory CSF manometry. The hallmark of diagnosis is to establish rise in CSF pressure in absence of any mass lesion or CNS infection. Diagnostic criteria of IIH were first established by Dandy in 1937. Modified Dandy criteria used for diagnosis of IIH till 2002 (Box 3). As there are recent advances in brain imaging a revision of the 2002 criteria done in 2013 (Box 4).

Red flags in the diagnosis of IIH include:
- Atypical demographic profile
- Cranial nerve palsies other than a 6th nerve palsy
- Alterations in level of consciousness
- Focal neurologic sings apart from a sixth nerve palsy

Box 3: Modified Dandy criteria for diagnosing idiopathic intracranial hypertension

1. If symptoms present, they may only reflect those of generalized intracranial hypertension or papilledema
2. If signs present, they may only reflect those of generalized intracranial hypertension or papilledema
3. Elevated intracranial pressure 25 cmH$_2$O measured in the lateral decubitus position
4. Normal CSF composition
5. No evidence of hydrocephalus, mass, structural, or vascular lesion on MRI or contrast-enhanced CT for typical patients, and MRI and MR venography for all others
6. No other cause of intracranial hypertension identified

Note: Definite IIH: Criteria 1–6 must be fulfilled.

CSF, cerebrospinal fluid; CT, computed tomography; IIH, idiopathic intracranial hypertension; MR, magnetic resonance; MRI, magnetic resonance imaging.

- Abnormal CSF profile
- Explosive onset of symptoms
- Rapid development of visual loss and progression of symptoms
- Global ophthalmoplegia

Evaluation of a patient of suspected IIH should therefore include:
- Fulfillment of Dandy criteria
- Ruling out secondary causes: Drug history, hemogram, thyroid profile, electrolytes, HIV

> **Box 4: Most recent revised diagnostic criteria for idiopathic intracranial hypertension**
>
> **Required for the diagnosis of idiopathic intracranial hypertension:**
>
> A diagnosis of idiopathic intracranial hypertension is definite if the patient fulfills criteria A–E
>
> The diagnosis is considered probable if criteria A–D are met, but the measured CSF pressure is lower than specified for a definite diagnosis
>
> A. Papilledema
> B. Normal neurologic examination except for cranial nerve abnormalities
> C. Neuroimaging: Normal brain parenchyma without evidence of hydrocephalus, mass, or structural lesion and no abnormal meningeal enhancement on MRI, with and without gadolinium, for typical patients (obese women), and MRI, with and without contrast, and MRV for others; if MRI is unavailable or contraindicated, contrast-enhanced CT may be used
> D. Normal CSF composition
> E. Elevated lumbar puncture CSF opening pressure [250 mmH$_2$O in adults and 280 mmH$_2$O in children (250 mmH$_2$O if the child is not sedated and not obese)] in a properly performed lumbar puncture
>
> **Diagnosis of idiopathic intracranial hypertension without papilledema**
>
> In the absence of papilledema, a diagnosis of idiopathic intracranial hypertension can be made if B–E from above are satisfied, and in addition the patient has a unilateral or bilateral abducens nerve palsy
>
> In the absence of papilledema or sixth nerve palsy, a diagnosis of idiopathic intracranial hypertension can be suggested, but not made, if B–E from above are satisfied, and in addition at least 3 of the following neuroimaging criteria are satisfied:
>
> 1. Empty sella
> 2. Flattening of the posterior aspect of the globe
> 3. Distention of the perioptic subarachnoid space with or without a tortuous optic nerve
> 4. Transverse venous sinus stenosis
>
> CSF, cerebrospinal fluid; CT, computed tomography; IIH, idiopathic intracranial hypertension; MRI, magnetic resonance imaging; MRV, magnetic resonance venography.

- serology, cortisol, creatinine, serum calcium, phosphate, markers for hypercoagulable states
- Neuroimaging: CT/MRI/MR angiogram and venogram
- Visual evaluation: Acuity, field charting, contrast sensitivity testing, and stereoscopic fundus photography.

The evaluation of IIH includes the history, physical examination, blood test, brain imaging, and a lumbar puncture particularly for opening pressure. In a patient with headache and papilledema urgent brain imaging is required to exclude secondary causes of raised ICP. A lumbar puncture is performed to document an opening pressure and for routine CSF examination after exclusion of secondary causes of intracranial hypertension particularly Space Occupying Lesions.

Ophthalmologic evaluation for fundus examination and documentation of the severity of optic nerve involvement and monitoring treatment response.

A complete blood count and general chemistry analysis should be done to exclude anemia or lymphoproliferative causes that may be associated with raised ICP.

Neuroimaging

Primary purpose of brain imaging is to exclude secondary causes of raised ICP. Magnetic resonance imaging brain with MR venography (MRV) is the preferred test. CT scan particularly contrast enhanced CT scan of brain may be done in patients with contraindications to MRI. In both cases contrast study is better as it increases sensitivity for subtle intracranial masses (e.g., gliomatosis cerebri) and meningeal-based pathologies as secondary intracranial hypertension can have a similar clinical presentation to IIH.

Contrast MRV is a more sensitive test than standard MRI for the detection of cerebral venous abnormality and cerebral venous thrombosis. Narrowing of the transverse venous sinus is seen in 65–90% of patients with IIH and suggests increase intracranial pressure. Although very common in IIH, transverse sinus stenosis is not specific of IIH.

Grossly, brain parenchyma and ventricles appear normal on MRI or CT in patients with IIH but, some subtle MRI abnormalities may be seen as follows:

- Flattening of the posterior sclera (43–80%)
- Distension of perioptic subarachnoid space (45–67%)
- Enhancement (with gadolinium) of the prelaminar optic nerve (7–50%)
- Empty sella (25–80%)

- Intraocular protrusion of the prelaminar optic nerve (3–30%)
- Vertical tortuosity of the orbital optic nerve (40%)
- Tonsillar ectopia
- Narrowing of the Meckel's cave and cavernous sinuses
- Widening of the foramen ovale.

These are not diagnostic, rather suggestive and their absence doesn't exclude the diagnosis.

Lumbar Puncture

Elevated opening pressure on lumbar puncture is an essential element of the diagnosis of IIH. Lumbar puncture and CSF manometry is essential to establish a CSF pressure of more than 250 mm of H_2O.

Ideal position of patient during lumbar puncture for CSF manometry: Patient should be relaxed and lying in the lateral decubitus position with legs extended. Falsely elevated ICP may be seen in prone, sitting position, anxiety, pain, and the use of sedating medications.

Falsely low opening pressure may be seen after multiple lumbar puncture attempts or in the setting of hyperventilation and treatment with intracranial pressure lowering medications.

If first lumbar tap fails to show elevated pressure, a second tap to be performed after 48 hours. In negative cases, where there is a strong suspicion, 24–48 hours continuous CSF pressure monitoring is required to establish the diagnosis. The CSF should have normal cytology and biochemistry. Any deviation from normal values should prompt the physician to look for additional pathologies. Repeated lumbar puncture (except as a therapeutic measure) and measurement of CSF pressure serve no purpose in following the course of the disease and planning management. The CSF pressure may remain raised long after disc edema has disappeared.

In addition to measuring the opening pressure, CSF is analyzed for cell count and differential, glucose, protein and CSF cytology, antigen testing (e.g., CSF VDRL if clinically suggested) CSF composition (protein, cells, glucose) is normal in patients with IIH.

Ophthalmologic Evaluation

Ophthalmological evaluation is essential for all patients with suspected IIH. A complete ocular examination includes formal visual field examination, dilated fundus examination and optic nerve photographs. In doubtful cases orbital ultrasound and fluorescein angiography may be done.

Visual field testing (Goldmann kinetic perimetry and the computer-assisted static perimetry) is essential in IIH to assess and documentation of the severity of optic nerve involvement and monitoring response to treatment.

The most common findings on perimetry in the Idiopathic Intracranial Hypertension Treatment Trial were a partial arcuate defect with an enlarged blind spot followed by generalized constriction of visual field. Less commonly, central, paracentral, arcuate, and altitudinal scotomas may occur.

Visual acuity and field testing should be the guide for decision making regarding surgical intervention and for this ophthalmologist and neurologist should work together in the care of these patients.

Fluorescein Angiography

Fluorescein angiography is an incompletely reliable test particularly in doubtful cases though it may be helpful in the detection of early papilledema, showing dye leakage, disc vascularity, and excess early and late disc fluorescence.

Optical Coherence Tomography (OCT)

Optical coherence tomography though not fully reliable may be useful to monitor the swelling of the nerve and also to clarify the effect upon and changes within the surrounding retina. It is operator dependent and is prone to error. However, modern technology (spectral rather than time based) has improved reliability.

DIFFERENTIAL DIAGNOSIS

Papilledema suggests elevated ICP, which can have many secondary causes in addition to IIH. Unilateral or bilateral pseudopapilledema that looks like optic disc swelling which can have a

Box 5: Differential diagnosis of papilledema

Bilateral disc abnormalities:
- Increased intracranial pressure
- Pseudopapilledema
- Malignant hypertension
- Diabetic papillopathy
- Others (hyperviscosity, toxins)

Unilateral disc abnormalities:
- Anterior ischemic optic neuropathy
- Papillitis, neuroretinitis
- Sarcoidosis
- Central retinal vein occlusion
- Papillophlebitis
- Malignancy
- Leber's hereditary optic neuropathy
- Other causes (low intraocular pressure, ocular injury, radiation)

TABLE 1: Treatment options in idiopathic intracranial hypertension

Lifestyle/Suppression of risk factors	Weight loss
Medical management	Acetazolamide
	Topiramate
	Furosemide
	Corticosteroid
Intervention	Repeated lumbar puncture
	Cerebral transverse sinus stenting
Shunts	Ventriculoperitoneal
	Lumboperitoneal
	Lumbar drain
	Optic nerve fenestration

similar appearance to papilledema should be ruled out (Box 5).

Secondary Intracranial Hypertension

Any entity that increases ICP may lead to papilledema. These include:
- Intracranial mass lesions (tumor, abscess)
- Obstruction of venous outflow or venous hypertension
  - Common causes:
    – Venous sinus thrombosis
    – Jugular vein compression
    – Neck surgery
  - Rare causes:
    – Transverse sinus septum causing sinus stenosis
    – Osteopetrosis of the jugular foramen
    – Depressed skull fracture
    – Stenosis of the superior sagittal sinus
    – Cerebral arteriovenous malformations
    – Dural arteriovenous malformations
    – Arteriovenous fistulas
    – Increased right heart pressure and superior vena cava syndrome
- Obstructive hydrocephalus
- Decreased CSF absorption, e.g., arachnoid granulation adhesions after bacterial or other infectious meningitis, subarachnoid hemorrhage
- Increased CSF production, e.g., choroid plexus papilloma
- Malignant systemic hypertension.

Optic Disc Abnormalities

There are many causes of an elevated optic nerve head. Papilledema is the conditions where elevated optic disc heads as a consequence of increased intracranial pressure.

MANAGEMENT (TABLE 1)

Treatment of patients with IIH are best managed jointly by neurologists and ophthalmologists, although a multidisciplinary approach, involving clinical psychologists, personal trainers and dieticians, may be of use in certain cases. Successful treatment requires motivation and an understanding that permanent visual loss is likely if ICP is poorly controlled.

Idiopathic intracranial hypertension is usually a benign condition and may remit by itself. Asymptomatic papilledema may persist for weeks to months without any serious complications.

Lifestyle Modification/Suppression of Risk Factors

As IIH is more common in obese patients, weight reduction might be effective in lowering CSF pressure. Several studies proved that increased CSF pressure in IIH may be due to obesity and lowering of body weight leads to disappearance of papilledema. Weight reduction by 6% was associated with improved visual function and papilledema in IIH patients. Weight reduction can be achieved by dietary restriction, exercise, or surgical methods.

Newborg first documented that dietary restriction improves IIH symptoms. In her study, patients were given low calorie low salt diet; the resultant weight loss (13–38%) was associated with improvement of papilledema and IIH symptoms. Some other case reviews also support this result.

There is class IV evidence for bariatric surgery as an effective treatment for IIH in obese patients, both in terms of symptom resolution and visual outcome.

Medical Management

Medical treatment of IIH consists of carbonic anhydrase inhibitor, loop diuretics, osmotic agents and steroids. Of these, carbonic anhydrase inhibitor like acetazolamide (1–2 g daily) and loop diuretics like frusemide (40–80 mg daily) is the mainstay.

Acetazolamide

Acetazolamide is considered as the mainstay of pharmacological management in IIH. It acts by reducing CSF production and secretion by choroid plexus by inhibiting the enzyme, carbonic anhydrase.

Acetazolamide (1–4 g/day) can be used in divided doses, two times a day or three times a day. Although, it improves papilledema and vision, it is believed to have a limited effect on the management of headaches.

Paresthesias due to hyponatremia and hypokalemia are the most common adverse effects. In such a situation, treatment can be continued with potassium supplementation and close monitoring. Other adverse effects are fatigue, nausea, diarrhea, and vomiting. Adverse effects such as rash, crystalluria, kidney stones, bone marrow depression, thrombocytopenia, and hemolytic anemia require discontinuation of the treatment.

In a study by Ball et al. in the UK, combination of weight loss and acetazolamide use in mild IIH showed clinical improvement.

In IIHTT the Neuro-Ophthalmologic Research Disease Investigator Consortium (NORDIC) enrolled 166 participants to determine the efficacy of acetazolamide compared with placebo in IIH, with both arms also receiving a supervised weight-reduction, low sodium diet. The initial dosing of acetazolamide was 500 mg twice a day with a schedule to increase the dose by 250 mg every 6 days up to a maximum of 4 g daily. Participants who could not tolerate the study drug could decrease the dosage to a minimum of 125 mg/day. All participants received a specific dietary plan and lifestyle modification program.

The IIHTT provides class I evidence that acetazolamide use provides a modest improvement of symptoms including visual field function in patients with IIH.

Topiramate

Topiramate also shows significant improvement in symptoms of IIH. Topiramate has been demonstrated to be effective in the treatment of IIH and should be used in patients who are refractory to acetazolamide or who cannot use the drug due to adverse effects. Daily 100–150 mg topiramate dosages that were initiated at 50 mg daily divided dosages were reported to be effective.

Topiramate use was first reported in a prospective open label study of 40 patients using both topiramate (daily dose range 100–150 mg) and acetazolamide daily (dose range 1000–1500 mg). A statistically significant improvement in visual symptoms was seen in topiramate group.

In patients with coexisting migraine-like headaches (68% at diagnosis) it may have additional benefit.

Side effects of topiramate: Cognitive impairment and exacerbation of depression (it is not recommended in severe depression).

Other Drugs

Other diuretics, such as furosemide, are used in IIH, when acetazolamide is contraindicated or not tolerated. It is postulated that furosemide reduces CSF production. Caution is advised when combining diuretics, as severe hypokalemia may result. Methazolamide can be used as an alternative to acetazolamide. Other drugs having controversial effects are:

- Octreotide, a somatostatin analogue improves papilledema in some cases
- Glycerol
- Mannitol
- Corticosteroids
- Indomethacin.

The osmotic agent glycerol in a dose of 0.25–0.5 mL/kg has been used, but the taste is unpalatable and procedure is cumbersome to recommend this as a routine treatment. Also it has a high calorie value which may lead to weight gain of already obese patients. Mannitol has never been used chronically to reduce CSF pressure in IIH.

The use of corticosteroids in the treatment should better be avoided. Although, corticosteroids may dramatically reduce disc edema, it rapidly returns once corticosteroids have been tapered off. Further, there is no evidence that steroids reduce CSF pressure. The reappearance of papilledema leads to prolonged use of steroids with emergence of adverse side effects. It is not unusual to see patients receiving steroids for more than 1 year.

Reasons for not routinely using corticosteroids:
- They do not lower CSF pressure
- Frequent recurrence of papilledema when withdrawn
- Further weight gain in an already obese patient
- Skin striae in a woman whose body image is already poor
- Depression in an anxious and depressed patient
- Rarely if ever are corticosteroids used in a short course.

Indomethacin: A cyclo-oxygenase inhibitors causes cerebral vasoconstriction, which reduces cerebral blood flow and has an ICP lowering effect. Infusion of 50 mg indomethacin over 1 minute causes significant reduction of ICP within minutes. However, rebound increase in ICP has been reported following discontinuation of indomethacin.

Management of Acute Idiopathic Intracranial Hypertension

Patients presenting with acute worsening of symptoms like increasing headaches or rapidly progressing visual disturbance need some treatment modalities for urgent reduction of ICP.

- A therapeutic lumbar puncture often helpful in ICP lowering. In some cases this can induce lasting remission as it can break the "cycle of self-sustained venous collapse". However, within hours CSF volume returns to almost normal level as 1 mL of CSF is produced approximately every 5 minutes
- Repeated lumbar puncture: Though long-term effect is controversial, very helpful in treating exacerbations during pregnancy. Complication of repeated lumbar puncture:
  - Uncomfortable in obese patients
  - Low-pressure headache
  - Cerebrospinal fluid leak or infection.
- Indomethacin injection: A short-term significant reduction (mean 14.4, range 8.0–20.0 cm CSF) in CSF opening pressure seen after a 50 mg infusion of indomethacin over 1 minute
- Invasive techniques: Cerebrospinal fluid shunting works directly by lowering CSF pressure and poses no direct risk to vision, while optic nerve sheath fenestration (ONSF) is less invasive and directly treats papilledema, but offers less headache relief.

Surgical Treatment of Idiopathic Intracranial Hypertension

Before Quincke described the syndrome of pseudotumor cerebri and soon after papilledema was first described, treatment of optic disc swelling was undertaken by a rather crude form of optic nerve sheath decompression. Surgical procedures have evolved from these early procedures and today a number of effective surgical methods are available.

Surgical treatment of IIH:
- Subtemporal decompression
- Lumboperitoneal shunt
- Ventriculoperitoneal shunt
- Optic nerve sheath surgery
- Surgical reduction of fat (bariatric surgery).

Before discussing with the relative merits and demerits of individual surgical methods, it will be prudent to outline the indications of surgical treatment in cases of IIH.

Indications for surgical treatment:
- Visual loss
- Disc swelling and visual loss despite medication
- Inability to tolerate medicine

- Unreliability of patient follow-up
- Inability to perform visual field.

Complications of subtemporal decompression:
- Seizures
- Hemiparesis
- Infection
- Cosmetic unsightliness
- Risk of brain trauma.

Methods of Surgical Intervention and their Complications

Subtemporal decompression

While the first method used to decompress the swollen disk was a form of optic nerve sheath decompression, the standard method of decompression is the subtemporal or suboccipital craniotomy. It is very effective in decompressing swollen optic discs. Its success depends on the fact that the dura is incised and the subarachnoid space comes into contact with the galea which works as an absorptive surface.

Lumboperitoneal shunts

Lumboperitoneal shunts use the peritoneum as the CSF absorptive surface. The silicone shunts are better tolerated. Even with these advances, lumboperitoneal shunts have a great many serious complications when used to preserve vision in patients with papilledema. All patients with shunts need close monitoring. Failure of a shunt when one is shunt dependent may be heralded by headache or other symptoms that had been the initial presenting complaints.

Complications of lumboperitoneal shunts:
- Continued visual loss
- Sciatica
- Arachnoiditis
- Scoliosis and hyperlordosis
- Limited spinal flexion
- Transient back pain
- Symptomatic tonsillar herniation
- Acquired cervical syringomyelia
- Herniation and posterior cerebral artery occlusion with stroke
- Infections: Meningitis, peritonitis, intervertebral discitis
- Headache: High pressure, low pressure
- Hindbrain herniation
- Abducens nerve palsy
- Intra-abdominal sequestration of the catheter
- Viscus perforation by or migration of the catheter
- Herniation and vascular occlusion with stroke.

Thus anyone who is likely to be noncompliant in follow-up should not be considered for lumboperitoneal shunts as the surgical method of treatment.

Other shunting procedures include ventriculoperitoneal and ventriculoatrial shunts, obviously effective for patients with papilledema due to hydrocephalus.

Optic nerve sheath decompression

This procedure was the first treatment of the swollen optic disc; it antedates subtemporal decompression and lumbar peritoneal shunting by over 20 years.

The presumed mechanism of the optic nerve sheath decompression is the absorption of CSF by orbital tissues. Suggestions that the site seals down and prevents pressure from being directed in the immediate retrolaminar optic nerve have not been borne out in the few postmortem studies that have been done. Neuroimaging and orbital echography in a few cases suggest a functioning filtering cyst. This also improves the circulation to optic nerves, which has been proved by pre and postoperative Doppler scanning.

The long-term follow-up of large numbers of cases has yet to appear, but late progression of visual loss and continued visual deterioration, despite repeated surgical decompression, have been reported.

Complications of optic nerve sheath decompression:
- Diplopia
- Continued loss of vision
- Infection
- Persistent papilledema
- Tonic pupil, partial, or complete
- Retrobulbar hemorrhage
- Hemorrhage into the optic nerve
- Transient blindness.

The unilateral optic nerve sheath decompression is effective in reducing disc swelling in both eyes in about half of the cases. As a rule one begins with a unilateral procedure followed by surgery on the second eye if papilledema fails to regress or if visual loss progresses.

Sheath decompression is also effective in reducing headache in 50–75% of reported patients.

Progressive visual loss and late visual failure usually occur in patients who have had severe compromise of visual field and/or visual acuity prior to surgery. This demonstrates the need for constant vigilance in the management of patients with papilledema of whatever cause. The development of substantial arcuate defects or field constriction in the presence of medical therapy and normal visual acuity should he the cue that substantial axonal loss has already occurred. Return of visual function is rare if surgery is delayed until the disc is gliotic or atrophic.

Venous pressure and venous stenting

Studies beginning with Foley's allusion to "otitic hydrocephalus" showed that intracranial pressure could be elevated by intracranial venous sinus occlusion.

There have been recent reports of intracranial venous stenting as a treatment for IIH. Success with this must be weighed against long-term effectiveness and complications and until more data is available use of venous stents must be considered experimental.

Surgically-induced weight loss (bariatric surgery): A treatment of papilledema due to idiopathic intracranial hypertension

Surgical procedures to reduce weight include liposuction, panniculectomy, gastric stapling, and bypass procedures. Such procedures are not recommended casually or for moderate weight gain, but should be done for morbid obesity.

This form of treatment of optic disc swelling is limited to patients with morbid obesity and IIH. It occurs predominantly in obese women although disc swelling may occur in a symptomatic form in morbidly obese patients with Pickwickian syndrome with CO_2 retention. It is these patients, the morbidly obese, who can benefit from bariatric surgery. Bariatric surgical procedures are not recommended for the patient who is rapidly losing vision.

Complications of bariatric surgery:
- Stomal stenosis
- Upper gastrointestinal bleeding due to marginal ulcer
- Incisional hernia
- Recurrent small bowel obstruction
- Anastomotic leaks
- Peripheral neuropathy
- Wernicke's encephalopathy.

Summary of Surgical Treatment

Subtemporal decompression, lumboperitoneal and other shunts and optic nerve sheath decompression are all techniques that work to reduce optic disc swelling from ICP. Each has its indications, contraindications, complications, advocates, and detractors. Papilledema is a cause of visual loss whether due to hydrocephalus, venous sinus occlusion, intracranial mass lesions, infections, spinal cord tumors, or IIH. One of these procedures should be contemplated for any patient who is losing vision due to papilledema. The procedure of choice appears to be optic nerve sheath decompression, but more prospective studies of efficacy are needed.

COMPLICATIONS OF IDIOPATHIC INTRACRANIAL HYPERTENSION

Long-term consequences of IIH:
- Visual loss
- Visual field abnormalities
- Recurrence of IIH
- Cerebrospinal fluid otorrhea and rhinorrhea
- Psychosocial impact.

Visual Loss

Although, most IIH patients after appropriate medical management have satisfactory visual outcomes, visual loss is the serious complication in up to one-fourth patients.

Visual loss in IIH is irreversible and due to progressive optic neuropathies in the setting of chronic papilledema, results in disruption of the axonal flow. Uncommonly, loss of vision may be due to extension of papilledema to the maculae or associated hemorrhage, edema, and exudates in maculae.

Visual Field Abnormalities

Almost half of patients show visual field defects. The most common visual field defect is an enlarged blind spot. Other visual field defects are:

- Arcuate defects
- Generalized constriction of the visual field
- Central loss of vision
- Altitudinal visual field defects or temporal visual field defects.

Recurrence of Idiopathic Intracranial Hypertension

Up to 50% of patients with IIH after improvement relapsed after additional weight gain. The BMI in those with disease recurrence was significantly higher than at diagnosis.

Cerebrospinal Fluid Otorrhea and Rhinorrhea

Chronically raised ICP lead to osseous erosion of the skull base and widening of the foramen ovale which lead to CSF otorrhea and rhinorrhea. Patients with spontaneous CSF leak are commonly middle-aged, obese and of female gender and sometimes fulfill the criteria for IIH. So, there is a probable link between these two.

Psychosocial Impact

A major morbidity of IIH is reduced quality of life, increased rate of anxiety and depression. Visual symptoms mostly associated with this psychosocial impact.

DISEASE COURSE AND PROGNOSIS

Disease course in IIH is poorly defined. Those with milder course with early management appear to stabilize early with or without occasional relapses, while those with severe onset and rare fulminant course and also delayed treatment develop more progressive disease and frequent relapse.

Those without papilledema generally have less risk of visual loss and good prognosis.

Follow-up

Regular ophthalmological examinations including visual acuity, fundoscopy, and automated perimetry should be done in all cases.

Ophthalmological examinations should be repeated after 2 weeks. More frequent follow-up required in those with deterioration of vision.

Subsequent examinations to be undertaken at intervals of 1 month. If the patient remains stable the interval of visual testing may be increased to 3 months till papilledema completely regresses.

Assessment of the nerve fiber layer and degree of optic nerve injury can be monitored by OCT which gives statistically valid and reproducible results.

The Idiopathic Intracranial Hypertension Treatment Trial

The Neuro-ophthalmological Research Disease Investigator Consortium (NORDIC) recruited 166 IIH patients with mild visual loss in the IIHTT. This multicentric, randomized, double-blind, placebo-controlled study compared two groups: One with diet control coupled with acetazolamide and another with dieting and placebo in IIH patients. The outcome measured were visual perimetry, change in papilloedema grade, ICP measurements, other visual field measurements and quality of life measures. The primary outcome is improvement in visual perimetry from baseline to 6 months. Analysis indicated that dieting and lifestyle modifications have resulted in 6% weight loss in almost half of patients recruited. High-doses of acetazolamide also appeared to be safe and well tolerated if given twice daily with food, although 2% of patients developed kidney stones. In IIHTT acetazolamide use provides a modest improvement of symptoms including visual field function in patients with IIH.

There are many unanswered questions regarding the pathogenesis of IIH which this trial hopes to address by studying proteomic and genetic risk factors in IIH patients compared to controls.

SPECIFIC SITUATIONS

Fulminant Idiopathic Intracranial Hypertension

Visual loss is typically insidious in IIH, but may have a fulminant course, characterized by rapid and devastating visual loss. These patients generally have severe papilledema and very high CSF opening pressure.

Fulminant IIH may be defined as: (i) The acute onset of symptoms and signs of intracranial hypertension (less than 4 weeks between onset of initial symptoms and severe visual loss) and (ii) rapid worsening of visual loss over few days.

Fulminant IIH is uncommon and seen in less than 3% of IIH patients. Hence, secondary causes of raised ICP should always be ruled out. Fulminant IIH is a medical emergency and should be recognized and managed as early as possible to avoid irreversible visual loss. Generally, an emergent CSF diversion procedure with serial LPs or lumbar drain needed followed by the definitive surgery.

Idiopathic Intracranial Hypertension and Pregnancy

Idiopathic intracranial hypertension in pregnant women is not uncommon. Prevalence of IIH among pregnant women is variable in different studies. It has been reported in up to 12%. Digre et al. found that 8.3% of IIH patients were pregnant on diagnosis and 14.7% were diagnosed with IIH while pregnant. In 2002, Huna-Baron and Kupersmith found that the prevalence was 5%.

Idiopathic intracranial hypertension can occur anytime from conception to 33 weeks, although it is usually more common during the first half of pregnancy, with 61% of the cases occurring during the first trimester.

Diagnosis of IIH during pregnancy is challenging. The discovery of papilledema during pregnancy prompts an emergent workup to exclude secondary causes particularly venous sinus thrombosis or eclampsia.

Measuring the opening pressure of CSF in a relaxed lateral recumbent position has no contraindication during pregnancy, rather essential for confirmation of raised ICP.

The major differential diagnosis of IIH in pregnancy is venous thrombosis.

In patients carrying the diagnosis of IIH prior to pregnancy, no specific changes in the management of pregnancy or the delivery are required.

Regarding the treatment of IIH during pregnancy, use of acetazolamide is controversial, generally used with caution (category C). The safety of prescribing topiramate to pregnant women with IIH is limited, and it is therefore not recommended.

If the patient has only mild symptoms, acetazolamide may be stopped during the first trimester. Serial lumbar punctures can also be used as needed until delivery.

Surgical intervention is recommended for patients with severe or progressive visual loss despite medical management. The current surgical approach consists of ONSF and CSF shunting (lumboperitoneal or ventriculoperitoneal shunts).

The coexistence of IIH and pregnancy does not increase the risk of relapse, worsen the prognosis of IIH, or affect perinatal outcome. Visual outcomes for pregnant and nonpregnant women with IIH are identical. As the most worrisome features of IIH are visual loss, patients should be followed throughout their pregnancy.

Subsequent pregnancies do not increase the risk of recurrence of IIH above the risk of recurrence in any other woman with IIH. There is no contraindication for women with IIH who wish to become pregnant. There are also no demonstrated fertility problems in these patients.

There is no reason to terminate a pregnancy for a woman diagnosed with IIH. The increase in ICP that occurs during labor and delivery is only transient and does not cause any harm to the mother or the baby.

Pediatric Idiopathic Intracranial Hypertension

Idiopathic intracranial hypertension, though occurs at any age is a rare neurological disorder in children.

Pediatric IIH has several distinctive features as follows:
- Idiopathic intracranial hypertension in adolescents share the same demographics as adults, but in children, the sex ratio is closer to 1:1
- Obesity is less frequently seen in prepubertal children with IIH
- Regarding the diagnosis, the cut-off for elevated CSF pressure has been set at 280 mmH$_2$O in the 2013 criteria based on a recent evaluation of CSF opening pressure in children.

In young children (<8 years), the upper limit of normal CSF opening pressure is considered to be 280 mmH$_2$O, and 250 mmH$_2$O in children who were not sedated or obese.

Other distinctive features include:
- A higher proportion of secondary intracranial hypertension

- Frequent absence of papilledema in children with open sutures
- Slowly resolving papilledema over months despite satisfactory ICP control.

Management of Pediatric Idiopathic Intracranial Hypertension

The best approach to manage IIH in children is through a multidisciplinary team that includes a pediatrician, pediatric neurologist, ophthalmologist, nutritionist, and neurosurgeon. In milder cases, like asymptomatic patients with normal vision and mild papilledema, only serial ophthalmological evaluation is required. Treatment is indicated when there is an evidence of visual loss, moderate to severe papilledema, or persistent headaches.

The treatment is not different from that of adults, except that repeat lumbar punctures are often not as well-tolerated in children.

KEY POINTS

Clinical profile suggestive of IIH should be evaluated thoroughly and quickly.
- Be certain the patient has elevated CSF pressure (lumbar puncture) before treating
- Investigate for treatable conditions (especially venous sinus occlusion) in all patients who are not obese women. This includes thin women patients, all men, and children
- Enlist the assistance of an ophthalmologist to do visual fields and fundus photography and to examine the eye carefully
- Treat headache as one would treat ordinary migraine. Repeat lumbar puncture for headache management should be at the patient's request only
- Visual loss is the only serious permanent complication and it is due to disc swelling
- Treat systemic hypertension very cautiously in the patient with swollen optic nerves. Sudden drops in blood pressure may infarct already swollen nerves
- Neurologic findings other than sixth nerve palsy should be viewed with suspicion
- Follow patients with repeat visual fields and not with repeated lumbar puncture. CSF pressure is chronically elevated in most patients with IIH and CSF pressures do not provide information on which one may make a surgical decision
- Surgical intervention should be considered early rather than late, loss of visual acuity is an ominous sign of serious visual dysfunction
- Patients who appear to be at higher risk for visual loss are men and patients with hypertension and/or elevated intraocular pressure (glaucoma)
- If visual fields begin to deteriorate on medical therapy, do not change medications, do a surgical procedure
- If the patient has renal failure and IIH with visual loss, do an optic nerve sheath decompression before subjecting the patient to repeated dialysis.

Patients who are obese frequently have sleep apnea and this may play a part in progression of visual loss despite shunting or optic nerve sheath decompression. All efforts should be made to improve visual symptoms and prevent visual loss.

CONCLUSION

Idiopathic intracranial hypertension, was earlier thought as a benign condition; however, it is not benign as having potential complication like irreversible visual loss. With global obesity epidemic, the incidence of IIH is likely to rise, more in females, also in males and children.

Currently, the pathophysiology of IIH is better understood with better identification of visual risk factors allowing better monitoring of patients' risk profiles, better description of atypical forms of IIH, including fulminant IIH and CSF leaks and recent advances in MRI technology revealing more findings specific to increased ICP.

In rapidly progressive cases and in those poorly respond to conservative management present a particular problem to neurologists and ophthalmologists and require neurosurgical intervention, which is often unsatisfactory in the long-term.

So, new clinical trials need for more treatment options including proper timings of surgical intervention to minimize long term complication.

SUGGESTED READINGS

1. Acheson JF. Idiopathic intracranial hypertension and visual function. Br Med Bull. 2006;79-80:233-44.
2. Andrews LE, Liu GT, Ko MW. Idiopathic intracranial hypertension and obesity. Horm Res Paediatr. 2014;81:217-25.
3. Avery RA, Shah SS, Licht DJ, et al. Reference range for cerebrospinal fluid opening pressure in children. N Engl J Med. 2010;363(9):891-3.
4. Badve M, McConnell MJ, Shah T, et al. Idiopathic intracranial hypertension in pregnancy treated with serial lumbar punctures. Int J Clin Med. 2011;2:9-12.
5. Baheti NN, Nair M, Thomas SV. Long-term visual outcome in idiopathic intracranial hypertension. Ann Indian Acad Neurol. 2011;14:19-22.
6. Ball AK, Howman A, Wheatley K, et al. A randomised controlled trial of treatment for idiopathic intracranial hypertension. J Neurol. 2011;258:874-81.
7. Ball AK, Sinclair AJ, Curnow SJ, et al. Elevated cerebrospinal fluid (CSF) leptin in idiopathic intracranial hypertension (IIH): Evidence for hypothalamic leptin resistance? Clin Endocrinol (Oxf). 2009;70:863-9.
8. Barness LA, Opitz JM, Gilbert-Barness E. Obesity: Genetic, molecular, and environmental aspects. Am J Med Genet A. 2007;143:3016-34.
9. Beri S, Gosalakkal JA, Hussain N, et al. Idiopathic intracranial hypertension without papilledema. Pediatr Neurol. 2010;42:56.
10. Bhardwaj A, Ulatowski JA. Hypertonic saline solutions in brain injury. Curr Opin Crit Care. 2004;10:126.
11. Biousse V, Bruce BB, Newman NJ. Update on the pathophysiology and management of idiopathic intracranial hypertension. J Neurol Neurosurg Psychiatry. 2012;83:488-94.
12. Bono F, Giliberto C, Mastrandrea C, et al. Transverse sinus stenoses persist after normalization of the CSF pressure in IIH. Neurology. 2005;65:1090-3.
13. Bret PH, Lapras CI, Twose G, et al. Lumbo-peritoneal shunt. Indications and results about 80 cases. Neuro Chir Paris. 1982;28:13-20.
14. Brourman MD, Sppor TC, Ramocki JM. Optic nerve sheath decompression for pseudotumor cerebri. Arch Ophthalmol. 1988;106:1378-83.
15. Buchheit W A, Burton C, Haag B, et al. Papilledema and idiopathic intracranial hypertension. N Engl J Med. 1969;280:938-42.
16. Bullock R, Clifton G. Guidelines for the Management of Severe Brain Injury, Brain trauma foundation/ American Association of Neurologic Surgeons, New York 1995.
17. Butros SR, Goncalves LF, Thompson D, et al. Imaging features of idiopathic intracranial hypertension, including a new finding: Widening of the foramen ovale. Acta Radiol. 2012;53:682-8.
18. Celebisoy N, Gokcay F, Sirin H, et al. Treatment of idiopathic intracranial hypertension: Topiramate vs. acetazolamide, an open label study. Acta Neurol Scand. 2007;116:322-7.
19. Celebisoy N, Seçil Y, Akyürekli O. Pseudotumor cerebri: Etiological factors, presenting features and prognosis in the western part of Turkey. Acta Neurol Scand. 2002;106:367-70.
20. Chari C, Rao NS. Benign intracranial hypertension–its unusual manifestations. Headache 1991;31:599-600.
21. Chumas PD, Kulkarni AV, Drake JM, et al. Lumboperitoneal shunting: A retrospective study in the paediatric population. Neurosurgery. 1993;32:376-83.
22. Cinciripini GS, Donahue S, Borchert MS. Idiopathic intracranial hypertension in prepubertal pediatric patients: Characteristics, treatment, and outcome. Am J Ophthalmol. 1999;127:178-82.
23. Corbett JJ, Savino PJ, Thompson HS, et al. Visual loss in pseudotumor cerebri. Follow-up of 57 patients from five to 41 years and a profile of 14 patients with permanent severe visual loss. Arch Neurol. 1982;39:461-74.
24. Corbett JJ, Thompson HS. The rational management of idiopathic intracranial hypertension. Arch Neurol. 1989;46:1049-51.
25. Cosar E, Cosar M, Ko¨ken G, et al. Polycystic ovary syndrome is related to idiopathic intracranial hypertension according to magnetic resonance imaging and magnetic resonance venography. Fertil Steril. 2008;89:1245-6.
26. Cunningham FG. Drugs commonly used in pregnancy. In: Swils A, ed. Williams Obstetrics. 21st ed. New York: McGraw Hill; 2001:1020-31.
27. D'Amico D, Curone M, Ciasca P, et al. Headache prevalence and clinical features in patients with idiopathic intracranial hypertension (IIH). Neurol Sci. 2013;34(Suppl 1):S147-9.
28. Dandy WE. Intracranial pressure without brain tumor: Diagnosis and treatment. Ann Surg. 1937;106:492-513.
29. Daniels AB, Liu GT, Volpe NJ, et al. Profiles of obesity, weight gain, and quality of life in idiopathic intracranial hypertension (pseudotumor cerebri). Am J Ophthalmol. 2007;143:635-41.
30. Davidoff LM, Dyke CG. Hypertensive meningeal hydrops: A syndrome frequently following infection in the middle ear or elsewhere in the body. Am J Ophthalmol. 1937;20:908-27.
31. De Simone R, Ranieri A, Bonavita V. Advancement in idiopathic intracranial hypertension pathogenesis: Focus on sinus venous stenosis. Neurol Sci. 2010;31(Suppl 1):S33-9.
32. De Wecker L. On incision of the optic nerve in cases of neuro-retinitis. Int Ophthalmol Congress Rep. 1872;4:11-14.
33. Dennis LJ, Mayer SA. Diagnosis and management of increased intracranial pressure. Neurol India. 2001;49 Suppl 1:S37.

34. Digre KB, Corbett JJ. Idiopathic intracranial hypertension (pseudotumor cerebri): A reappraisal. Neurologist. 2001;7:2-67.
35. Digre KB, Varner MW, Corbett JJ. Pseudotumor cerebri and pregnancy. Neurology. 1984;34:721-9.
36. Digre KB. Neuro-ophthalmology and pregnancy: what does a neuro-ophthalmologist need to know? J Neuroophthalmol. 2011;31(4):381-7.
37. Dubourg J, Javouhey E, Geeraerts T, et al. Ultrasonography of optic nerve sheath diameter for detection of raised intracranial pressure: A systematic review and meta-analysis. Intensive Care Med. 2011;37:1059-68.
38. Falardeau J, Lobb BM, Golden S, et al. The use of acetazolamide during pregnancy in intracranial hypertension patients. J Neuroophthalmol. 2013; 33(1):9-12.
39. Farb RI, Vanek I, Scott JN, et al. Idiopathic intracranial hypertension: The prevalence and morphology of sinovenous stenosis. Neurology. 2003;60:1418-24.
40. Förderreuther S, Straube A. Indomethacin reduces CSF pressure in intracranial hypertension. Neurology. 2000;55:1043-5.
41. Foley J. Benign forms of intracranial hypertension: "toxic" and "otitic" hydrocephalus. Brain 1955;78:1-41.
42. Foley KM. Is benign intracranial hypertension a chronic disease? Neurology. 1977;27:388.
43. Fraser CL, Biousse V, Newman NJ. Minocycline-induced fulminant intracranial hypertension. Arch Neurol. 2012;9:1067-70.
44. Friedman DI, Rausch EA. Headache diagnoses in patients with treated idiopathic intracranial hypertension. Neurology. 2002;58:1551-3.
45. Friedman DI, Jacobson DM. Diagnostic criteria for idiopathic intracranial hypertension. Neurology. 2002;59(10):1492-5.
46. Friedman DI, Jacobson DM. Idiopathic intracranial hypertension. J Neuroophthalmol. 2004;24:138-45.
47. Friedman DI, Liu GT, Digre KB. Revised diagnostic criteria for the pseudotumor cerebri syndrome in adults and children. Neurology. 2013;81(13):1159-65.
48. Geeraerts T, Launey Y, Martin L, et al. Ultrasonography of the optic nerve sheath may be useful for detecting raised intracranial pressure after severe brain injury. Intensive Care Med. 2007;33:1704-11.
49. Geeraerts T, Merceron S, Benhamou D, et al. Non-invasive assessment of intracranial pressure using ocular sonography in neurocritical care patients. Intensive Care Med. 2008;34:2062-7.
50. Giuseffi V, Wall M, Siegel PZ, et al. Symptoms and disease associations in idiopathic intracranial hypertension (pseudotumor cerebri): A case-control study. Neurology. 1991;41:239-44.
51. Greenfield DS, Wanichwecharungruang B, Liebmann JM, et al. Pseudotumor cerebri appearing with unilateral papilledema after trabeculectomy. Arch Ophthalmol. 1997;115:423-6.
52. Han Y, McCulley TJ, Horton JC. No correlation between intraocular pressure and intracranial pressure. Ann Neurol. 2008;64:221-4.
53. Headache Classification Committee of the International Headache Society (IHS). The International Classification of Headache Disorders, 3rd edition (beta version). Cephalalgia 2013;33(9):629-808.
54. Huna-Baron R, Kupersmith MJ. Idiopathic intracranial hypertension in pregnancy. J Neurol 2002;249:1078-81.
55. Jacobson DM, Berg R, Wall M, et al. Serum vitamin A concentration is elevated in idiopathic intracranial hypertension. Neurology. 1999;53:1114-8.
56. Jensen K, Ohrström J, Cold GE, et al. The effects of indomethacin on intracranial pressure, cerebral blood flow and cerebral metabolism in patients with severe head injury and intracranial hypertension. Acta Neurochir (Wien). 1991;108:116-21.
57. Johnson LN, Krohel GB, Madsen RW, et al. The role of weight loss and acetazolamide in the treatment of idiopathic intracranial hypertension (pseudotumor cerebri). Ophthalmology 1998;105:2313-17.
58. Johnston I, Owler B, Pickard J. The pseudotumor cerebri syndrome: Pseudotumor cerebri, idiopathic intracranial hypertension, benign intracranial hypertension and related conditions. Cambridge (United Kingdom): Cambridge University Press; 2007. P. 1-356.
59. Karnik S, Kanekar A. Childhood obesity: A global public health crisis. Int J Prev Med. 2012;3:1-7.
60. Kaye AH. Brain tumors: An Encyclopedic Approach, 2nd, Churchill Livingstone, New York 2001. P. 205.
61. Keltner JL. Optic nerve sheath decompression. How does it work? Arch. Opthalmol. 1988;106:1365-9.
62. Kesler A, Kliper E, Assayag EB, et al. Thrombophilic factors in idiopathic intracranial hypertension: A report of 51 patients and a meta-analysis. Blood Coagul Fibrinolysis. 2010;21:328-33.
63. Kesler A, Kliper E, Shenkerman G, et al. Idiopathic intracranial hypertension is associated with lower body adiposity. Ophthalmology. 2010;117:169-74.
64. Kidron D, Pomeranz S. Malignant pseudotumor cerebri. Report of two cases. J Neurosurg 1989;71:443-5.
65. Kimberly HH, Shah S, Marill K, et al. Correlation of optic nerve sheath diameter with direct measurement of intracranial pressure. Acad Emerg Med. 2008;15:201-4.
66. Kirk T, Jones K, Miller S, Corbett J. Measurement of intraocular and intracranial pressure: Is there a relationship? Ann Neurol. 2011;70:323-6.
67. Kirkham TH, Sanders MD, Sapp GA. Unilateral papilledema in benign intracranial hypertension. Can J Ophthalmol. 1973;8:533-8.
68. Ko MW, Chang SC, Ridha MA, et al. Weight gain and recurrence in idiopathic intracranial hypertension: A case-control study. Neurology. 2011;76:1564-7.

69. Ko MW, Liu GT. Pediatric idiopathic intracranial hypertension (pseudotumor cerebri). Horm Res Paediatr. 2010;74(6):381-9.
70. Krishna R, Kosmorsky GS, Wright KW. Pseudotumor cerebri sine papilledema with unilateral sixth nerve palsy. J Neuroophthalmol. 1998;18:53-5.
71. Krishnakumar D, Pickard JD, Czosnyka Z, et al. Idiopathic intracranial hypertension in childhood: Pitfalls in diagnosis. Dev Med Child Neurol. 2014;56:749-55.
72. Kuensting LL. A 15-year-old with blurred vision, nausea, back pain, and abdominal pain. J Emerg Nurs. 2003;29:171-3.
73. Kupersmith MJ, Gamell L, Turbin R, et al. Effects of weight loss on the course of idiopathic intracranial hypertension in women. Neurology. 1998;50:1094-8.
74. Kupersmith MJ, Sibony P, Mandel G, et al. Optical coherence tomography of the swollen optic nerve head: Deformation of the peripapillary retinal pigment epithelium layer in papilledema. Invest Ophthalmol Vis Sci. 2011;52:6558-64.
75. Lam BL, Siatkowski RM, Fox GM, et al. Visual loss in pseudotumor cerebri from branch retinal artery occlusion. Am J Ophthalmol. 1992;113:334-6.
76. Lampl Y, Eshel Y, Kessler A, et al. Serum leptin level in women with idiopathic intracranial hypertension. J Neurol Neurosurg Psychiatry. 2002;72:642-3.
77. Lashutka MK, Chandra A, Murray HN, et al. The relationship of intraocular pressure to intracranial pressure. Ann Emerg Med. 2004;43:585-91.
78. Lee AG, Golnik K, Kardon R, et al. Sleep apnea and intracranial hypertension in men. Ophthalmology. 2002;109:482-5.
79. Lee AG, Pless M, Falardeau J, et al. The use of acetazolamide in idiopathic intracranial hypertension during pregnancy. Am J Ophthalmol. 2005;139(5):855-9.
80. Lessell S. Pediatric pseudotumor cerebri (idiopathic intracranial hypertension). Surv Ophthalmol. 1992;37:155-66.
81. Li Z, Maglione M, Tu W, et al. Meta-analysis: pharmacologic treatment of obesity. Ann Intern Med. 2005;142:532-46.
82. Libien J, Blaner WS. Retinol and retinol-binding protein in cerebrospinal fluid: Can vitamin A take the "idiopathic" out of idiopathic intracranial hypertension? J Neuroophthalmol. 2007; 27:253-7.
83. Liu GT, Glaser JS, Schatz NJ. High-dose methylprednisolone and acetazolamide for visual loss in pseudotumor cerebri. Am J Ophthalmol. 1994;118:88-96.
84. Marcelis J, Silberstein SD. Idiopathic intracranial hypertension without papilledema. Arch Neurol. 1991; 48:392-9.
85. Marcus DM, Lynn J, Miller JJ, et al. Sleep disorders: A risk factor for pseudotumor cerebri? J Neuroophthalmol. 2001;21:121-3.
86. Mathew NT, Ravishankar K, Sanin LC. Coexistence of migraine and idiopathic intracranial hypertension without papilledema. Neurology. 1996;46:1226-30.
87. McCarthy KD, Reed DJ. The effect of acetazolamide and furosemide on cerebrospinal fluid production and choroid plexus carbonic anhydrase activity. J Pharmacol Exp Ther. 1974;189:194-201.
88. McCluskey G, Mulholland DA, McCarron P, et al. Idiopathic intracranial hypertension in the northwest of northern Ireland: Epidemiology and clinical management. Neuroepidemiology 2015;45:34-9.
89. Moretti R, Pizzi B, Cassini F, et al. Reliability of optic nerve ultrasound for the evaluation of patients with spontaneous intracranial hemorrhage. Neurocrit Care. 2009;11:406-10.
90. Moretti R, Pizzi B. Optic nerve ultrasound for detection of intracranial hypertension in intracranial hemorrhage patients: Confirmation of previous findings in a different patient population. J Neurosurg Anesthesiol. 2009;21:16-20.
91. Mortazavi MM, Romeo AK, Deep A, et al. Hypertonic saline for treating raised intracranial pressure: Literature review with meta-analysis. J Neurosurg. 2012;116:210-21.
92. Newborg B. Pseudotumor cerebri treated by rice reduction diet. Arch Intern Med 1974;133:802-7.
93. Nonne M. Über, Fälle vom. Symptomkomplex 'tumor cerebri' mit Ausgang in Heillung (Pseudotumor cerebri). Über Letal Verlaufene Fälle von 'Pseudotumor Cerebri' mit Sektionsbefund. Dtsch Z Nervenheilkd. 1904;27:169-216.
94. Piper RJ, Kalyvas AV, Young AM, et al. Interventions for idiopathic intracranial hypertension. Cochrane Database Syst Rev. 2015;8:CD003434.
95. Quattrone A, Bono F, Fera F, et al. Isolated unilateral abducens palsy in idiopathic intracranial hypertension without papilledema. Eur J Neurol. 2006;13:670-1.
96. Quincke H, Ueber meningitis serosa and verwandlte Zustande. Dtscb Z Nervenheilk. 1897;9:149-168.
97. Quincke H. Ueber meningitis serosa: Sammlung linische Vortra 67. Inn Med. 1893;23:655-94.
98. Radhakrishnan K, Ahlskog JE, Cross SA, et al. Idiopathic intracranial hypertension (pseudotumor cerebri). Descriptive epidemiology in Rochester, Minn, 1976 to 1990. Arch Neurol. 1993;50:78-80.
99. Radhakrishnan K, Thacker AK, Bohlaga NH, et al. Epidemiology of idiopathic intracranial hypertension: A prospective and case-control study. J Neurol Sci. 1993;116:18-28.
100. Rangwala LM, Liu GT. Pediatric idiopathic intracranial hypertension. Surv Ophthalmol. 2007;52:597-617.
101. Raoof N, Sharrack B, Pepper IM, et al. The incidence and prevalence of idiopathic intracranial hypertension in Sheffield, UK. Eur J Neurol. 2011;18:1266-8.

102. Rasmussen M. Treatment of elevated intracranial pressure with indomethacin: Friend or foe? Acta Anaesthesiol Scand. 2005;49:341-50.
103. Rohr A, Bindeballe J, Riedel C, et al. The entire dural sinus tree is compressed in patients with idiopathic intracranial hypertension: A longitudinal, volumetric magnetic resonance imaging study. Neuroradiology. 2012;54:25-33.
104. Round R, Keane JR. The minor symptoms of increased intracranial pressure: 101 patients with benign intracranial hypertension. Neurology. 1988;38:1461-4.
105. Rudnick E, Sismanis A. Pulsatile tinnitus and spontaneous cerebrospinal fluid rhinorrhea: Indicators of benign intracranial hypertension syndrome. Otol Neurotol. 2005;26:166-8.
106. Saito J, Kami M, Taniguchi F, et al. Unilateral papilledema after bone marrow transplantation. Bone Marrow Transplant. 1999;23:963-5.
107. Salman MS, Kirkham FJ, MacGregor DL. Idiopathic "benign" intracranial hypertension: Case series and review. J Child Neurol. 2001;16:465-70.
108. Schmoker JD, Shackford SR, Wald SL, et al. An analysis of the relationship between fluid and sodium administration and intracranial pressure after head injury. J Trauma. 1992;33:476-81.
109. Selhorst JB, Kulkantrakorn K, Corbett JJ, et al. Retinol binding protein in idiopathic intracranial hypertension (IIH). J Neuroophthalmol. 2000;20:250-2.
110. Shah VA, Kardon RH, Lee AG, et al. Long-term follow-up of idiopathic intracranial hypertension: The Iowa experience. Neurology. 2008;70:634-40.
111. Sheeran P, Bland JM, Hall GM. Intraocular pressure changes and alterations in intracranial pressure. Lancet. 2000;355:899.
112. Sibony P, Kupersmith MJ, Rohlf FJ. Shape analysis of the peripapillary RPE layer in papilledema and ischemic optic neuropathy. Invest Ophthalmol Vis Sci. 2011;52:7987-95.
113. Sismanis A, Butts FM, Hughes GB. Objective tinnitus in benign intracranial hypertension: An update. Laryngoscope. 1990;100:33-6.
114. Skau M, Milea D, Sander B, et al. OCT for optic disc evaluation in idiopathic intracranial hypertension. Graefes Arch Clin Exp Ophthalmol. 2011;249:723-30.
115. Smith ER, Madsen JR. Cerebral pathophysiology and critical care neurology: Basic hemodynamic principles, cerebral perfusion, and intracranial pressure. Semin Pediatr Neurol 2004;11:89-104.
116. Smith MB, Griffiths EA, Thompson JE, et al. High pseudotumor cerebri incidence in tretinoin and arsenic treated acute promyelocytic leukemia and the role of topiramate after acetazolamide failure. Leuk Res Rep. 2014;3:62-6.
117. Soler D, Cox T, Bullock P, et al. Diagnosis and management of benign intracranial hypertension. Arch Dis Child 1998; 78:89-94.
118. Stienen A, Weinzierl M, Ludolph A, et al. Obstruction of cerebral venous sinus secondary to idiopathic intracranial hypertension. Eur J Neurol. 2008;15:1416-8.
119. Sureda B, Alberca R. Pregnancy and benign intracranial hypertension. An Med Interna. 1991;8:8-10.
120. Symonds CP. Otitic hydrocephalus. Brain. 1931;54:55-71.
121. Szewka AJ, Bruce BB, Newman NJ, et al. Idiopathic intracranial hypertension: Relation between obesity and visual outcomes. J Neuroophthalmol. 2012;33:4-8.
122. Tabassi A, Salmasi AH, Jalali M. Serum and CSF vitamin A concentrations in idiopathic intracranial hypertension. Neurology. 2005;64:1893-6.
123. Tang RA, Dorotheo EU, Schiffman JS, et al. Medical and surgical management of idiopathic intracranial hypertension in pregnancy. Curr Neurol Neurosci Rep. 2004;4:398-409.
124. Thambisetty M, Lavin PJ, Newman NJ, et al. Fulminant idiopathic intracranial hypertension. Neurology. 2007;68:229-32.
125. The Organization for Economic Co-operation and Development (OECD). Obesity and the economics of prevention: Fit not fat – Canada key facts, 2010 [cited 2018 August 21]. Available from: http://www.oecd.org/els/healthpoliciesanddata/obesityandtheeconomicsofpreventionfitnotfat-canadakeyfacts.htm
126. Tranmer BI, Iacobacci RI, Kindt GW. Effects of crystalloid and colloid infusions on intracranial pressure and computerized electroencephalographic data in dogs with vasogenic brain edema. Neurosurgery. 1989;25:173-8.
127. Vieira DS, Masruha MR, Gonçalves AL, et al. Idiopathic intracranial hypertension with and without papilloedema in a consecutive series of patients with chronic migraine. Cephalalgia. 2008;28:609-13.
128. Wall M, George D. Idiopathic intracranial hypertension. A prospective study of 50 patients. Brain. 1991;114:155-80.
129. Wall M, Dollar JD, Sadun AA, et al. Idiopathic intracranial hypertension. Lack of histologic evidence for cerebral edema. Arch Neurol. 1995;52:141-5.
130. Wall M, Kupersmith MJ, Kieburtz KD, et al. The idiopathic intracranial hypertension treatment trial: Clinical profile at baseline. JAMA Neurol. 2014;71:693-701.
131. Wall M, McDermott MP, Kieburtz KD, et al. NORDIC Idiopathic Intracranial Hypertension Study Group Writing Committee. Effect of acetazolamide on visual function in patients with idiopathic intracranial hypertension and mild visual loss: the idiopathic intracranial hypertension treatment trial. JAMA. 2014;311:1641-51.
132. Wall M, White WN 2nd. Asymmetric papilledema in idiopathic intracranial hypertension: prospective interocular comparison of sensory visual function. Invest Ophthalmol Vis Sci. 1998; 39:134-42.
133. Wall M. Idiopathic intracranial hypertension and the idiopathic intracranial hypertension treatment trial. J Neuro-Ophthalmol 2013;33:1-3.

134. Wang SJ, Silberstein SD, Patterson S, et al. Idiopathic intracranial hypertension without papilledema: A case-control study in a headache center. Neurology. 1998;51:245-9.
135. Warman R. Management of pseudotumor cerebri in children. Int Pediatr. 2000;15:147.
136. Warner JE, Larson AJ, Bhosale P, et al. Retinol-binding protein and retinol analysis in cerebrospinal fluid and serum of patients with and without idiopathic intracranial hypertension. J Neuroophthalmol. 2007;27:258-62.
137. Warner JEA, Bernstein PS, Yemelyanov A, et al. Vitamin A in the cerebrospinal fluid of patients with and without idiopathic intracranial hypertension. Ann Neurol. 2002;52:647-50.
138. Welch K. The intracranial pressure in infants. J Neurosurg. 1980;52:693.
139. Wong R, Madill SA, Pandey P, et al. Idiopathic intracranial hypertension: the association between weight loss and the requirement for systemic treatment. BMC Ophthalmol 2007;7:15.
140. Yri HM, Rönnbäck C, Wegener M, et al. The course of headache in idiopathic intracranial hypertension: A 12-month prospective follow-up study. Eur J Neurol 2014;21:1458-64.

22 CHAPTER

Eye and Headache

Koushik Pan, Ambar Chakravarty

Ophthalmologists are often the first physicians to evaluate patients with headaches, eye pain, and headache-associated visual disturbances. Although ophthalmic causes are sometimes diagnosed, most eye pain and many types of visual disturbances are neurologic in origin. This article reviews the primary as well as secondary and systemic headache disorders and focuses on their ophthalmic manifestations.

INTRODUCTION

Eye and brain are developmentally related. The eye develops from the optic vesicle which comes out of the developing forebrain vesicle. The forebrain vesicle develops as the cerebral hemispheres and the optic vesicle as the eye with the connecting stalk developing as the optic nerve. Naturally the sensory nerves carrying pain sensations from these two organs are very similar. Eye pains are referred to the head and pain of central origin often are referred to the eyes.

Sensory pain pathways are as follows.

Brain

- Brain is itself, just as any solid viscera in the body, insensitive to pain
- Head pain arises from the coverings of brain, e.g., skull, scalp, dura, walls of dural sinuses, meninges, walls of blood vessels, and cranial nerves including optic nerve: pain pathways involve trigeminal nerve (NV).

Eye

All pain fibers travel by ophthalmic division of NV:
- Meeting points of pain fibers from eye and brain: NV ganglion (Gasserian) and trigeminal nuclear complex (TNC) in brain stem
- Convergence of sensory pain paths (NV): Referred headache from eye diseases
- Autonomic supply to eye arises from brain: Symphathetic and parasympathetic.

EVALUATION OF EYE/HEAD PAIN

- Onset: Abrupt/insidious
- Location
- Severity: Mild/moderate/severe
- Pattern: Periodic/nonperiodic
- Precipitating factors: Eye movement, sounds/lights etc., position
- Relieving factors: Sleep, dark room, vomiting, and position
- Radiation
- Nature: Throb, dull, shock-like, and stab/jab
- Duration: Seconds, minutes, hours, and days
- Associated symptoms: Red/white eye, visual loss/dimness, autonomic features, diplopia, photophobia/phonophobia, eye discharge, lacrimation, and nose block
- Field defect: Restricted to one eye or both eyes involved
- Family history.

EXAMINATION

- Visual acuity (VA): Headaches associated with visual disturbances may be due to associated with refractive errors, papilledema, idiopathic intracranial hypertension, field loss retinal migraine, optic neuritis, or giant cell arteritis (GCA). Only refractive errors are a rare cause of headache. This is best expressed by the English adage "Hands full of glasses syndrome". Headaches related to refractive errors need to be classified as secondary headaches.

According to the definition of secondary headaches by the International Headache Society (ICHD-3, 2013), such headaches should "resolve within 2 weeks of appropriate treatment of the alleged cause" in this case meaning prescription of appropriate spectacles or perhaps laser keratoplasty. Unfortunate total resolution of headache with glasses occur only in small number of subjects. Most such subjects are ultimately diagnosed to have been suffering from migraine
- Eye appearance: A white eye is a rare cause of headache. In most eye diseases causing headache, the eyes look congested. On the other hand, primary headache disorders like trigeminal autonomic cephalgias (TACs) present with autonomic manifestations in the eye like ptosis, lacrimation, conjunctival injection, Horner's syndrome, and eyelid edema
- Pupils: Pupillary abnormalities accompanying headaches can be a manifestation of cluster headache with Horner's syndrome, Adie's pupil, parasellar neoplasms or aneurysms, internal carotid dissection or occlusion, and Tolosa–Hunt syndrome. Headache with a dilated and unreactive pupil may indicate the presence of life-threatening posterior communicating artery aneurysm
- Fundoscopy: Looking for papilledema, optic atrophy, deep cupping, or a normal fundus
- Head and neck examination:
  - Scalp tenderness and condition of scalp arteries
  - Extracranial arteries including neck arteries
  - Trochlear tenderness (only in some special circumstances)
  - Temporomandibular joints
  - Paranasal sinuses—tenderness
  - Blood pressure measurement
  - Cranial/orbital auscultation.

Headache: When to go to an Ophthalmologist?

- All patients with painful red eye with fall in VA (to rule out glaucoma)
- All patients with "bizzare" visual field defects not conforming to any known neurological disease (to rule out glaucoma and psychogenic)
- To differentiate early papilledema from papillitis
- Suspicion of central retinal vein occlusion and neuroretinitis.

Periorbital Headaches

See table 1.

Eye Pain: The Red Flags for the Clinician

- Recent change in VA/visual field
- Relative afferent pupillary defect
- Ocular palsy/ptosis
- Proptosis
- Redness: Conjunctival/circumcorneal
- Corneal haziness
- Pupillary abnormalities
- Fundoscopic changes (papilledema, subhyaloid hemorrhage)
- Recent ocular trauma

Table 1: Periorbital Headaches

Ocular	Extraocular	Secondary
- Acute angle closure glaucoma - Uveitis - Posterior scleritis - ? Severe refractive error - Strabismus/Orthoptic errors? - Optic neuritis (pain with eye movements and phosphenes) - Corneal/conjunctival Inflammation - Trochleitis	All primary headaches – especially migraine, TACs (CH, PH, SUNCT, SUNA, HC)	- Giant cell arteritis - Carotid dissection - Nasopharyngeal carcinoma - Sinus disease (?) - Tolosa–Hunt Syndrome - Orbital myositis - Cavernous sinus disease - Mucormycosis

TACs, trigeminal autonomic cephalgias; CH, cluster headache; PH, paroxysmal hemicranias; SUNCT, short-lasting unilateral neuralgiform headache attacks with conjunctival injection and tearing; SUNA, short-lasting unilateral neuralgiform headache attacks with cranial autonomic symptoms; HC, hemicrania continua.

A White Eye is An Uncommon Cause of Headache: What are the Exceptions?

- Intermittent angle closure glaucoma
- Intermittent raised intraocular pressure (IOP) in open angle glaucoma
- Uveitis and posterior scleritits
- Intraocular/intraorbital tumors
- Optic neuritis
- Orbital myositis (?except Cysticercus).

Eye Strain Headache: Does it Exist?

- Commonly found in those who work on computer for several hours, while looking in dark for long, reading fine print
- Overuse of muscles of eyelid, face, and jaw resulting headache
- Extended visual task leads to less blinking that results in dryness of ocular surface and ultimately a dry eye.

The inability to make both eyes work together in a binocular fashion as occurs in phorias and squints may also generate the symptoms of eye strain in people with phorias. In the authors experience, subjects who had been diagnosed to have eye strain headache, ultimately turn to have been suffering from a primary headache disorder most commonly migraine without aura. However, most individuals who have limited or no binocular vision have no such symptoms. All ocular structures are supplied by the NV which carry pain sensation as well. Hence, pain sensations carried from taut ocular muscles are apt to cause headache.

PRIMARY HEADACHE DISORDERS WITH OPHTHALMIC MANIFESTATIONS

Migraine

Migraine refers to a primary headache disorder commonly characterized by severe, unilateral (alternating hemicranias), throbbing pain with associated nausea, photophobia, phonophobia, and preceding aura. Positive, negative, autonomic, or efferent symptoms and signs are associated with migraine. Positive and negative symptoms are part of migraine aura, whereas autonomic and efferent symptoms often occur before or during the headache phase. Migraine can occur more commonly without aura of course. The eyes are generally white during acute migraine attacks. Varying proportion of migraine patients (40–60%) may develop autonomic symptoms as well, but they are generally bilateral (as opposed to TACs where they are unilateral) and are generally mild. Children often have a different location, nature, and duration of migraine headaches. However, it is in children that the diagnosis is missed most often and mistaken for refractive errors or sinus diseases.

Trigeminal Autonomic Cephalalgia

The TACs are characterized by unilateral pain in the distribution of the ophthalmic division of the NV and cranial autonomic activation. Cluster headache is the most common TAC; SUNCT (short-lasting unilateral neuralgiform headache attacks with conjunctival injection and tearing), SUNA (short-lasting unilateral neuralgiform headache attacks with cranial autonomic symptoms) and paroxysmal hemicrania (PH) occur infrequently. Hemicrania continua (HC) is not very uncommon, but correct diagnosis is often missed. Most TACs are primary, but secondary ones are not too infrequent and hence appropriate neuroimaging is mandatory.

Cluster Headache

- Commonly occurs in men
- Characterized by unilateral attacks of severe pain persisting for 15–180 minutes
- Pain is so severe that patient may awaken from sleep
- Usually patients are restless
- There is associated autonomic symptoms like conjunctival injection, eyelid edema, and lacrimation. Nasal congestion or rhinorrhea and forehead/facial flushing and sweating
- Periodicity is hallmark.

Paroxysmal Hemicranias

- Women are more commonly affected compared to men
- Pain is severe in intensity, throbbing or stabbing in character, lasting for 2–120 minutes, shorter compared to cluster headache
- More frequent occurrence usually several times a day

- Patients may either lie down or sometimes they sit quietly holding their head.

SUNCT AND SUNA
- Rare form of TAC
- Paroxysmal severe, unilateral pain lasting 5–300 seconds, with a maximum duration of 2 hours
- The attack frequency varies, as high as 100 attacks can occur
- Neck movement often precipitate the attack
- Autonomic features like nasal congestion, rhinorrhoea often associated
- No refractory period in contrast to trigeminal neuralgia
- The SUNA is similar to SUNCT, but the attacks last between 2 seconds and 10 minutes, with an attack frequency of one or more per day and has only one autonomic nervous system feature
- SUNCT in fact is a subtype of SUNA
- The differential diagnosis of SUNCT includes posterior fossa abnormalities, such as arteriovenous malformations and other structural malformations, and HIV/AIDS. Magnetic resonance imaging (MRI) is warranted to exclude a secondary cause.

Hemicrania Continua

Persistent, strictly unilateral headache, associated with ipsilateral conjunctival injection, lacrimation, nasal congestion, rhinorrhoea, forehead and facial sweating, miosis, ptosis and/or eyelid edema, and/or with restlessness or agitation. The headache is absolutely sensitive to indomethacin. Present for more than 3 months, with exacerbations of moderate or greater intensity. May be associated with a sense of restlessness or agitation, or aggravation of the pain by movement. In an adult, oral indomethacin should be used initially in a dose of at least 150 mg daily and increased if necessary up to 225 mg daily. The dose by injection is 100–200 mg. Smaller maintenance doses are often employed. A small percentage of patients unresponsive to indomethacin have been and designated as non-indomethacin responsive HC (NIRCH). Brain imaging studies show important overlaps between all disorders included here, notably activation in the region of the posterior hypothalamic grey. In addition, the absolute response to indomethacin of HC is shared with paroxysmal hemicrania.

OTHER CAUSES OF HEADACHE AND PERIOCULAR PAIN

Orbital and Ocular Etiologies

Keratitis Sicca (Dry Eye)
- Another common disorder of adulthood
- Commonly found in Sjögren's syndrome, thyroid eye disease that affects lacrimal gland, parkinsonian disorders where there is decreased blink rate
- Common symptoms include—monocular diplopia or polyopia, a foreign body sensation in the eye, eye irritation, redness, and tearing. Corneal damage can occur in severe cases
- Drugs which are used to treat headache like tricyclic antidepressants, propranolol, phenothiazines, metoclopramide, and muscle antispasmodics, and decreases tear production, hence cautious use needed.

Trochlear Pain
- Site of pain in the superomedial part of the orbit
- Exacerbated with eye movement specially looking down or reading
- Some patients experience diplopia and erythema near the superior oblique insertion
- The pain can be manually reproduced by palpating the trochlear region. Injection of local anesthetic and hydrocortisone relieves pain
- The condition is sometimes associated with rheumatoid arthritis
- Contrast enhanced MRI often shows enhancement of the offending trochlea (Fig. 1).

Angle-closure Glaucoma

Sudden onset may resemble a stroke or even a TAC syndrome. Commonly occur where there is shallow anterior chamber, detected by gonioscopy. It produces rapid rise of IOP because of blockage of the trabecular meshwork by the iris resulting in impaired drainage of the aqueous humour. Acute

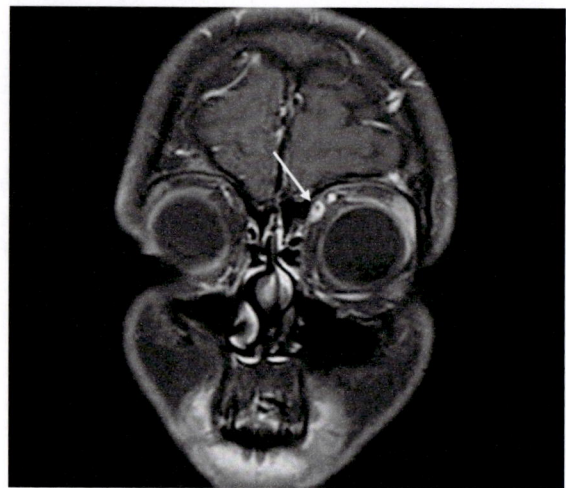

FIG. 1: Enhancement of trochlea in a case of trochleaitis.

angle closure glaucoma can present with pain, blurred vision, rainbow- colored halos around lights, nausea, and vomiting. Examinations reveal high IOP, a mid-dilated and sluggishly reactive pupil, corneal edema, dilated conjunctival blood vessels, and a shallow anterior chamber. Topiramate and acetazolamide, may precipitate angle-closure glaucoma. Anticholinergics and antidepressants may produce attacks in predisposed individuals. Subacute angle-closure glaucoma may mimic migraine or a TAC, producing episodes of ocular or periocular pain, halos, and blurred vision. The attacks are often precipitated by rapid miosis, while emerging from a dark theatre into daylight. Sleep often relieves the symptoms due to mydriasis of pupil during sleep, which is commonly mistaken as migraine, because migraine pain is relieved by sleep also.

Inflammatory Orbital Disease

Closest differential are connective tissue diseases, neoplasm, congenital malformations, infectious disease like bacterial, tubercular and fungal, and trauma. It can present in various ways depending on involvement of the orbital structures, including the extraocular muscles (myositis), sclera (scleritis, episcleritis), aqueous or vitreous (uveitis), lacrimal gland (dacryoadenitis), and uncommonly, the retinae or optic nerves. Common presentation include unilateral or bilateral symptoms of diplopia, pain, proptosis, conjunctival injection, photophobia, and periorbital edema.

The pain is very severe and can be precipitated by manually retropushing the globe under closed eyelids.

Tolosa-Hunt syndrome is a painful ophthalmoplegia syndrome which had been discussed elsewhere in this volume.

Cervical arterial dissection causes acute neck and ipsilateral eye pain and often accompanied with ipsilateral postganglionic Horner's syndrome. This is a diagnosis which often demands a high index of suspicion.

Marfan's syndrome, Ehlers-Danlos syndrome, and fibromuscular dysplasia, are common predisposing factors.

Vertebral artery dissection: The pain often precedes the neurologic symptoms and is localized to the ipsilateral trapezius, posterior neck, occiput, or cervical nerve roots. Sometimes, there is frontal headache. It can manifest either in the form of transient ischemic attack or stroke; although, sometimes there is no neurologic symptoms. Rarely spinal cord infarction can occur. The classic intracranial syndrome of cervical vertebral artery dissection is posterior inferior cerebellar artery syndrome of Wallenberg. The details had been discussed elsewhere in this volume in relation to ocular movements.

Intracranial aneurysms may cause eye and head pain and cranial nerve palsies. This had been discussed earlier in relation to ocular motor palsies.

Giant Cell Arteritis

Temporal arteritis or GCA is a disease of the elderly population. It is found among people aged 50 years or older and is commoner in females and people of north European origin. It is less common in Hispanics, African Americans and people of Asian origin. The authors have encountered only around 70 cases in our department and private clinics in the last 35 years only one of whom developed visual problem. Incidence of disease increases with the age of the population. Although the disease is named as temporal arteritis it is not restricted to the superficial temporal arteries. It can involve the extracranial portion of the carotid artery and several of its branches. The vertebrobasilar system may be involved in a significant number of cases. The subclavian, brachial, and axillary arteries may be affected leading to steal syndromes and upper limb claudication. The lower limb arteries like the iliac, femoral, and popliteal arteries may be involved in a small number of cases and need to be differentiated from atherosclerotic changes. The aorta is often involved leading to aortic dilatation, aneurysm, and dissection. Periodic imaging of the aorta is necessary to monitor for these changes, but the modality and frequency is not well defined. Widespread involvement of the aorta may mimic Takayasu disease.

Giant cell arteritis is also a systemic disease and patients may have constitutional symptoms like fever, malaise, joint pain, and muscle soreness. Some patients may only have these constitutional symptoms and are labelled as polymyalgia rheumatica. These patients often require a higher dose of steroids and it may be very difficult to taper off the dose.

The most dreaded complication of this disease is painless visual loss. This is often irreversible and early steroid therapy is needed to save the fellow eye which may be involved in less than a week. The visual loss is due to arteritic anterior ischemic optic neuropathy (AION). This is differentiated from more common demyelinating optic neuritis by the lack of pain and from the nonarteritic form of AION by the presence of more florid retinal changes. Some patients may also have central or branch retinal artery occlusion or arteritic posterior optic neuropathy. A small set of patients may have diplopia due to ischemia of the external ocular muscles.

Jaw claudication or pain when chewing tough solid food is considered characteristic and may be associated with tongue claudication or tongue infarction in a small number of cases. Patients may have pain over the nape of the neck or shoulder girdle or interscapular muscles. Proximal lower extremity muscles may be sore and painful. There is no joint swelling or inflammation. Only constitutional features with muscle pain is termed polymyalgia rheumatica and most consider it to be a different manifestation of the same disease process.

The temporal arteries may be thickened, nodular, and tender and superficial temporal artery pulsation may be weak or absent.

The headache in temporal arteritis lacks any special character and may be holocranial, pulsatile, throbbing, tight-band like or even boring. Any new headache in an elderly or change in character of headache should raise suspicion.

Temporal arteritis is an inflammatory process and associated with a rise in erythrocyte sedimentation rate (ESR). This is usually above 50 mm by the Westergren method and often above 100 mm. C-reactive protein (CRP) is also elevated. Simultaneous rise of ESR and CRP is more suggestive of GCA. Some recent observers have noted a rise in the platelet count and have suggested that thrombocytosis may also be an important marker.

The gold standard for the diagnosis is temporal artery biopsy. The segment has to be at least 5 mm in length and is to be taken from an involved site. A lengthy specimen and bilateral biopsies may increase the diagnostic yield as temporal arteritis is characterized by skip lesions where a large segment of the artery may be uninvolved. The positive biopsy specimen is characterized by transmural inflammation and by the presence of lymphocytes, other inflammatory cells, and giant cells. The giant cells are considered to be pathognomonic. Color duplex ultrasonography may complement temporal artery biopsy. There is a hypoechoic halo surrounding the area of inflammation. This finding is operator dependent at present. However, this method can help to identify areas of involvement and help in the area which would give a greater diagnostic yield during biopsy. Computed tomography angiography and magnetic resonance angiography can also be complementary, but in itself is still not considered diagnostic. Positron emission tomography studies with appropriate tracers can also pick up sites of inflammation.

Therapy should not be delayed for conducting the biopsy and for confirmatory reports, as delay may cause irreversible damage to the eyes and results of biopsy continue to be positive up to several days after starting corticosteroids. Prednisone is started at a dose of 60–80 mg daily and continued for at least 1 month. Drug taper must be very slow and for any re-emergence of either constitutional or visual symptoms, one must revert to the initial dose. The total duration of therapy is about 2 years, but may be longer up to 5 years in some cases. Such a long duration of steroids often leads to unacceptable side effects like infections, bony changes such as osteoporosis, vertebral fractures and avascular necrosis of the femoral neck, diabetes, and peptic ulcers. Steroid sparing agents such as azathioprine and methotrexate have been largely unsuccessful. A recent monoclonal antibody tocilizumab directed against a critical inflammatory marker interleukin-6 has shown a lot of promise. It has been found useful in the acute phase and also in the long-term treatment to reduce the total steroid burden.

Idiopathic intracranial hypertension and pituitary apoplexy are two important conditions presenting with headache where the eyes are also involved. Both these conditions had been discussed elsewhere in this volume.

Idiopathic Intracranial Hypertension and Increased Intracranial Pressure

- Idiopathic intracranial hypertension (IIH) is characterized by raised intracranial pressure without any detectable cause like a mass, ventriculomegaly, etc.
- Obese women of childbearing age are frequently affected, although it may occur in children and men
- The most common symptom is headache which can be retro-orbital, bifrontal, unilateral, or posteriorly located accompanying photophobia, phonophobia, nausea, and vomiting. The pain may be throbbing or steady, constant or intermittent, and is generally severe. Children, have more prominent neck and back pain than headache
- There may be transient visual obscurations, often precipitated by postural change and reflect papilledema. Other symptoms include visual loss, pulsatile tinnitus, diplopia, radicular pain, and ataxia
- The diagnosis can be easily clinched by papilledema, although it is not universally present and some cases asymmetrical.

Pituitary Apoplexy

- Pituitary apoplexy is a rare condition caused by a hemorrhage into or infarction of the pituitary gland. Often there is a pre-existing pituitary tumor. The headache is acute, severe (thunderclap), and retro-orbital or frontal in location
- When there is upward expansion of the pituitary gland from the hemorrhage, it result in compression of the visual apparatus causing unilateral or bilateral vision loss
- Lateral expansion into the cavernous sinus may produce unilateral or bilateral, single or multiple ocular motor cranial neuropathies
- The MRI is investigation of choice in a suspected case of pituitary apoplexy
- Management involves urgent neurosurgical decompression of the optic chiasm and medical therapy of the hypopituitarism.

Optic Neuritis

- Vision loss typically develops over a period of hours to days, peaking within one to 2 weeks
- Eye pain: The onset of pain generally coincided with the VA loss and improved along with it. Ipsilateral pain with eye movement, ipsilateral aching head pain
- An afferent pupillary defect always occurs in optic neuritis if the other eye is uninvolved and otherwise healthy
- The visual field defect in optic neuritis is typically characterized as a central scotoma
- Photopsias (flickering or flashes of light) are often precipitated with eye movement
- Loss of color vision out of proportion to the loss of VA is specific to optic nerve pathology
- Papillitis with hyperemia and swelling of the disk, blurring of disk margins, and distended veins.

CONCLUSION

Awareness of these various conditions is essential to achieve the correct diagnosis and management. Many of these conditions require a multidisciplinary approach. Early detection and prompt investigations may preserve vision or save the patient's life.

SUGGESTED READINGS

1. Bhatti MT. Orbital syndromes. Semin Ophthalmol. 2007;27:269-87.
2. Caplan LR. Dissections of brain-supplying arteries. Nat Clin Pract Neurol. 2008;4:34-42
3. Danesh-Meyer HV, Savino PJ. Giant cell arteritis. Curr Opin Ophthalmol. 2007;18:443-9.
4. Engelter ST, Brandt T, Debette S, et al. Antiplatelets versus anticoagulation in cervical artery dissection. Stroke. 2007;38:2605-11.
5. Flis CM, Jäger HR, Sidhu PS. Carotid and vertebral artery dissections: Clinical aspects, imaging features and endovascular treatment. Eur Radiol. 2007;17:820-34.
6. Gilbert ME, Friedman D. Migraine and anisocoria. Surv Ophthalmol. 2007;52:209-12.
7. Gilbert ME, Sergott RC. Intracranial aneurysms. Curr Opin Ophthalmol. 2006;17:513-8.
8. Gladstone JP. An approach to the patient with painful ophthalmoplegia, with a focus on Tolosa-Hunt syndrome. Curr Pain Headache Rep. 2007;6:129-47.
9. Gordon LK. Orbital inflammatory disease: A diagnostic and therapeutic challenge. Eye 2006;20:1196-1206.
10. Grosberg BM, Solomon S, Lipton RB. Retinal migraine. Curr Pain Headache Rep 2005;9:268-71.
11. Headache Classification Subcommittee of the International Headache Society. The International Classification of Headache Disorders. Cephalalgia. 2004;24(Suppl 1):1-151.
12. Jacobson DM. Benign episodic unilateral mydriasis. Clinical characteristics. Ophthalmology. 1995;102:1623-7.
13. Leone M, Proicetti Cecchini A, Mea E, et al. Functional neuroimaging and headache pathophysiology: New findings and new prospects. J Neurol Sci. 2007;28:S108-13.
14. Liu GT, Schatz NJ, Galetta SL, et al. Persistent positive visual phenomena in migraine. Neurology. 1995;45:664-8.
15. Markl M, Uhl M, Wieben O, et al. High resolution 3T MRI for the assessment of cervical and superficial cranial arteries in giant cell arteritis. J Magn Reson Imaging. 2007;24:423-7.
16. May A, Leone M, Áfra A, et al. EFNS guidelines on the treatment of cluster headache and other trigeminal autonomic cephalgias. Eur J Neurol. 2006;13:1066-77.
17. McMillan HJ, Keene DL, Jacob P, et al. Ophthalmoplegic migraine: Inflammatory neuropathy with secondary migraine? Can J Neurol Sci. 2007;34:349-55.
18. Melson MR, Weyland CM, Newman NJ, et al. The diagnosis of giant cell arteritis. Rev Neurol Dis. 2007;4:128-42
19. Niederkohr RD, Levin LA. Management of the patient with suspected temporal arteritis: A decision-analytic approach. Ophthalmology. 2005;112:744-56.
20. Pareja JA, Sánchez del Río M. Primary trochlear headache and other trochlear painful disorders. Curr Pain Headache Rep. 2006;10:316-20.
21. Queseshi AI, Janardhan V, Hanel RA, et al. Comparison of endovascular and surgical treatments for intracranial aneurysms: An evidence-based review. Lancet Neurol. 2007;6:816-25.
22. Rangwalla LM, Liu GT. Pediatric idiopathic intracranial hypertension. Surv Ophthalmol 2007;52:597-617.
23. Rozen TD, Saper JR, Sheftell FD, et al. Clomiphene citrate as a new treatment for SUNCT (hormonal manipulation for hypothalamic influenced trigeminal autonomic cephalgias). Headache. 2005;45:754-6.
24. Schwedt TJ, Dodick DW, Caselli RJ. Giant cell arteritis. Curr Pain Headache Rep 2006;10:415-20.
25. Stiebel-Kalish H, Kalish Y, Setton A, et al. Presentation, natural history, and management of carotid cavernous aneurysms. Neurosurgery. 2005;57:850-7.
26. Umasankar U, Carroll TJ, Famuboni A, et al. Vertebral artery dissection: Not a rare cause of stroke in the young. Age Ageing. 2008;37:345-6.
27. Williams MH, Broadley SA. SUNCT and SUNA: Clinical features and medical treatment. J Clin Neurosci. 2008;15:526-34.

Problem Oriented Neuro-Ophthalmology: Pearls and Pitfalls

CHAPTER 23

Koushik Pan, Ambar Chakravarty

INTRODUCTION

The present chapter would highlight on common and some uncommon neuro-ophthalmic problems where both neurologists and ophthalmologists alike tend to make mistakes both in diagnosis and management. The topics are categorized as symptoms as well as physical findings. It is true that several aspects discussed earlier in various chapters are repeated; but recapitulation is always helpful for both students and practitioners.

VISUAL LOSS-NEUROLOGICAL OR OCULAR?

- Visual loss due to aberration of ocular media (cataract/corneal disease) is described as blurring while the visual loss of optic nerve dysfunction is more often experienced as dimming or darkening of vision often with color desaturation. In contrast to patients with disorders of media, those with retinal or optic nerve disease often report missing "pieces" or areas of vision
- Alteration of object shape or size (metamorphopsia, micropsia, macropsia) usually indicate retinal disease and never caused by optic neuropathy. Prominent degradation of vision in dim or bright light is who characteristic of retinal disease
- Photostress test measures the time it takes to recover central visual function, i.e., acuity, following exposure to bright light and is very helpful for distinguishing maculopathy from optic neuropathy. Recovery times are prolonged in variety of macular disorders, but are normal in optic neuropathies
- Amsler grid test is an objective way to assess alteration of object shape and size, characteristic of macular disease
- Sorting out ocular disease early in the course of evaluation is important for avoiding unnecessary and expensive investigation.

UNEXPLAINED VISUAL LOSS

Cases of visual loss with normal imaging, with clear ocular media and normal pupillary response strongly suggest nonorganic visual loss. In most cases of nonorganic visual loss, specific examination techniques can disclose the nature of disorder (see Chapter 20). Patient is asked to navigate in the room/reach the objects despite claimed blindness; intact central visual field in the face of severe loss of acuity is a helpful clue to diagnose nonorganic visual loss.

Sudden Monocular Visual Loss with Normal Fundus

Compressive/Infiltrative optic nerve lesion should be in the differential, although abrupt onset is unusual. Optic neuritis is a possibility, but elderly age may be atypical for demyelinating disease.

Acute painless monocular visual loss in a patient age more than 50 years most often is ischemic in origin. In the large majority of patients it affects most anterior portion of nerve, termed Anterior Ischemic Optic Neuropathy. So disc edema is seen acutely. Apart from neurologic causes, retinal artery occlusion produces acute, painless, monocular visual loss. Patients with retinal artery occlusion, often describe just what they are doing when visual loss occurred. Permanent visual loss due to retinal artery occlusion is sometimes preceded by episodes of transient monocular visual loss lasting less than 5 minutes often with altitudinal pattern, described as curtain descending over vision.

Fundus appearance depends upon time of examination. In the hyperacute phase, there is obvious attenuation and segmentation of blood column within renal arteries and the responsible embolus may be visible. If the embolic material has moved on through retinal circulation and flow has already been restored, the retina may have completely normal appearance. This phase lasts up to 24 hours. As edema develops, areas of central whitening appear. This may take the form of cotton wool spots. In a hyperacute retinal artery occlusion, the retina may have a normal appearance (Chapter 10).

Central Blurring of Vision and Optic Disc Pallor

This scenario is often encountered in common entities like optic neuropathy (demyelinating optic neuritis, ischemic optic neuropathy which may be compressive, infiltrative, and inflammatory in origin). Glaucoma is such a disease that should be included in the differential diagnosis of any patient with unexplained optic neuropathy. This disease has a predilection for arcuate fibers, which produces progressive loss of neural rim starting at superior and inferior pole of optic disc and causes vertical elongation of cup.

Asymmetry of cup:disc ratio in two eyes, may be the first sign of this condition. An interocular cup:disc asymmetry of 0.1 or more may be significant. Single splinter hemorrhage in disc margin known as Drance hemorrhage is often seen.

Glaucomatous versus Nonglaucomatous Cupping

Glaucomatous disc rim generally maintains normal hue, even in advanced cases when the degree of excavation of disc is disproportionately greater than severity of rim pallor. In contrast, rim pallor is a prominent feature of nonglaucomatous cupping.

Focal thinning of temporal retinal rim is more characteristic of nonglaucomatous damage, whereas diffuse obliteration of neural rim and peripapillary atrophy usually reflects glaucomatous damage.

Episodic Monocular Blur

History of episodic visual loss prompts consideration of neurovascular mechanism. The most common vascular cause of transient monocular visual loss is retinal embolism. Typically it has an abrupt onset and offset, often described as curtain/shade descending over vision. Episodes are spontaneous and not accompanied by pain. The source of retinal emboli is commonly internal carotid artery, sometimes heart and rarely great vessels of neck.

Transient monocular visual loss also occurs in ocular ischemic syndrome (OIS). Ocular ischemia most often occurs in the setting of high grade carotid stenosis/occlusion and occasionally secondary to giant cell arteritis. Visual loss in OIS is of more gradual onset and of longer duration compared to embolic visual episode and often lasting minutes to hours.

Apart from neurologic causes, visual disturbance due to corneal dystrophy produces sufficient fluctuation to suggest vascular disorder. The stereotypic timing of visual loss associated with awakening even before arising from bed is quite characteristic of corneal disorder. Corneal decompensation is often worse, first thing in morning because of lid closure during night preventing normal oxygenation and evaporation. In contrast OIS, visual loss begins only upon arising from bed. In both the OIS and corneal disorder the patient may experience pain. Pain associated with corneal disease is described as foreign body sensation, whereas OIS is associated with deep eye/brow ache. Patients with visual loss due to corneal disease describe seeing halos, monocular diplopia, ghost images, whereas in OIS vision is dim, sometimes blotchy.

So, transient visual loss due to ocular disease can often be distinguished from retinal ischemic disease based on history.

Optic Neuropathy with Persistent Pain and Progression of Visual Loss

When this presentation is encountered by a neurologist, possibility of optic perineuritis (OPN) rather than optic neuritis needs to be considered. Optic perineuritis is inflammation of optic nerve sheath. The natural history often includes stabilization of vision and improvement of pain within two weeks of onset.

Although OPN shares some similarities with demyelinating optic neuritis, there are several clinical differences:

- Optic neuritis typically causes decreased visual acuity, whereas in patients with OPN, acuity is often spared or loss delayed
- In contrast to the self-limiting nature of optic neuritis, pain, and visual loss in OPN continue to progress
- Unlike optic neuritis, patients with OPN show a dramatic response to steroids; however, it may recur if steroids are discontinued too early
- Optic neuritis visual loss is central; in OPN it is often paracentral/arcuate
- Hence, severe and persistent pain is atypical for optic neuritis and suggest the possibility of OPN.

Sequential Visual Loss without Pain and No Improvement in Due Course

This often points towards bilateral optic neuropathy. Acute onset of unilateral optic neuropathy in a young adult is most often due to idiopathic (demyelinating) optic neuritis. In acute stage, optic disc is either swollen or normal. Lack of visual improvement in due course is atypical for idiopathic optic neuritis and along with involvement in fellow eye, generally points to alternative diagnosis like NMO. Absence of pain at the onset of such a patient's visual loss would be highly atypical for idiopathic optic neuritis. In a patient who seems to have optic neuritis but without pain, it is important to consider alternate possibility, including ischemic optic neuropathy, neuroretinitis, compressive optic neuropathy, Leber's hereditary optic neuropathy (LHON), etc. The LHON is characterized by acute to subacute onset of painless central visual loss. Visual loss usually occurs sequentially and deteriorates over several months before stabilisation. Second eye involvement occurs in most cases within weeks to months after first eye.

Optic disc appearance is variable. Hyperemic swelling of disc along with circumpapillary telangiectasia is characteristic. Sometimes the disc is completely normal. In some cases optic atrophy has already developed by the time the patient is evaluated. The LHON should be included in the differential diagnosis of any patient with acute painless optic neuropathy, regardless of age and gender.

Headache and Elevated Disc

Elevated disc is not always pathological. Pseudopapilledema can usually be distinguished from acquired disc edema based on ophthalmoscopic appearance (Chapter 3). The most sensitive and specific indicator of acquired disc edema is opacification of nerve fiber layer.

Examination of retinal vessels can provide additional clues. In true papilloedema, the capillaries on disc surface are usually hyperemic and the retinal veins become tortuous, distended and nonpulsatile. In addition branching pattern of retinal vasculature is normal in papilloedema, anomalous in pseudopapilledema.

Disc drusens are bilateral in 75% of cases. However, visual acuity is rarely reduced because the defect usually involves arcuate/redial nerve fiber bundles rather than papillomacular bundle. Observing the size of physiologic cup is also helpful. In most eyes with pseudopapilloedema, the cup is absent. In contrast, filling in of the physiologic cup is a late event in evolution of papilledema. Disc hemorrhage in papilloedema is in nerve fiber layer, whereas in pseudopapilledema, it is usually deep.

Ancillary investigations like visual field, optical coherence tomography (OCT) and fluorescein angiography are often needed.

Headache with Bilateral Disc Edema

This presentation is often seen in day-to-day clinical practice and usually clinicians seriously think of alarming causes like brain tumor, cerebral venous thrombosis, etc. However, it is very commonly seen in malignant hypertension.

A pronounced and sudden rise in blood pressure beyond the compensatory capacity can result in vascular leakiness and widespread end organ dysfunction affecting brain, heart, and kidney. Retinal changes are the earliest. Hemorrhage can be intraretinal (dot/blot) or in nerve fiber layer (flame/splinter hemorrhage). Occlusion of choroidal vessels may cause areas of secondary retinal detachment. Macular alteration include edema, formation of microcyst and exudate. Nerve fiber layer infarcts appear as cotton wool spot.

Malignant hypertension with disc edema and macular star formation are sometimes mistakenly diagnosed as bilateral neuroretinitis. Although neuroretinitis rarely affects both eyes simultaneously and does not cause more widespread retinal abnormalities.

Optic disc swelling in malignant hypertension is multifactorial, sometimes as a part of retinopathy, some cases representing ischemia of optic nerve head, in others reflecting raised intracranial pressure. Clinical features and fundus findings are nonspecific and may resemble several other conditions. Careful measurement of blood pressure should be included in the evaluation of any patient with bilateral optic disc edema. With timely diagnosis and treatment, clinical manifestations are often reversible. However, rapid lowering of blood pressure is not recommended as it can cause devastating infarction of optic nerve.

Homonymous Hemianopia with Negative Neuroimaging

Regarding homonymous hemianopia presentation, clinician often think of stroke/tumor of parieto-occipital region or of internal capsular lesions. However, if neuroimaging is normal, then it poses great difficulty to reach the diagnosis.

Common diseases that produce focal occipital dysfunction without magnetic resonance imaging (MRI) change are nonketotic hyperglycemia, Alzheimer's disease, Creutzfeldt–Jakob disease (CJD), complicated migraine, hypoxic ischemic encephalopathy, and occipital seizure.

Sporadic CJD to be considered in differential. In one particular form of it, the brunt of the disease process affects the posterior cerebral hemisphere causing homonymous defect, cortical blindness, and a variety of higher cortical visual deficit. This form is referred as Heidenhain variant. It has a more rapidly progressive course. Cortical ribbon may be detected in a MRI flair sequence.

Unexplained Visual Loss with Bilateral Centrocecal Scotoma with Normal Magnetic Resonance Imaging

This visual field pattern is unusual for functional visual loss. This pattern indicates disease process involving papillomacular bundle. Specific forms of optic neuropathy that produce bilateral centrocecal scotoma include certain toxins, nutritional deficiency, hereditary optic neuropathy, and demyelinating disease. It is extremely unusual for this pattern of visual loss to be produced by a mass lesion.

The possibility of vitamin B12 deficiency also needs to be considered in the above scenario, as visual loss in vitamin B12 deficiency is bilaterally symmetric, painless, and gradually progressive. Loss of color vision, decreased acuity, and central/centrocecal scotoma are characteristic. The optic disc may be normal, hyperemic acutely, pale and atrophic later. Visual loss and other neurologic manifestations occur well in advance of hematologic change.

Inferior Altitudinal Visual Field Defect

Patients with inferior altitudinal visual field defect along with optic disc pallor or blurring, point to optic neuropathy of ischemic origin. Careful fundus examination to be done as sometimes maldeveloped optic discs often look pale.

Optic nerve hypoplasia is a congenital anomaly, where there is inferior altitudinal field defect. With maldeveloped optic disc which looks like pale disc, the classic fundus picture is double ring/halo sign. Optic nerve hypoplasia may occur as an isolated anomaly or may be associated with other abnormalities. The most common of these are absence of septum pellucidum and agenesis of corpus callosum. Optic nerve hypoplasia sometimes is associated with panhypopituitarism which may lead to growth retardation and developmental delay.

A specific form of partial optic nerve hypoplasia that affects offsprings of insulin dependent diabetic mothers has been termed superior segmental hypoplasia/topless disc syndrome. It is rarely present in patients who do not have a history of maternal diabetes.

Progressive Visual Difficulty, Homonymous Hemianopia and Normal Magnetic Resonance Imaging and Nondominant Parietal Lobe Syndrome

The three cardinal features here are progressive visual difficulty, homonymous hemianopia nondominant parietal lobe syndrome with normal MRI. Patients in whom the brunt of disease affects right posterior parietal lobe typically present with visual symptoms relating to spatial disorganization. In the late state of disease, when both posterior hemispheres are involved, patients have more profound visual difficulty, including inability to attend to more than one visual stimulus at a time termed simultanagnosia. When accompanied by optic ataxia and apraxia of gaze, this is termed Balint's syndrome, and indicates bilateral damage to the posterior visual association areas and dorsal stream.

Alzheimer's disease, is such a disease that often manifests in above fashion (posterior cortical atrophy). Recognition of these visual presentations of Alzheimer's disease is challenging, as cognitive function is often unimpaired and routine neuroimaging is normal.

In addition to these higher cortical deficit, other mechanisms affect the vision in Alzheimer's disease. Progressive retinal ganglion cell loss affecting M cell pathways would result in impairment of spatial organization. The MRI is normal not because the lesion is small or overlooked but because these degenerative process do not generally produce visible change on MRI, OCT is often helpful.

The CJD can also present in above manner. This can be differentiated from Alzheimer's disease on the basis of disease course and other parameters like electroencephalography and cerebrospinal fluid (CSF) study. Functional imaging studies like positron emission tomography may also help.

Pseudobitemporal Defect

Most common pattern of visual loss associated with chiasmal lesion is bitemporal hemianopia.

Certain ocular conditions when bilateral, can cause simultaneous temporal field losses. These include papilloedema, disorders of outer retina, retinal degeneration, macular disease, congenital disc anomalies, and glaucoma. The bitemporal visual field defects found in these ocular disorders do not strictly respect the vertical meridian, and hence sometimes referred to as pseudo-bitemporal field defect.

Isolated Unilateral Mydriasis

Acute unilateral mydriasis raises the possibility of third nerve palsy due to posterior communicating artery aneurysm. Other causes include small perimesencephalic hemorrhage affecting the fascicular pathway of NIII and transtentorial herniation. However, apart from thinking the above mentioned serious causes, more common causes like Adie's tonic pupil, pharmacologic blockade and direct damage to iris sphincter muscle need also to be kept in the differential. Adie's tonic pupil is a 2-fold process. Acute denervation followed by reinnervation. There is denervation supersensitivity of iris sphincter to weak cholinergic agonist. Following instillation of 1/8% of pilocarpine, there is pupillary constriction.

Painful Mydriasis

When a patient presents with painful mydriasis, clinicians often think of posterior communicating artery aneurysm or other alarming cause like transtentorial herniation, although it is often associated with alteration of consciousness and focal neurologic deficit.

Presence of isolated, nonreactive pupil in an awake patient should be considered indication of ocular disease. History should be taken regarding any halos which can occur due to corneal edema secondary to angle closure glaucoma. Angle closure glaucoma patients present with severe face/head pain along with blurred vision and halos. Pain is usually localized around the eye but may extend to maxillary region.

As there is often conjunctival injection during an attack, it often mimics trigeminal autonomic cephalgia. Prone position, dim light, prolonged near work, sneezing, and physical stress often precipitate angle closure. Sometimes pain is excruciating and accompanied by vasovagal reaction and vomiting mimicking intracranial pathologies like subarachnoid hemorrhage.

Diagnosis is essentially clinical and confirmed by gonioscopy or ultrasound biomicroscopy. Neurologists, therefore, should keep possibility of acute angle closure glaucoma in the differential diagnosis of painful isolated mydriasis and seek urgent ophthalmic referral.

Tonic Pupil versus Pharmacologic Mydriasis

Acute postganglionic denervation of iris sphincter (Adie's tonic pupil) as well as exposure to atropine like agent, over time, may lead to a denervated pupil. Cholinergic supersensitivity, light-near dissociation (LND), and tonicity develop later. Thus in the acute state, the only examination feature that effectively distinguishes denervation injury from pharmacologic mydriasis is the presence of sectoral palsy of iris sphincter. Sectoral palsy visible as demarcation between areas of functioning and nonfunctioning iris sphincter rules out pharmacologic blockade and localizes the site of damage to peripheral short ciliary nerve, but needs examination with a slit lamp microscope. This is because pharmacologic agent act diffusely on iris sphincter and cannot produce sectoral paralysis.

Direct injury to iris can result in similar focal paralysis of sphincter muscle. In such cases, however there is history of trauma, or intraocular inflammation or ocular surgery.

Sectoral sphincter palsy persists in the chronic phase of Adie's pupil and remains an extremely valuable clinical sign. It is important to remember that the demonstration of cholinergic supersensitivity is neither completely sensitive nor specific. About 20% of patients with tonic pupil fail to demonstrate enhanced sensitivity.

Chronic Tonic Pupil versus Argyll Robertson Pupil

Both of these can present with LND. In patients with normal vision, LND is often due to dorsal midbrain damage. Afferent signals arising from dorsal midbrain and periaqueductal region mediate pupillary light reflex. In contrast, afferent signals mediating pupillary near response approach Edinger–Westphal Nucleus ventrally.

Central LND results from an injury to midbrain that selectively interrupts more dorsally situated fibers mediating pupillary light reflex. In case of Argyll Robertson pupil there is selective deafferentation of pupillomotor center due to periaqueductal inflammation and gliosis.

A completely different mechanism is seen with tonic pupils. The initial event is acute injury to short ciliary nerves, the fibers that carry postganglionic parasympathetic impulses to iris sphincter and ciliary body. An acute Adie's tonic pupil is large, over time its size tends to diminish. The mechanism for this change is related to the amount of aberrant reinnervation of iris sphincter. However, short ciliary nerves contain a far greater number of accommodative fibers compared to light reflex fibers so in the process of regeneration and reinnervation, the iris sphincter becomes increasingly innervated with accommodative fibers. So, near response is restored but light reflex is absent.

The speed of pupillary movement is an important differential. Tonic pupil have a delayed, slow constriction to near effort and more importantly also demonstrate sustained constriction and a similarly slow redilation upon distance refixation. In contrast Argyll Robertson pupil constrict to near effort with the briskness of normally innervated pupil and promptly redilates after release of near effort.

Intermittent Diplopia: Ocular or Neurological?

Intermittent monocular diplopia presentation in a patient although rarely can be found in cerebral polyopia but mostly it occurs due to aberration of ocular media. Common causes include refractive error, corneal disease, cataract and macular distortion. Symptoms are more often noticeable in dim illumination and at night time. Less often in brightly lit room because of resulting pupillary constriction producing a pinhole like effect. Pinhole relieves monocular diplopia.

At the same time cerebral polyopia is a visual illusion due to parietal lobe dysfunction, in which subjects are seen as multiple in each eye. Cerebral polyopia can be distinguished from monocular diplopia by the following: Cerebral polyopia is present in both eyes, not relieved by pin hole and often associated with homonymous visual field defect.

Hence, before embarking on a neurologic evaluation for diplopia it is important to verify that diplopia is truly binocular. Diplopia that is present with one eye viewing and relieved by pinhole is not due to neurologic disease.

Fatigable Ptosis

Fatigable ptosis refers to the demonstration of weakness of levator that increases with prolonged use of the muscle and is a classic sign of myasthenia. However, one thing needs to be kept in mind that individuals with aponeurotic ptosis which represents disinsertion of levator aponeurosis to tarsal plate, often report worsening of ptosis later in day.

To differentiate it from myasthenic ptosis, levator function needs to be assessed. Levator function is measured as excursion of upper lid from extreme downgaze to extreme upgaze (normal range 12–17 mm).

Aponeurotic ptosis is a form of acquired ptosis which is caused by thinning and disinsertion of levator aponeurosis. The most important risk factor for aponeurotic dehiscence is increasing age. The key diagnostic feature in ptosis due to levator dehiscence is preservation of levator function. In contrast levator function decreases in neurogenic and myopathic disease.

Second helpful feature for distinguishing is position of eyelid crease. A higher eyelid crease on the side of ptosis and deepening of superior lid sulcus are suggestive of aponeurotic ptosis.

Third observation that is often helpful is comparison of lid position in upgaze, primary position and downgaze. In aponeurotic dehiscence, ptotic lid is lower than normal lid, not only in primary position, but also in downgaze. In contrast, myopathic or neurogenic ptosis, the lid position is normal on downgaze, compared to healthy side.

Painless Ptosis with Diplopia with Normal Magnetic Resonance Imaging, and Negative Myasthenia Screen

This presentation often brings confusion to neurologists regarding the diagnosis of myasthenia.

Diagnosing ocular myasthenia on the basis of anti-acetylicholine receptor antibody is really not ideal. In contrast to generalized disease, who harbor automate bodies in 90% or more of cases, fewer than half of patients with ocular myasthenia have positive antibody test. Blocking and modulating antibodies are positive in only 8% of patients, in whom binding antibodies are negative and musk antibodies are rarely positive in ocular myasthenia.

Repetitive nerve stimulation test similarly is normal in most patients with myasthenia limited to ocular muscles. For the diagnosis of ocular myasthenia, edrophonium test remains the gold standard. A history of cardiac arrhythmia, use of atrioventricular nodal blockers, bronchospastic disease are relative contraindication. Falsely positive edrophonium tests are rare.

Another test is the ice test, an ice pack is placed on the ptotic lid for 1–2 minutes. Ptosis improving after ice pack application is considered positive for myasthenia as there is enhanced transmission at neuromuscular junction at lower temperature (Chapter 14).

Painful Ptosis and Diplopia

Painful ptosis and diplopia often point towards either cavernous sinus or superior orbital fissure syndrome.

Apart from these two causes orbital disease should be kept in mind and if pain is exacerbated by eye movement then, it is most likely orbital disease rather than an intracranial process.

Idiopathic orbital inflammatory disorder, known as orbital pseudotumor is a nongranulomatous inflammation of orbital structure with no known local/systemic cause. Pain is the most common feature; those with extraocular muscle involvement also produce diplopia. Accompanying signs of orbitopathy such as periorbital edema, lid swelling, conjunctival injection, proptosis, and chemosis are present in most patients.

Postcontrast computed tomography of orbit shows enlargement of one or more extraocular muscles. The tendons are frequently thickened, leading to tubular configuration. It is a diagnosis of exclusion, hence thorough evaluation of systemic inflammatory disorder is required. Biopsy is reserved for those with atypical finding, lack of steroid responsiveness and recurrence following treatment.

Headache with Third Nerve Palsy (Pupil Involving) with Normal MRI and MR angiography

The very acute onset of third nerve palsy goes against a skull base tumor or infiltrative process such as nasopharyngeal carcinoma or chronic meningitis. A brainstem stroke can cause third nerve palsy, but most cases are not accompanied by pain. The etiologies should be addressed most urgently in this case are posterior communicating artery aneurysm, pituitary apoplexy and carotid dissection.

On the background of negative MRI and magnetic resonance angiography (MRA) clinicians often think of vasculopathic and inflammatory etiology. However, one thing to be kept in mind is that acute, painful, pupil involving third nerve palsy in a young/middle aged adult with no vascular risk factor, is so strongly suggestive of posterior communicating artery aneurysm, that clinicians must pay extra attention to exclude it. Conventional noninvasive angiogram even if it is negative, catheter angiography is necessary to exclude aneurysm.

The ability of MRA or computed tomography angiography (CTA) to detect an aneurysm approaches 100% for aneurysm larger than 5 mm; however, the risk of aneurysmal rupture for aneurysm smaller than 5 mm can approach 10%.

So, neither MRA nor CTA fully replaces conventional arteriography in the investigation of possible cerebral aneurysm. The extra benefit of subtraction CTA needs to be assessed fully.

Painful Progressive Third Nerve Palsy with All Negative Investigations: Beware of Nasopharyngeal Carcinoma

When patient presents with such a clinical feature, clinicians consider ischemic, infective, noninfective inflammatory, immunologic causes, or malignant skull base tumors. However, in the background of normal MRI, MRA, and CSF study most of these above mentioned etiologies become less likely.

Progressive and painful course suggest inflammatory or neoplastic process but neuroimaging is negative in this case. Vasculopathic cranial nerve palsy is also unlikely when it is progressive along with negative vasculitic profile.

Take home message in this case is when all conventional investigations reveal negative results, then ear, nose and, throat evaluation should be done. Nasopharyngeal carcinoma is notorious for infiltrating skull base and picking up cranial nerves while remaining below the "radar screen" on radiographic testing.

Another setting in which repeated neuroimaging may be negative despite progressive cranial nerve palsy is the patient who develops a sixth nerve palsy one or 2 years after excision and radiation treatment of a head/neck tumor. In the face of negative diagnostic studies, radiation damage is often considered. Unlike the afferent visual pathways, however, the ocular motor nerves are relatively resistant to radiation necrosis. These patients almost invariably turn out to have recurrent tumor at the skull base, despite scans that purportedly "ruled out" this process.

Abduction Deficit without Diplopia

An abduction deficit that is acquired to produce diplopia, when it does not, a congenital anomaly should be suspected. In that case, carefully look for palpebral fissure and globe retraction. Then this indicates Duane syndrome.

Despite loss of abduction, patient with Duane syndrome usually remain well aligned in primary position. This clinical feature is extremely helpful for distinguishing this condition from acquired sixth nerve palsy which typically produces esotropia.

Adduction Deficit

Regarding this clinical presentation neurologists often think of internuclear ophthalmoplegia (INO). But possibility of myasthenia also to be kept as medial rectus muscle is frequently affected in myasthenia and thus the clinical picture of bilateral pseudo INO is not uncommon.

Slowing of medial rectus saccade is the most sensitive and specific sign of INO, demonstrable even in the absence of an adduction deficit. Such slowing can be demonstrated for both large and small amplitude eye movement. In contrast in adduction deficit due to myasthenia, small amplitude medial rectus saccade exhibit a normal/supra normal velocity, due to increased firing rate in paramedian pontine reticular formation designed to overcome the neuromuscular blockade, because myasthenia can affect just one/two muscles. It often resembles cranial nerve palsy or supranuclear gaze disturbance.

Bilateral Sixth Nerve Palsy with Normal Magnetic Resonance Imaging, Normal Cerebrospinal Fluid and Normal Blood Tests

This is often encountered in day-to-day practice. While vasculopathic cranial neuropathy is the most common cause of sixth nerve deficit in individuals age more than 50 years, such palsies are unilateral.

Investigation of unexplained bilateral sixth nerve palsy should include critical evaluation of clivus region as two abducens nerves travel along clivus, where they are prone to tumorous expansion. Recurrent sixth nerve palsy may be an early feature of clivus chordoma. If a skull base tumor is suspected, adequate radiographic investigations may require both MRI and CT with bone windows as well as contrast study.

Painful Sixth Nerve palsy

Confusion arises whether there is an intracranial cause or it is due to orbital pathology. The presence of pain with eye movement indicate orbital pathology. Preservation of saccadic velocity in the presence of a functional deficit suggest orbital restrictive disease.

In case of orbital inflammation, inflammatory swelling of opposing medial rectus has caused lateral rectus to lose its normal elasticity, thus limiting abduction. Orbital MRI needs to be done for confirmation which often shows enlargement and enhancement of medical rectus muscle.

Acute Isolated Sixth Nerve Palsy in an Elderly Individual with Normal Investigations

Etiologies of acute sixth nerve palsy include tumor, stroke. demyelinating disease, intracerebral hemorrhage, meningeal disease, increased intracranial pressure, trauma and a variety of infectious, inflammatory and immunologic disorders. Considering normal investigations, microvascular sixth nerve palsy is a common cause in this scenario. Microvascular ischemia of the peripheral portion of nerve is commonly referred to as vasculopathic cranial neuropathy. Such palsies are usually accompanied by ipsilateral headache or retrobulbar pain that precede the palsy by a day or two and usually remits in 7–10 days. The motor deficit in vasculopathic cranial neuropathies often shows initial progression for a few days.

Assessment of vascular risk factors (blood pressure, plasma glucose, and lipid profile) should be undertaken and in patients older than 60 years, additional tests for giant cell arteritis are needed. In patients without associated pain, an edrophonium test may be performed. Spontaneous recovery is the clinical feature that best defines this syndrome.

Continued progression beyond 2 weeks, failure to show improvement by 8 weeks or significant residual nerve palsy after 3 months needs prompt evaluation by additional testing.

This restrained approach to the evaluation of sixth nerve palsy applies to an acute event. In contrast, any patient with chronic ocular motor palsy should be thoroughly evaluated for compressive lesion at skull base (especially nasopharyngeal carcinoma), meningeal infiltration, and increased intracranial pressure.

Intermittent Vertical Diplopia

Common causes of vertical diplopia include cranial nerve palsy (N III or N IV), skew deviation, restrictive orbitopathy, and myasthenia. The most common cause of acquired fourth nerve palsy is trauma. However, the most common nontraumatic mechanism is congenital anomaly of superior oblique muscle/its tendon.

Congenital fourth nerve palsy often presents in midlife rather than childhood, not because of worsening muscle weakness, but rather due to progressive loss of fusion. The range of fusional capacity is variable and tends to decline over a lifetime. Individuals with congenital fourth nerve palsy initially have sufficiently large fusional capacity to maintain ocular alignment. Such fusional capacity may diminish as a part of normal ageing process.

In a nutshell, when the fusional capacity becomes inadequate, the congenital fourth nerve palsy is said to be decompensated and patient experience diplopia. Because of this apparent variability, patients with decompensated congenital fourth nerve palsy often are misdiagnosed as myasthenia.

Clinicians should look for head tilt from old photographs. While these findings are supportive, the most definitive clinical feature is demonstration of greater than normal vertical fusional amplitude. Normal vertical fusional amplitude range from 2–4 diopters but occasionally are a bit larger in patients with long standing acquired muscle imbalance. In contrast, patients with congenital phoria often have huge fusional amplitude (see Chapter 15).

Recurrent Headache and Impairment of Upgaze

Limitation of elevation can occur from neuromuscular junction disease, supranuclear disorder of gaze and bilateral third nerve palsy (superior recti and inferior oblique). Apart from these causes, restrictive orbitopathy can mimic neurologic ocular motor disorder. Restrictive orbitopathy is characterized by loss of normal elasticity of an eye muscle, causing limited eye movement in the direction opposite to the action of the involved muscle.

Restrictive orbitopathy can occur with or without trauma. Ocular motility deficit may be present in absence of external signs of trauma. Normal ocular alignment in primary position and normal saccadic velocity in the direction of paresis suggest restrictive orbitopathy, even in the absence of typical orbital signs/symptoms.

Horizontal and Vertical Gaze Limitation with Slow Saccade

The debate lies whether it is a case of progressive supranuclear palsy (PSP), some form spinocerebellar ataxia (SCA 2 and 3 specially) or chromic progressive external ophthalmoplegia (CPEO/Kearns–Sayre syndrome). The status of reflex eye movements [vestibulo-ocular reflex (VOR)] help differentiate these conditions.(see Chapter 16)

The range of eye movement improved with reflex maneuver in case of PSP. In contrast, in CPEO, range of eye movement does not improve with reflex maneuver. The VOR is preserved in PSP, whereas in ocular myopathy/CPEO, ocular excursions are no greater with caloric testing. Decreased blink rate and general paucity of facial expression also go in favor of PSP.

Acute Esotropia with Bilateral Abduction Deficit

The debate lies between convergence spasm and bilateral sixth nerve palsy. The near reflex is a normal synkinesis of convergence, accommodation and pupillary constriction that serves to keep a near target in fovea. Spasm of near reflex occurs when this reflex is inappropriate for visual task or excessively strong for a near target. Esotropic convergence spasm is accompanied by miosis but not in bilateral sixth nerve palsy.

Another helpful examination technique for identification of convergence spasm is comparison of ocular motility with binocular versus monocular viewing. Tested with both eyes open, the patient with convergence spasm demonstrates variable esotropia and apparent (usually bilateral) abduction deficit. When one eye is patched; the same patient will often demonstrate a strikingly normal range of abduction. In addition, there is often a disparity between eye movements when tested normally (refixation saccade and pursuit movement).

Wernicke's Encephalopathy versus Brainstem Stroke

Both these conditions may present as bilateral ptosis, limitation of gaze, slow upward saccade, upbeat nystagmus, and mild ataxia.

Wernicke's encephalopathy is a treatable cause of neurologic morbidity. The key to making this diagnosis is a high index of suspicion based an awareness of risk factors—persistent vomiting from any cause (e.g., hyperemesis gravidarum), nutritional deficiency state such as chronic alcoholism, malignancy, etc. Another group of patients having high risk is obese patients undergoing gastric surgery (e.g., bariatric surgery).

Ocular motor dysfunction is the earliest sign. This may be subtle as small amplitude horizontal end gaze nystagmus or slowing of saccade. Abduction weakness is common. Conjugate gaze palsy may be horizontal, vertical or both. Upbeat nystagmus is characteristic.

When the onset of symptoms is abrupt, Wernicke's encephalopathy can be mistaken for stroke syndrome. In this clinical setting, emperic trial of thiamine may have both diagnostic and therapeutic value. Patients with Wernicke's encephalopathy typically experience rapid clearing of mental status with resolution of esotropia, whereas patients with stroke show no beneficial response.

Diagnosis is confirmed by MRI. Lesions are often symmetric with predilection for mammillary bodies, periventricular region of third ventricle, medial thalamus, periaqueductal grey and midbrain tegmentum.

Brainstem Syndrome Resembling One-and-Half Syndrome With Normal MRI

Most commonly this occurs in demyelinating disease. However, normal MRI can be accounted for if the lesion is below the resolving power of current MRI scan. Despite continued advances in neuroimaging, some pathologic process, even when focal, elude radiographic detection. The FLAIR images are most sensitive sequence of detection of demyelinating disease. In cases with topically localizing neurologic deficit, clinical diagnosis triumphs over the scan.

Ocular Manifestations of VP Shunt Dysfunction: Dorsal Midbrain Syndrome

Upgaze palsy, poorly reacting pupil, light near dissociation are components of dorsal midbrain syndrome. Dorsal midbrain syndrome is most often caused by mass lesion, either by direct compression from a pineal region tumor or due to intrinsic tectal tumor.

In patients with intraventricular shunt, the appearance of signs and symptoms of dorsal mid brain syndrome is an early clinical sign of shunt malfunction. Ventricles are often not enlarged, giving the false impression that shunts are working properly. Despite the absence of radiographic change, these patients exhibit clinical manifestation of shunt malfunction like headache, vomiting, gait problem, or alteration of sensorium. Shunt revision to be considered in this scenario.

Photopsia

This is a form of positive visual phenomenon that can arise anywhere along afferent visual pathway. Photopsia evoked by eye movement indicate disorder of anterior part of visual system usually due to vitreous traction, retinal detachment or optic neuritis. The last of these three conditions is associated pain and visual impairment, whereas vitreous and retinal detachments are painless. In case of spontaneous photopsia, pattern of visual loss suggest the correct localization.

Occipital disorders are a frequent source of positive visual phenomena, including photopsia. The three main diagnostic considerations are migraine, transient ischemic attack (TIA), and occipital seizure. Migraine visual aura consists of scintillation that are geometric and achromatic lasting not more than 20–30 minutes usually.

The TIA affecting vertebrobasilar circulation produces negative visual symptoms but occasional attacks include positive visual element. Occipital seizure may resemble migraine but generally are of shorter duration, lasting 5 min or less, often consist of colored circle rather than achromatic zigzag pattern of migraine. This is not the case in diseases of outer retina. Any metabolic failure involving photoreceptors or retinal pigmentary epithelial cells can result in positive phenomena like flashing light, shimmers, which can persist continuously.

So, in case of photopsia apart from neurologic cause, disease of outer retina to be kept in mind if there is continuous photopsia.

Photopsia, Nyctalopia with Scotoma in Temporal Field but Normal Acuity

This pattern of field loss suggest a disorder of photoreceptors rather than optic nerve/chiasmal lesion. This patient's history of nyctalopia and photopsia are also consistent with diagnosis of photo-receptor disease. About 90% of axons in optic nerve and chiasm subserve the central 10° of visual field. Therefore the earliest visual field change in chiasmal compression involves macular vision, i.e. central field. However, bitemporal defect rather suggests retinal disorder, specially involving photoreceptor. The diagnosis of retinal dystrophy needs to be confirmed by electroretinogram.

Case of Atrial Fibrillation with Continuous Sparkling and Twinkling with Left Occipital Infarct

In this scenario patient has suffered an embolic stoke secondary to atrial fibrillation. The infarct might produce cortical irritability in the form of focal seizure that led to positive visual symptoms. However, the continuous nature of photopsia is unusual.

So, in this scenario, this positive visual symptoms could be due to digitalis toxicity, as most patients with atrial fibrillation receive digitalis as antiarrhythmic drug. Digitalis toxicity has a widespread visual symptoms like blurred vision, alteration of color, positive phenomena like flashes/sparkles, flickering, and scintillations. Consistent with a predilection for causing cone dysfunction, visual symptoms of digitalis are most prominent in bright light, and are often accompanied by positive visual phenomena and photosensitivity and central scotoma that are bilateral and symmetric. Toxicity may occur without a change in dose or the addition of another medication; even toxicity can occur in doses within therapeutic range.

The positive visual phenomena of digitalis toxicity sometimes are wrongly attributed to other mechanisms such as vitreous detachment, migraine, seizure or TIA. This diagnosis should be considered in any patient on digitalis who have unexplained visual loss or positive visual symptoms. The visual manifestations of digitalis are reversible upon stopping the medication or lowering the dose.

Episodic Scintillating Scotoma of Migraine

Most cases of migraine visual aura are followed or accompanied by the characteristic headache. However, migraine visual aura without headache is a well-recognized entity. The temporal and spatial characteristics of the visual episode are much more helpful. Migrainous visual phenomena are usually positive and usually include quality of motion (shimmering/sparkling) These migrainous scintillations often start adjacent to fixation and spread to periphery on one side over 20 minutes. This slow spread or march corresponds to the speed of the spreading cortical depression that underlies an attack and generally considered pathognomonic of migraine.

Rare cases in which characteristic pattern of scintillation have been associated with structural lesion (occipital arteriovenous malformation/tumor) are believed to be due mechanical stimulus that has provoked an episode of migraine. Indication for neurodiagnostic investigations in a patient with suspected migraine should include– prolonged visual field defect, or other persistent focal neurologic deficit or attacks always localized to same area.

Sudden Difficulty in Reading with all Ocular and Neuro-diagnostic Findings Normal

This is a curious problem. Unilateral lesion at the tip of the occipital lobe produces a congruous central homonymous hemianopic scotoma within the central 10° degrees. The visual disturbance is most noticeable when fine visual discrimination is required such as reading. The visual defect is less bothersome or even in apparent while driving or watching television because when viewing large objects at a distance, the missing information or scotoma is compensated by information from the rest of the visual field. Visual acuity also is generally unaffected as the lesion is retrogeniculate and unilateral. Such a small lesion is often missed in the MRI scan as well. It is often overlooked in routine visual field testing.

The Amsler grid testing (Chapter 1) is perhaps the only test to ascertain such a small lesion.

Postovarian Cancer Surgery for 7 Hours with Hypotensive Spell: Complaining of Bilateral Visual Loss with Normal Pupils and Fundi

This story would have gone very well with a bilateral Posterior Ischemic Optic Neuropathy save for the normal pupillary reaction. Hence, the lesion must be retrochiasmal/retrogeniculate. Careful inspection of the visual field would be needed. Inspection of the contours of the central scotoma should give the correct localization. In case of lesion of the occipital tip produces matched, bilateral, homonymous hemianopic scotoma in central field with a small vertical step between the two sides. This region is the overlap zone of supply of the posterior cerebral and middle cerebral arteries. Perioperative hypotension probably caused a bilateral watershed infarcts at the occipital tips. Very careful field charting would be useful. Diffusion weighted MRI showed the bilateral occipital tip infarcts.

Chronic Pink Eye

Chronic pink eye gives impression of conjunctivitis and treated by antibiotic eye drop. However, a chronic red eye, that fails to respond to treatment for inflammation should raise suspicion of dural arteriovenous fistula and the patient should be questioned about pulsatile tinnitus.

Dural arteriovenous fistula occurs when a defect involves meningeal branch of external/internal carotid artery, resulting low flow communication with cavernous sinus.

Traumatic direct carotid-cavernous fistula shunt blood flow anteriorly through superior and inferior ophthalmic veins causing orbital venous congestion resulting in proptosis, chemosis, lid edema and conjunctival injection. When orbital signs are prominent, the main differentials are thyroid eye disease, orbital cellulitis, pseudotumor of orbit, and cavernous sinus thrombosis.

Increased orbital pressure causes an increase of episcleral venous pressure resulting in dilated and tortuous episcleral vessels giving a classic corkscrew appearance. Occasionally drainage is directed posteriorly through superior and inferior petrosal sinuses causing cranial nerve palsies.

Visual loss can occur due to glaucomatous change in disc, compression of intracranial optic nerve and ischemia of optic nerve.

Uncommonly signs and symptoms can be bilateral or even contralateral to fistula due to prominent intercavernous venous connection.

Appendix 1

Dynamic Visual Acuity: A Simple Test for Vestibular Function

Arnab Biswas

Objective, clinical, and diagnostic tests, such as bi-thermal caloric tests, low frequency rotatory chair tests in darkness, and vestibular evoked myogenic potentials (VEMPs), provide good, relatively direct measures of vestibular function. These tests are good indicators of vestibular impairment. However, these tests do not indicate how well patients use their vestibular function in daily life. For purposes of screening people for vestibular impairments quickly, bithermal caloric tests, rotatory chair tests and VEMP may take too long and may require too much expense and space-occupying equipment. Tests of dynamic visual acuity (DVA), the ability to see clearly while moving, provide a bridge between classical, objective diagnostic testing and clinical, subjective observation of functional motor behavior. Such tests usually take only a few minutes, are not nauseogenic, and are objective.

The DVA is an indirect indicator of vestibulo–ocular reflex (VOR) function. It is a functional test of whole body integration that includes the requirement of good VOR function. It is impaired in patients with bilateral loss. It may also be impaired in unilateral vestibular impairment during unpredictable head movements. Changes in DVA might indicate development of compensatory mechanisms after vestibular impairment. Therefore DVA may be useful for screening. It may also be a useful indicator of compensation

Some experts have recommended screening patients with DVA. Goebel has suggested using passive head shaking while the patient reads a Snellen's chart. A drop in VA by more than is indicative of vestibular dysfunction. The Snellen's chart; however, presents some perceptual disadvantages and passive head shaking presents an uncontrolled stimulus so that results may not be comparable across trials or subjects. Peters and Bloomberg developed a DVA test that used a Landholt C, which appeared in various sizes and orientations on a computer screen, and was tested during treadmill locomotion which provides an active perturbation to the head during each step. Passive movement of the head as part of a vestibular testing paradigm has a long history in clinical vestibular science. Passive, and therefore unpredictable, head motion avoids the potential problem of generating predictive saccades and smooth pursuit during predictable head rotations. Vital et al. developed a DVA test using the Landholt C and either active movement by the patient or passive head thrusts given by the examiner standing behind the patient. Active head movements may confound testing by allowing the patient to predict the position of the head and thus make corrective saccades. Passive head thrusts probably vary across trials, patients, and examiners. Also, that stimulus does not occur in daily life.

Appendix 2

Strabismus Terminology

Pushpita Sahu, Ambar Chakravarty

Ductions		The rotational movements of one eye:
	Abduction	Outward (lateral) movement
	Adduction	Inward (medial) movement
	Elevation	Upward movement (also supraduction, sursumduction)
	Depression	Downward movement (also infraduction, deorsumduction)
	Intorsion	Inward torsional movement—upper pole of eye rotates medially (also incycloduction)
	Extorsion	Outward torsional movement—upper pole of eye rotates laterally (also excycloduction)
Version		The rotational movement of both eyes in the same direction. Commonly referred to as "gaze", e.g. right gaze, left gaze, upgaze, and downgaze
Primary position		For clinical purposes, the eye position when viewing a distant target straight ahead
Secondary positions		Eye positions along the meridians, i.e. adduction, abduction, elevation, and depression
Tertiary positions		Oblique positions, i.e. adduction and elevation, adduction and depression, abduction and elevation, and abduction and depression
Tropia		Misalignment of the eyes relative to each other during binocular viewing (also heterotropia or manifest strabismus, ocular deviation, or squint)
	Exotropia	Outward deviation
	Esotropia	Inward deviation
	Hypertropia	Upward deviation
	Hypotropia	Downward deviation. Note that, by convention, hypertropia is the preferred term for a vertical deviation of one eye relative to the other, regardless of the side of the "paretic" eye
	Incyclotropia	Upper poles of eyes deviated inward
	Excyclotropia	Upper poles of eyes deviated outward
	Orthotropia	No deviation during binocular viewing
Phoria		Misalignment of the eyes relative to each other only during monocular viewing or other disruption of binocular fusion (also heterophoria or latent strabismus, deviation, or squint)
Comitant		Refers to an ocular deviation that is the same in all gaze positions (also concomitant)
Incomitant		Refers to an ocular deviation that varies in size according to gaze position (also nonconcomitant)

Continued

Continued

Paralytic strabismus	Incomitant deviation caused by extraocular muscle weakness
Horizontal diplopia	Diplopia in which images are separated horizontally
Vertical diplopia	Diplopia in which images are separated vertically
Oblique diplopia	Diplopia in which images are separated obliquely
Crossed diplopia	Horizontal diplopia in which each image comes from the contralateral eye. Signifies an exotropia (crossed = X = exotropia)
Uncrossed diplopia	Horizontal diplopia in which each image comes from the ipsilateral eye. Signifies an esotropia

Appendix 3

A Note on Ocular Motor Disorders in Multiple Sclerosis

Angshuman Mukherjee, Ambar Chakravarty

Most CNS lesions in MS are not associated with identifiable clinical findings. This is perhaps related to a high predilection of tissue damage within non-eloquent zones of cerebral white matter, including the cerebral periventricular zones, the centrum semiovale, and corona radiata. By contrast, there are discrete neuroanatomically eloquent sites where the pathological process in MS results in stereotyped and easily recognized syndromes, such as internuclear ophthalmoplegia.

Nystagmus

Pathological nystagmus on eccentric gaze, gaze-evoked nystagmus, refers to a "jerk" nystagmus with a slow drift in one direction and a resetting saccade in the other. This commonly indicates failure of the neural integrators. Not surprisingly, gaze-evoked nystagmus is common in MS because of the high number of brainstem lesions.

Pendular nystagmus (nystagmus in which there is a back and forth slow-phase oscillation) can also arise from disturbances in the neural integrators, usually involving critical feedback pathways that interconnect brainstem networks and the cerebellum. Pendular nystagmus is especially common in MS, and is also particularly distressing because it can severely disrupt vision (primarily via retinal slip). Examples include elliptical nystagmus and the ocular oscillations associated with palatal myoclonus (now called ocular palatal tremor). Pendular nystagmus may arise, in part, from increases in conduction time on demyelinated fibers. Another contributing factor to pendular nystagmus may be visual loss. Pendular nystagmus can also arise from lesions in the Guillian–Mollaret triangle (dentate nucleus, superior cerebellar peduncle, red nucleus, central tegmental tract, inferior olive, inferior cerebellar peduncle) and may be associated with palatal tremor (previously referred to as palatal myoclonus).

Saccadic Intrusions

Disorders of pause-cell neurons, which are located in the pontine raphe between the abducens nuclei and tonically inhibit saccadic premotor burst neurons in the paramedian reticular formation of the pons and midbrain, may produce impaired fixation due to extraneous saccades. The most common of these are square-wave jerks, characterized by 1–5 degrees eye movements away and back from the neutral position, and punctuated by an intrasaccadic latency. Larger movements of 10–40 degrees in excursion are referred to as macrosquare-wave jerks. Large to-and-fro eccentric movements across the midline represent macrosaccadic oscillations.

Ocular flutter is a saccadic intrusion characterized by horizontal back-to-back saccades without an intersaccadic latency (by contrast with square-jerks in which there is an intersaccadic interval). Opsoclonus is similar but is characterized by both horizontal and vertical back-to-back saccades. Finally, microsaccadic flutter is a binocular condition with similar back-to-back saccades. These movements, however, are generally seen only on ophthalmoscopy or on eye-movement recordings. Patients typically complain of shimmering, jiggling, or wavy vision. This disorder should be differentiated from superior oblique myokymia, which is strictly monocular and characterized by a strong torsional component. Patients with MS will on occasion experience steady fixation interrupted by paroxysmal episodes of diplopia.

Cerebellar Regulation of Eye Movements

The dorsal vermis and the posterior fastigial nuclei are key cerebellar structures concerned with the control of saccadic accuracy by calibration of the size of the saccadic pulse. Saccadic dysmetria can occur after demyelinating lesions within these structures and is characterized by hypermetric (if the deep nuclei are involved) or hypometric (if the vermis alone is involved) saccades. Macrosaccadic oscillations (large repetitive, back-and-forth saccades that cross the point of attempted fixation) are an extreme example of saccadic hypermetria. Demyelinating lesions within the cerebellar peduncles can produce hypermetric saccades toward the side of a lateral medullary lesion, involving the pathways through the inferior cerebellar peduncle (ipsipulsion) or hypermetric saccades away from a lesion localized to the Hook bundle region near the superior cerebellar peduncle. Floccular (and parafloccular—(the tonsils in human beings) lesions produce horizontal gaze-evoked nystagmus, primary-position downbeat nystagmus, impaired (low gain) pursuit requiring corrective saccades, rebound nystagmus (e.g., a transient jerk nystagmus that occurs on returning the eyes to straight ahead after sustained attempted eccentric gaze-holding with the slow phase of rebound nystagmus is in the direction of prior attempted lateral gaze-holding), post-saccadic drift (glissades), and a loss of vestibulo-ocular reflex cancellation. All of these are commonly seen in patients with MS.

Internuclear Ophthalmoplegia

Internuclear ophthalmoplegia is characterized by slowing or limitation of the adducting eye during horizontal saccades and is the result of damage to the MLF within the dorsomedial pontine or midbrain tegmentum, adjacent to the fourth ventricle and cerebral aqueduct, respectively. During horizontal saccades, the burst cells in the paramedian reticular formation of the pons innervate the abducens nucleus, which contains two distinctive sets of neurons. Axons from abducens motor neurons innervate the ipsilateral lateral rectus muscle and the axons of abducens interneurons cross the midline to become the MLF and subsequently innervate the medial rectus subnucleus of the occulomotor complex (cranial nerve nucleus III). Despite adduction weakness, convergence is generally intact, consistent with integrity of the vergence pathways. If the lesion is sufficiently rostral to involve the vergence circuitry or medial rectus motor neurons themselves, then convergence is compromised, potentially producing divergence of the eyes and bilateral internuclear ophthalmoplegia (wall-eyed bilateral internuclear ophthalmoplegia).

In the most subtle form of internuclear ophthalmoplegia, the range of adduction is normal whereas only the velocity is reduced. With infrared oculography one can validate the presence of internuclear ophthalmoplegia. Internuclear ophthalmoplegia is commonly associated with a lesion within the MLF at the level of the dorsal pons or midbrain.

Abduction Nystagmus in Internuclear Ophthalmoplegia

The discrepant movement of the two eyes in internuclear ophthalmoplegia during saccades results in a break in binocular fusion that can lead to visual confusion, transient oscillopsia, diplopia, reading fatigue, and loss of stereopsis. There is also a horizontal dissociated nystagmus that is most prominent in the abducting eye. The most likely mechanisms for abducting nystagmus (either of which, or both, can be present in an individual patient) are an adaptive response to overcome the weakness of the contralateral medial rectus and a dissociated gaze-evoked nystagmus.

Vertical Eye Movements in Internuclear Ophthalmoplegia

The white-matter myelinated pathways involved in the regulation of vertical pursuit, vertical vestibular, and otolithic mediated eye movements or vertical alignment are contained within the MLF. Many patients with bilateral internuclear ophthalmoplegia consequently show characteristic patterns of disorganized vertical eye movements, such as diminished vertical-gaze holding, inadequate vertical vestibulo-ocular reflex, and abnormal optokinetic and pursuit responses. Vertical and torsional types of nystagmus can occur on the basis of disruption of the semicircular canal pathways. Many patients with MS and internuclear ophthalmoplegia have a skew deviation, which is characterized by a supranuclear vertical misalignment and changes in ocular torsion of the two eyes.

One-and-a-Half Syndrome

A gaze palsy in one direction and internuclear ophthalmoplegia on attempted gaze contralaterally is referred to as the one-and-a-half syndrome. This syndrome is produced by a lesion that damages either the paramedian reticular formation of the pons or abducens nucleus (or both) together with the MLF on the same side. An ipsilateral internuclear ophthalmoplegia and cranial-nerve-VI fascicle lesion can produce paralysis of both adduction and abduction in one eye (monocular horizontal gaze paralysis).

Skew Deviation and Vestibular Abnormalities

Skew deviation is a supranuclear vertical ocular misalignment with the higher eye most commonly on the side of the lesion in midpontine and midbrain lesions, and the lower eye on the side of the lesion in medullary lesions. It can occur in isolation or in conjunction with internuclear ophthalmoplegia. In addition to change in alignment, the higher eye is usually intorted while the lower eye extorted, though not necessarily by the same amounts. Many patients have a head tilt away from the high eye and may also perceive a deviation of the subjective visual vertical. Taken together, these features are referred to as the ocular tilt reaction. On occasion, MS patients will present with positional vertigo. The most common cause of vertigo (and its corresponding nystagmus) in MS is benign paroxysmal positioning vertigo. Demyelinating plaques within the eighth cranial nerve entry zone at the pontomedullary junction and in the medullary tegmentum can also produce vertigo that can mimic an acute peripheral vestibulopathy.

Abnormal Suppression of the Vestibulo-ocular Reflex and Impaired Smooth Pursuit

Suppression of the vestibulo-ocular reflex is the ability to cancel the reflex during combined smooth eye and head movements. When abnormal, the characteristic feature is "catch up" saccades that are needed to maintain fixation of the target moving with the head because the reflex normally drives the eyes in a direction opposite from head movement. This is elicitable during a head thrust test and sometimes elicitable in MS patients where the plaque lies at the root entry zone of the eighth cranial nerve. Abnormal vestibulo-ocular-reflex suppression typically parallels abnormalities in smooth pursuit tracking.

Vertical Saccadic Abnormalities

When demyelinating lesions occur in the dorsal midbrain, Parinaud's syndrome may occur and is characterized by diminished upward saccades, convergent retraction nystagmus on attempted upward saccades (often best elicited when viewing a downward-moving optokinetic-nystagmus tape), and near-light dissociation. Other features can include skew deviation, fixation instability (square-wave jerks), convergence spasm or divergence paralysis, irregular pupils (correctopia), pseudoabducens palsy (a slower moving abducting eye during horizontal saccades perhaps related to convergence excess), downward gaze preference (setting sun sign), downbeat nystagmus, and abnormalities of vertical smooth pursuit and the vertical vestibulo-ocular reflex.

Nuclear and Fascicular Lesions

Nuclear and fascicular cranial nerve syndromes have been described in MS. Sixth nerve paresis is the most common.

Involvement of the abducens nucleus produces a gaze palsy to the side of the lesion; involvement of the abducens nerve produces only an ipsilateral lateral rectus palsy. Bilateral horizontal gaze palsy secondary to a midline pontine lesion has been reported in MS.

Isolated oculomotor (cranial nerve III) palsies can occur in MS and partial fascicular (upper and lower division) and nuclear lesions have also been reported. Trochlear nucleus and nerve lesions are rare. A unique ocular motor syndrome combines an internuclear ophthalmoplegia with a contralateral hyperdeviation secondary to superior oblique weakness. Neuroanatomically, the lesion is localized to the caudal midbrain involving the MLF and trochlear nucleus and may also be associated with Horner's syndrome.

Ptosis from a brainstem lesion can be unilateral or bilateral. When caused by oculomotor dysfunction, fascicular lesions give rise to unilateral ptosis, whereas nuclear lesions produce bilateral ptosis owing to involvement of the central caudal subnucleus of cranial nerve III. This nucleus is unpaired and contains cells that project to both levator palpebre superioris muscles.

An unusual eyelid abnormality—blepharoclonus—has been reported in MS and is characterized by paroxysms of forced eye closure that can be triggered by eccentric eye movements or spontaneously while looking straight ahead.

FURTHER READINGS

1. Frohman EM, Frohman TC, Zee DS, et al. The neuro-ophthalmology of multiple sclerosis. Lancet Neurol. 2005;4(2):111-21.
2. Frohman EM, Zhang H, Kramer PD, et al. MRI characteristics of the MLF in MS patients with chronic internuclear ophthalmoparesis. Neurology. 2001;57:762-8.
3. Leigh RJ, Wolinsky JS. Keeping an eye on MS. Neurology. 2001;57:751-2.
4. Newman NJ. Multiple sclerosis and related demyelinating diseases. In: Miller NR, Newman NJ, editors. Walsh and Hoyt's Clinical Neuro-Ophthalmology. 5th ed. Baltimore: Williams and Wilkins; 1998. pp. 5539-76.
5. Zee DS, Hain TC, Carl JR. Abduction nystagmus in internuclophthalmoplegia. Ann Neurol. 1987;21(4):383-8.

INDEX

Page numbers followed by *b* refer to box, *f* refer to figure, *fc* refer to flowchart, and *t* refer to table.

A

Abduction deficit 261
   bilateral 263
   causes of 142*b*
Abscesses 110, 233
Acephalgic migraine 51
Acetazolamide 233, 234, 250
Achromatopsia 123
Acquired cervical syringomyelia 236
Acuity test, near 2
Acupuncture 211
Addison's disease 226
Adduction deficit 261
Adenomas, adrenal 100
Adie's tonic pupil 33-35, 36*f*, 258, 259
Adjunctive therapy 75
Adrenocorticotropic hormone 100
   producing adenomas 100
Adrenoleukodystrophy 47, 110
Agnosia 113
Agraphia 114
Aicardi syndrome 18
Akinetopsia 114
Alcohol, direct neurotoxicity of 87
Alexander's law 193
Alexia 114
   syndrome of 107
Allbutt's seminal publication 68
Allesthesia 119
Altitudinal defects, superior 78
Alzheimer's disease 5, 41, 47, 109, 112, 114, 171, 172, 182, 183, 257, 258
Amaurosis fugax 48
Amblyopia 46, 102, 157
   anisometropic 157
   diagnosis of 46
Ambulation 219
Amenorrhea 95, 99
Amino acids 86
Amiodarone 226
Amoebicidal drug 86
Amsler grid test 3, 3*f*, 254
Ancillary test, major 61
Anemia 226
Aneurysms, intracranial 131*f*, 250
Angiogram 134

Angiography, conventional 226
Angiotensin-converting enzyme 213
Angle closure glaucoma 48, 52, 62, 249
   acute 247
   intermittent 248
Angular gyrus 112
Anhidrosis 37
Aniseikonia 118
Anisocoria 23, 33, 34
   episodic 33
   evaluation of 32
   simple 38
Anomalous discs, varieties of 11
Anorexia 70, 81
Antiamoebic drug 86
Antibody
   antinuclear 50
   antiphospholipid 50
Anticoagulants 79
Antiepileptic drugs 75
Antimyelin oligodendrocyte glycoprotein antibody 72
Antiplatelet agents 79
Antituberculosis agent 85
Anton syndrome 109
Apert syndrome 18
Aperture 115
Aphasia 24, 120
Apraxia, oculomotor 180
Aquaporin-4 antibodies 71, 72
Arachnoiditis 236
Arcuate defects 238
Arcuate scotoma 45
Areflexia 35
Argyll Robertson pupils 23, 34, 39, 39*f*, 259
Arrhythmia, cardiac 260
Arter, extracranial 247
Arteries 20*f*
Arteriovenous
   fistula, dural 266
   malformations 52, 120, 208
Arteritis, temporal 250, 251
Artery
   biopsy, temporal 81
   choroidal 9
   cilioretinal 10, 78*f*
   common carotid 131

Ataxia 144, 140
   telangiectasia 180
Atherosclerotic lesion 55
Atrial fibrillation 264
Atrophic papilledema 12
Atrophy
   ascending 15
   descending 15
   hemifacial 18
Attacks, acute 74
Auditory
   nerve 230
   reflexive saccades 163
Autoimmune disorders, organ-specific 71
Autoimmune thyroid disorders 71, 75
Autosomal dominant cerebellar ataxias 178
Azathioprine 74, 75, 211

B

Back pain 227
   low 228
   transient 236
Balint's syndrome 112*f*, 183
Bariatric surgery 235, 237, 263
   complications of 237
Basal ganglia, sign of 171
Basal meningitis, part of 65
Base-out prism test 219
Basifrontal fractures 89
Basilar syndrome 110
B-complex vitamins 87
Behçet's disease 65, 71, 226
Bell's phenomenon 30, 36
Benedikt's syndrome 145, 145*f*
Bergmeister's papilla 11
Bickerstaff's encephalitis 140
Bielschowsky head tilt 161
Bifoveal fixation 155
Big blind spot syndrome 62
Binasal field loss 23
Binocular illusions 119
Binocular perimetry 221, 222
Binocular peripapillary plethora 85
Binocular transient visual loss, causes of 49*b*

Binocular vision
  advantages of 153
  grades of 154
Biomicroscopic abnormalities 42
Biopsy 136
Birth injuries 201
Blepharitis 206
Blepharoptosis 199
Blepharospasm 199, 204
  diagnosis of 205
  drug therapy for 206
  essential 205
  secondary 205t
  treatment for 206
Blind spot 28
Blindness
  postfixational 221
  prefixational 222
  transient 236
Blood
  and thunder fundus 16
  count, complete 50, 213
  pressure measurement 247
  tests
    normal 262
    routine 60
Blurred disc margin 11
Body mass index 226
Bonnet-Dechaume-Blanc syndrome 18
Bortezomib 75
Botulinum toxin 206
Bowel disease, inflammatory 71
Bowel obstruction, recurrent small 237
Brain 71, 246
  gray matter 58
  parenchyma 231
  trauma, risk of 236
Brainstem 30, 128, 140, 143
  ptosis 202
  stroke 129, 142, 263
  syndrome 70, 264
Bromocriptine 101, 211
Brown's syndrome 141
Bruits, machine-like 214
Brun's nystagmus 194

C

Cajal, interstitial nucleus of 188
Calcium emboli 52
Campylobacter jejuni 140
Carbamazepine 75
Carbimazole 211
Carbon dioxide retention 227
Carcinomas 100
Caroticocavernous fistulae 89

Carotid angioplasty 54
Carotid artery 93
  giant intracavernous 132
  injury 89
  internal 94, 131
  intracavernous 131, 140
  supraclinoid internal 98
Carotid cavernous fistula 132, 213, 214
Carotid disease, asymptomatic 55
Carotid dissection 82, 247
Carotid fistula
  signs of 214
  symptoms of 214
Carotid occlusive disease, severe 79
Carotid stenosis
  management of 54
  symptomatic 54
Carotid sympathetic fibers 134
Carotid ultrasound 53
Carotids, computed tomography
  angiography of 53
Cataract 43, 118, 254
  congenital 157
  early traumatic 157
Catheter
  angiography 133
  intra-abdominal sequestration of 236
  migration of 236
Cavernous sinus 128, 129f, 140, 141, 143, 232
  disease 247
  enhancement of 129f
  fistulas 208
  symptoms 131, 162
  thrombosis, bilateral 129f
Cellular infiltration 73
Central nervous system 70, 134, 171
Central retinal
  artery 9
    occlusion 43, 62
  vein 10
    occlusion 14, 15, 62, 233
Cephalgia, attack of 138
Cerebellar
  artery syndrome, anterior inferior 145
  diseases 177
  dysfunction 139
  strokes 139
Cerebral
  achromatopsia 113
  angiography 51
  arteries
    anterior 53, 131
    posterior 131
  arteriovenous malformations 233

artery occlusion, posterior 25, 236
  cortex, part of 105
  cortical ganglia, sign of 171
  diplopia 119
  dysfunction 113
  hemisphere 182b
  infarction 109
  ischemia 215
  lesions, acute unilateral 172
  metamorphopsia 119
  origin, visual loss of 109
  polyopia 119, 120, 259
  substrates 115
  syndrome, symptomatic 70
  transverse sinus stenting 233
  venous thrombosis 226
  visual impairment, causes of 110
  visual loss 110
    causes of 110
Cerebrospinal fluid 12, 68, 69, 74, 97, 136, 211, 225, 226, 228, 230, 231, 258
  fistulae 89
  leak 235
  normal 262
  otorrhea 237, 238
  pressure 12f
  rhinorrhea 227, 237, 238
  studies 72
Cervical arterial dissection 250
Charles Bonnet syndrome 123
Chiari anomaly 192
Chiasmal
  disorders 93
  field defects 28
  syndrome 101
Cholesterol emboli 52
Choroid plexus papilloma 233
Ciliary artery
  posterior 10
  short 9
Ciliospinal reflex 32
  loss of 37
Claude's syndrome 145
Clinical activity score 209
Clioquinol 86
  neurotoxicity 86
  optic neuropathy 86
Closed-angle glaucoma, acute 33
Cogan's eyelid twitch sign 147
Cognitive activity, normal 117
Collagen vascular diseases 213
Colliculus, superior 166
Collier's sign 173, 182
Color anomia 113
Color vision 81, 83
Computed tomography 96, 230, 231
  angiography 261

Computer-assisted static perimetry 232
Conjunctival inflammation 247
Conjunctival injection 247
Conjunctival veins, arterialization of 214
Connective tissue diseases 73
Consciousness 230
Cornea 60, 115
Corneal
　breakdown 210
　disease 254
　haziness 247
　inflammation 247
　involvement 209
　opacity 157
　pregadolinium 96
Corrugator superciliaris 205
Corticosteroid 79, 233, 235
　intravenous 64
　replacement therapy 101
Corticotropin-releasing hormone 100
Cosmetic unsightliness 236
Cover test 155*f*, 161*f*
　alternate 155
Cover-uncover test 155
Coxsackie B virus infection 226
Cranial auscultation 247
Cranial autonomic symptoms 247
Cranial nerve 129*f*, 229
　deficits 229
　palsies 89, 230
Craniopharyngiomas 97, 97*f*, 101, 102
C-reactive protein 81, 251
Creatine phosphokinase 70
Creutzfeldt-Jakob disease 41, 47, 109, 110, 173, 174, 182, 257
Crohn's disease 65
Cushing's
　disease 95, 96, 100
　syndrome 100
Cyanopsia 118
Cysteine 86
Cystic craniopharyngioma 98*f*
Cystoid macular edema 214
Cysts, intrasellar 97
Cytomegalovirus 140

D

Dacryoadenitis 213, 250
Dandy criteria
　fulfillment of 230
　modified 230, 230*b*
Dandy-Walker syndrome 18
De Morsier syndrome 18

Degenerative disorders 192
Dementia 117, 123
Demyelinating disease 48
Demyelinating disorders 73, 110
Demyelination 128, 142
Deoxyribonucleic acid 149
Devic's disease 68, 87
Dextrodepression 154
Dextroelevation 154
Dextroversion 154
Diabetes 109
　insipidus 16, 89
Diabetic retinopathy study, early treatment 1
Diabetic third nerve palsy 129
Diaphragma sellae 93, 95, 97
Diencephalic syndrome, acute 70
Digital subtraction angiography 134
Dilated pupils, pharmacologically 23, 34
Diplopia 127, 153, 157, 178, 227, 228, 236, 261
　central 182*b*
　improvement of 159
　intermittent 259
　monocular 157
　painful 260
Disc 9
　abnormalities
　　bilateral 233
　　unilateral 233
　capillaries 11
　edema, bilateral 256
　swelling 12*f*, 235
　swollen 11
　vascular supply of 9
Discitis, intervertebral 236
Distal internal carotid artery 53
Doll's eye 170
Doll's head 176
　maneuver 177
Dorsal midbrain syndrome 182*b*, 264
Dorsolateral medulla 123
Dorsolateral prefrontal cortex 180, 181
Double ring sign 18
Double simultaneous stimulation 111
Double vision 32
Down syndrome 226
Doxycycline 226
Duane's syndrome 144, 261
Duochrome test 219
Dyschromatopsia 85
Dysplasia 119
　fibromuscular 53, 250
Dysthyroid optic neuropathy 210

Dystonia 84
Dystonic reaction 171

E

Eccentric gaze 50
Echocardiography 54
Eculizumab 75
Edinger-Westphal nucleus complex 30, 31*f*, 39
Edrophonium
　effects of 148
　injection of 147
　test 202
Ehlers-Danlos syndrome 133, 250
Eilepsy, benign childhood 52, 121
Electric shock-like sensation 70
Electroencephalography 258
Electroretinography 218, 220
Emotional disorders 96
Empty sella 227
　syndrome 97
Encephalitis 65, 128
Encephalopathy 144
　hypoxic ischemic 257
　inflammatory 123
Endoscopic trans-sphenoidal surgery 99
Enophthalmos 37, 212
Enzyme-linked immunosorbent assay 71
Epileptic seizures 182
Episcleral venous pressure 214
Episcleritis 250
Episodic monocular blur 255
Erythrocyte sedimentation rate 50, 81, 213, 251
Esotropia 160
Ethambutol 85
　optic neuropathy 85
European Group on Graves' Orbitopathy 210
Excyclophoria 154
Exophthalmos 209*f*
Exotropia 160
Exposure keratitis, evidence of 210
Extraocular muscle
　action of 157*t*, 159*f*
　cysts, treating 150
　enlargement of 214
Extrastriate cortex 108
Eye 5, 118, 246
　abducted 159
　appearance 247
　deviation, episodic horizontal 170
　displacement of 163
　dry 249
　evaluation of 246

field, supplementary 164, 180, 181
hypotropic 174
ipsilateral 159
movement 119, 184t
　abnormal 183b
　classes of 189
　conjugate 167
　disconjugate 167
　disorders, nonconjugate supranuclear 174, 182b
　downward 182
　in coma 176
　spontaneous 176, 184t
　upward 182
　vergence 167
muscle 149, 157-159
　analysis of 157
　topography 157
　weak 159
normal 9
pain 247
red painful 33
refractive 42
resting position of 176
strain headache 248
white 248
Eyelid 204
　edema 247
　excursion, measurement of 201f
　muscles, anatomy of 199f
　myokymia 206
　twitch, benign 206

F

Facial analgesia 145
Facial hypoesthesia, contralateral 145
Facial nerve 230
　injury 206
Fasciculus, medial longitudinal 146, 166, 188
Fast spin-echo technique 96
Feeding disorders, types of 70
Fetal
　alcohol syndrome 18
　hyaloid artery 11
Fever 134
Fisher's syndrome 183
Fistulas, arteriovenous 226, 233
Flickering lights 119
Fluorescein angiography 232
Focal lesions, effects of 181b
Focal neurologic sings 230
Folate deficiency 87
Foramen ovale, widening of 232
Forced duction test 149, 162

Fossa aneurysm, posterior 138
Fossa mass, posterior 141
Foster-Kennedy syndrome 13
Fourth cranial nerve 140
　palsy 127, 131, 141, 142
　　evaluation of 140
Fourth nerve palsy, causes of 140b
Foville's syndrome 145
Frenzel glass 189, 194
Frenzel lenses 189
Friedreich's ataxia 16, 195
Frisén scale 229
Frontal eye field 164, 180, 181
Frontalis muscles 205
Fulminant idiopathic intracranial hypertension 238
Fundoscopy 247
Fundus examination, dilated 6
Fungal sinusitis 65
Furosemide 233
Fusion 154

G

Gabapentin 75
Gadolinium 71
Gait, drunken 139
Galactorrhea 99
　syndrome 95
Ganglion cell 9
　axons 106
　ciliary 30, 34
　layer 6
Gastritis 70, 71
Gaucher's disease 173, 174
Gaze
　deficits 169, 171
　deviations, vertical 170
　disturbances 169, 183b
　holding 163
　palsy, vertical 110
　shifting 163
Geographic scotoma 21
Giant cell arteritis 10, 62, 78, 80, 138, 246, 247, 250, 251
Gigantic fingers 119
Glaucoma 21, 27, 27f, 255
Glaucomatous disc 255
Glial fibrillary acidic protein 72
Glioma 98
　chiasmatic 99f
Gliomatosis cerebri 231
Globus pallidus interna, lesions of 108
Glycerol 235
Goldmann perimetry 19, 21, 232
Granuloma, eosinophilic 137

Graves'
　disease 171
　myopathy 213
　ophthalmopathy 141, 143, 208, 209
Growth hormone 95, 101, 226
　secreting adenomas 101
Guillain-Barré syndrome 13, 65, 128, 139, 140, 143, 202, 204, 226
Guillain-Mollaret triangle 193

H

Haemophilus influenzae 140
Hallucinations 117, 119, 120, 122
　hypnagogic 123
Harlequin syndrome 35
Head
　impulse test 175
　pain, evaluation of 246
　tilt test 161
　trauma 50, 226
Headache 13, 81, 134, 227, 236, 246-249, 256, 260
　cluster 247, 248
　disorders, primary 248
　low pressure 235
　recurrent 263
　types of 122
Heart
　disease, atherosclerotic 109
　pressure 226, 233
Heidenhain variant 257
Hemangioma 212
　cavernous 211
Hematuria 13
Hemianopia
　bilateral homonymous 108f
　binasal 221, 222
　complete homonymous 24, 105
　contralateral homonymous 106
　homonymous 26f, 105, 106, 108, 222, 257
　incongruous homonymous 24
　temporal 45
Hemianopic visual field defects 45, 83
Hemicrania continua 247-249
Hemifacial spasm 206
Hemiparesis 24, 120, 236
Hemisensory loss 24
Hemisphere, superolateral surface of 112f
Hemispheric lesions, acute 182b
Hemorrhage 16, 128, 214, 226, 236
　peripapillary 80f
　subarachnoid 132, 226, 233
　subhyaloid 247

subretinal 11
Hernia, incisional 237
Herring's law 156, 160
Heteroplasmy 84
Hindbrain herniation 236
Holmes-Adie syndrome 35
Homonymous defect 105
Hormonal products 226
Hormone 95
Horner's syndrome 23, 34, 37, 38, 38*f*, 79, 131, 132, 145, 146, 201, 203, 247
  causes of 37*t*
  partial 38
Human immunodeficiency virus infection 226
Humphrey field analyzer 220
Humphrey perimetry 229
Huntington's disease 114, 171, 182, 183
Hutchinson's pupil 36
Hydroxyamphetamine test 38
Hydroxychloroquine toxicity 6
Hyperbaric oxygen 79
Hypercapnia 226
Hypercoagulable states 226
Hypercortisolism 95
Hyperemesis gravidarum 263
Hyperemia 11
Hyperhomocysteinemia 79
Hyperlordosis 236
Hyperopic discs 11
Hyperplasia, adrenal 100
Hyperprolactinemia 95, 99
Hypertension
  intracranial 233
  malignant 13, 47, 233, 256
Hypertensive meningeal hydrops 225
Hyperthyroidism 209*f*
Hypertrophy, left ventricular 129
Hypertropia 155, 160
  ipsilateral 146
Hyperviscosity 233
  syndrome 48
Hyphema 48, 52
Hypoalbuminemia 180
Hypocretin 70
Hypodense 97
Hypointense masses 97
Hypometria 171
Hypoparathyroidism 226
Hypopigmented discs 10
Hypoplasia, congenital 128
Hyporeflexia 35
Hypothalamic dysfunction 24
Hypotropia 155

I

Idiopathic intracranial hypertension 6, 225, 228*b*, 230, 230*b*, 230*f*, 231, 231*b*, 233, 233*t*, 237, 239, 240, 246, 252
  acute 235
  complications of 237
  diagnosis of 231
  pediatric 239
  recurrence of 238
  surgical treatment of 235
  treatment trial 6, 227, 232, 238
Idiopathic orbital inflammatory disorder 260
Immunoglobulins, intravenous 211
Incidentalomas 98
Incyclophoria 154
Indomethacin 235
Infarction 119, 128
Infection 236
Inflammations 119, 128, 221
Inflammatory demyelinating polyneuropathy, acute 74
International Classification of Headaches Disorder 228*b*
Intracranial hypertension, benign 225
Intracranial pressure 13, 225, 226*b*, 233, 252
Intracranial stenosis, treatment of 55
Intraocular pressure
  intermittent raised 248
  low 233
Ipsilateral eye pain, syndrome of 106
Iris
  congenital malformation of 33
  dilator muscle 31*f*
  neovascularization 214
  sphincter muscle 127
Ischemia 51
  acute 110
  anterior segment 214
Ischemic attack, transient 119, 228, 264
Ischemic optic neuropathy
  non-arteritic anterior 6, 6*f*
  posterior 77, 82
Isoniazid optic neuropathy 86

J

Jaw claudication 81, 251
Jaw-winking phenomenon 201
Jerk nystagmus 187
Jugular foramen, osteopetrosis of 233

Jugular vein
  compression 233
  thrombosis, bilateral 226

K

Kearns-Sayre syndrome 149, 203, 263
Keratitis sicca 249
Kernicterus 173
Kinetic Goldmann perimetry 22, 45
Kissel's patients 132
Klippel-Trénaunay-Weber syndrome 18

L

Lacrimal gland 213, 250
Laevodepression 154
Laevoelevation 154
Laevoversion 154
Lamina cribrosa 10, 15, 77
Lamina terminalis 93
Lanreotide 211
Lateral medullary syndrome, nystagmus of 194
Laurence-Moon-Biedl syndromes 16
Leber's congenital amaurosis 84
Leber's hereditary optic neuropathy 16, 84, 233, 256
Leigh's disease 172
Lens 115
Leptomeningeal carcinomatosis 128
Lesion
  retrochiasmal 24, 105
  unilateral 182
Leukoencephalopathy, bihemispheric 47
Levator function 260
  classification of 200
Levator palpebrae superioris 199
Levodopa 79
Lhermitte's sign 70
Lid 188
  lag 32, 209, 209*f*
  opening, apraxia of 201
  retraction 182, 208, 209, 209*f*, 211
    contralateral 201
Light-near dissociation 173, 259
Lithium 226
Little red discs 11
Liver failure 226
Liver function test 50
Long segment myelitis, acute 70
Low pressure syndromes 227
Lumbar
  drain 233
  puncture 134, 232, 233

Lumboperitoneal shunt 235, 236
  complications of 236
Lupus erythematosus 65
Lyme's disease 65, 88, 226
Lymphangiomas 212
Lymphoma 135, 213
Lymphoproliferative disorders 213

M

M cells 113
Macroadenoma 97, 99
Macropsia 254
Macrosaccadic oscillation 195
Macula 8, 214
Macular
  degeneration 3f
  edema 229
  exudates 229
  ischemia 214
  lesions 21
  photostress phenomenon 48
  sparing 106
  star appearance 62
Maculopathy 6, 214
Magnetic resonance 230
  angiography 53, 133, 261
  imaging 69, 71, 133, 210, 213, 230, 231, 257, 260
  techniques 96
  venography 226, 231
Magnocellular ganglion cells 58
Malaria 226
Mammillary bodies 93
Maple syrup urine disease 172
Marching paresthesia 121
Marcus-Gunn
  jaw-winking phenomenon 202
  pupil 59
Marfan's syndrome 250
Mass lesions, intracranial 233
Mastoid infection 226
Meckel's cave, narrowing of 232
Medial
  rectus muscles 157
  vestibular nucleus 166
Medullary syndrome, lateral 146, 174
Medullated nerve fibers 17
Meige's syndrome 205, 206
Memory deficits 110
Meningioma 135
  cavernous 214
Meningitis 128, 236
  bacterial 226
  chronic 260
  infectious 65, 233
  serosa 225

Meningoencephalitis, inflammatory 117
Mental state, abnormal 123
Mercury poisoning, chronic 110
Messenger ribonucleic acid 100
Metabolic disorders 183b
Metabolic encephalopathy 123
Metamorphopsia 117, 254
Metastatic tumor 212
Methanol optic neuropathy 85
Methazolamide 234
Methionine 86
Methyl prednisolone regime, intravenous 64fc
Methylprednisolone pulses 210
Meuromyelitis optica spectrum disorder 71
Mexaform 86
Meyer's loop 106
Microadenomas 97
Microcystic macular edema 72
Micropsia 117, 118, 254
Microsaccades 195
Microvascular ischemia 262
Midbrain
  lesions 181
  pupils 23, 34
  stroke 133
  syndromes 145f
Middle cerebral arteries 131
Migraine 51, 82, 119-121, 248, 257, 264
  cilioretinal 119
  dissociated 121
  episodic scintillating scotoma of 265
  features of 51b
  with aura 120
Migrainous visual phenomena 265
Millard-Gubler syndrome 145
Miller Fisher syndrome 139, 140, 143, 202
Mimicking classical migraine 122
Minamata disease 110
Minocycline 226
Miosis 30
Mirror movement 219
Mitochondria
  accumulate 149
  cytopathies 203
  disease 149
Mobius syndrome 172
Monocular
  alterations in color 118
  blindness, transient 48
  hallucinations 119
  illusions 118
  peripheral field loss 26

  silvery scintillations 119
  temporal hemianopia 221
  visual loss, transient 255
Mononuclear transient visual loss, causes of 48b
Mononucleosis, infectious 226
Moore's lightning flashes 119
Mucormycosis 214, 247
Müller's muscle 199
Multiple cranial nerve dysfunction, symptoms of 162
Multiple evanescent white dot syndrome 119
Muscle contraction, uncontrolled 204
Muscle
  ciliary 127
  extraocular 132, 133, 209, 213
  fatigue 146
  inferior oblique 157
  intraocular 127
Muscular dystrophy 203
Myalgia 81
Myasthenia 143, 147
  congenital 201, 202
  gravis 146, 147, 200, 202
  neonatal 201, 202
Mycobacterium tuberculosis 137
Mycophenolate mofetil 74, 75
Mycoplasma pneumonia 140
Mydriasis
  acute unilateral 258
  isolated unilateral 258
  painful 258
  pharmacologic 37, 258
Myelitis 69, 70, 73
Myelo-optic neuropathy, subacute 86
Myelopathy 86
Myocardial infarction 109
Myoneural junction 201
Myopathy, congenital 201, 202
Myositis 141, 213, 250

N

Nalidixic acid 226
Narcolepsy
  symptomatic 70
  syndrome of 70
Narrow angle glaucoma 8
Nasal fundus ectasia 11
Nasopharyngeal carcinoma 247, 260, 261
Nasotracheal intubation 37
Nausea 13
Neck
  arteries 247

surgery 233
Nelson's syndrome 95
Neovascularization, choroidal 229
Nerve
  fiber bundle defects 45
  fiber layer 9, 14
    infarction 81
  palsy, abducens 236
  peripheral portion of 262
Nervous system
  autonomic 30
  disorders, developmental 192
Neural disorders 117
Neural pathway lesion 42
Neurodegenerative disorders,
  progressive 183b
Neurofibromatosis 99f
Neurogenic palsy 142
Neuroimaging 105, 231
Neuromuscular junction disorder
  146
Neuromyelitis optica 65, 68, 73
  classification of 69t
  spectrum disorder 5, 68, 69t, 70,
    71, 73-76
  diagnosis of 72
Neurons, loss of 4
Neuro-ophthalmic
  disaster 23
  examination 48
  visual field 19
Neuro-ophthalmologic research
  disease investigator consortium
  234, 238
Neuropathy 87
Neuroradiological studies 136
Neuroretinitis 62, 233
Niemann-Pick disease 173, 174
Nitrofurantoin 226
Noises, intracranial 227, 228
Nonhemianopic defects, nonspecific
  45
Nonidiopathic orbital inflammations
  213
Noninflammatory pathologies,
  several 77
Noninvasive carotid imaging 79
Nonketotic hyperglycemia 257
Nonparetic left eye 160
Nothnagel syndrome 145
Nuclear and infranuclear
  lesions 127
  ophthalmoplegias 127
Nuclear ocular motor nerve
  syndromes 145
Nucleus
  lesions, lateral geniculate 25, 106
  prepositus hypoglossi 166

Nutritional deficiency optic
  neuropathy 87
Nyctalopia 264
Nystagmus 102, 187, 188, 190
  abduction 191
  acquired 192, 192t
    pendular 193, 196
  afferent 191
  caloric 190
  clinical types of 189
  congenital 191, 192, 192t
  convergent-divergent 193
  down-beat 176, 192
  drug-induced 190
  efferent 191
  epileptic 195
  evaluation of 188
  gaze-evoked 184, 194
  horizontal-torsional jerk 193
  latent 191
  of Maddox, see-saw 193
  optokinetic 190
  pendular 187
  periodic alternating 192
  positional downbeat 184
  pure torsional 192
  treatments for 196t
  types of 191
  upbeat 192
  vestibular 193
  voluntary 191

O

Obesity 70
  hypothesis 226
Oblique muscle, superior 127, 157
Oblique myokymia
  movements of superior 142
  superior 142, 196
Oblique nucleus, superior 166
Obstructive hydrocephalus 33, 233
Occipital arteriovenous
  malformation 265
Occipital paroxysms 121
Occipito-parieto-temporal
  lesions 119-121
  region 119
Occlusive arterial disease 48
Octreotide 211, 235
Ocular bobbing 196
Ocular cysticercosis 150
Ocular ductions 127, 159
Ocular dysmetria 195
Ocular flutter 195
Ocular injury 233
Ocular ischemia 50, 215
Ocular ischemic syndrome 255

Ocular misalignment, types of 160
Ocular motility disorders 127
Ocular motor
  abnormalities 177
  apraxia, acquired 182
  nerve palsies, evolution of 127
  system 163
Ocular movement affected, types
  of 171
Ocular muscles
  disorders of 149
  external 127
Ocular myasthenia 141-143, 146,
    162, 211, 260
  childhood 203f
Ocular neuromyotonia 196
Ocular oscillations 187, 195
  diagnosis of 197fc
  drug treatment for 196
  pathophysiology 187
Ocular perfusion, marginal 50
Ocular posture, maintenance of 187
Ocular Todd's paralysis 170
Ocular trauma 60
Ocular version 154, 159
Oculocephalic maneuver 169, 176
Oculomasticatory myorhythmia 193
Oculomotor nerve 93, 131f
  dysfunction 35
  palsy 33
Oculomotor nuclear complex 128f
Oculomotor nuclei, lesions of 202
Oculomotor palsy 23, 34
Oculopalatal tremor 193
Oculopharyngeal muscular
  dystrophy 203
Omnidirectional pursuit paresis 172
Omnipause cells 166
One-and-half syndrome 147, 182,
  264
Open angle glaucoma 248
Ophthalmic artery 53
Ophthalmoparesis 179, 191
Ophthalmoplegia 101, 143
  brainstem causes of 145
  chronic progressive external 149,
    263
  diabetic 129, 138
  internuclear 146, 147, 191, 261
  painful 134, 137b, 138, 138b
  restrictive 142
Ophthalmoplegic migraine 138
Ophthalmoscopy 8, 219
  dilated 8
  types of 8
Opsoclonus 195
  management strategies of 195
Optic atrophy 10, 15, 86, 87, 102

bilateral 87
causes of 15
postpapilloedemic 15
primary 15
Optic chiasm 23, 43, 93, 105
    masses around 94f
Optic disc 8, 9, 10f, 41, 81
    abnormalities 233
    anomalies 18
    appearance 256
    drusen 11
    edema 10, 52
    gliomas 17
    normal 9, 9f
    pallor 255
    swelling 257
        bilateral 13
        unilateral 14
Optic glioma 98f
Optic nerve 9, 9f, 21, 27, 41, 43, 58, 71, 77, 82, 88, 93, 188, 236
    and disk, blood supply of 78f
    anterior 21
    disease 109
        noninflammatory bilateral 88
    disorders 58
    drusen 8, 62
    dysfunction, retrobulbar 82
    enlargement 85
    fenestration 233
    head 21, 58, 59
    hypoplasia 257
    ischemia 214
    meningiomas 212
    pathogenesis of 89
    pathology 37
    prelaminar 232
    retrolaminar 10f
    sheath
        decompression 236
        fenestration 235
        meningioma 103f, 212
        surgery 235
    subclinical 46
    tumor 15, 102
        unilateral 102
    vascular supply of 9
Optic neuritis 5, 11, 14, 15, 45, 58, 59, 61, 62, 68-70, 77, 81, 81t, 246-248, 252, 256
    classical features of 59b
    demyelinating 14, 81, 255
    management of 64
    pediatric 63
    treatment trial 14, 60, 63
    visual loss 256
Optic neuropathy 45, 60, 84, 87, 255
    alcohol-related 86

anterior ischemic 10, 14, 21, 61, 77, 77b, 78f, 80f, 81f, 233, 251
bilateral posterior ischemic 265
causes of 77
chronic recurrent immune 65
compressive 15, 83
decompression trial 78
demyelinating 87
dominant 83
evidence of 210
fundus anterior ischemic 80f
hereditary 62, 83
immune 65
infective 65
infiltrative 15, 83
inflammatory 65
ischemic 11, 15, 77, 255
noninflammatory 77
recessive 84
tobacco-related 86
types of 6
Optic pathway 22, 31f, 107f
    glioma 99f, 212
Optic perineuritis 63, 255
Optic radiation, lesions of 24, 106
Optic tract 43, 46
    lesion 24, 106
Optical coherence tomography 4, 6f, 72, 232, 232, 256
    normal 5f
    role of 61
    uses of 5
Optical disorders 117
Optociliary shunt vessels 15
Optokinetic stimulus 219
Orbicularis
    oculi 205
    spasm 30
Orbit, postcontrast computed tomography of 260
Orbital auscultation 247
Orbital cellulitis 150, 213
Orbital decompression surgery 211
Orbital disease 138
    inflammatory 250
    signs of 143
    symptoms of 143
Orbital dysplasia 213
Orbital fissure, superior 128, 140, 143
Orbital hemorrhage, spontaneous 213
Orbital inflammatory disease 63
Orbital lymphoproliferative disorders 213
Orbital mass lesions 211, 213
Orbital myositis 143, 149, 247, 248

Orbital optic nerve, vertical tortuosity of 232
Orbital pain 79
Orbital pseudotumor 141, 149, 150, 213, 214
Orbital radiotherapy 210
Orbital trauma 141, 213
Orbital tumor 141
Orbitopathy, restrictive 263
Oromandibular dystonia 205
Orthoptic errors 247
Oscillopsia 124, 169
Osteogenesis imperfecta 18
Otitic hydrocephalus 225

P

P cells 113
Pain 81
    pathways 246
    persistent 255
Painless monocular visual loss, acute 254
Palinopia 120
Palinopsia 120
Paliopia 120
Palpebral fissure
    height 200
    width 203f
Panum's area 153, 154
Papilla 58
Papilledema 6, 11, 12f, 13, 14, 24, 229, 231, 233, 246, 247
    causes of 12
    differential diagnosis of 13, 13b, 233b
    evolution of 12
    grading 12
    persistent 236
    treatment of 237
Papillitis 14, 59, 233
Papillomacular
    bundle 87
    fibers 85
Papillopathy, diabetic 13, 233
Papillophlebitis 233
Paralysis 218
Paralytic pontine exotropia 146
Paralytic squint 156, 157
    result of 156
Paramedian pontine reticular formation 146
Paranasal sinus 214, 247
Paraneoplastic autoantibodies 71
Paraneoplastic retinopathy 119
Parasellar mass 96
Parasellar syndrome 138
    causes of 137, 137b

Parasympathetic paresis 33
Paresthesias 120, 228, 234
Parietal eye field 164, 180
Parietal lobe syndrome,
    nondominant 257
Parietal-occipito-temporal focus
    182
Parinaud's syndrome 182
Parkinson's disease 5, 108, 171, 172,
    183
Parkinsonian syndromes, atypical 5
Paroxysmal hemicranias 247, 248
Parvocellular ganglion cells 58
Pediatric idiopathic intracranial
    hypertension, management of
    240
Perimetry
    automated 21
    systems 21t
Periocular pain 249
Periorbital
    headaches 247, 247t
    swelling 213
Peripapillary disc area 9
Peripheral nasal retinal fibers 107
Peripheral nerve 58
    palsy 182
Peripheral neuropathy 86, 87, 237
Peripheral retina 60, 163
Peritonitis 236
Pernicious anemia 71
Phakomatoses 18
Phenylephrine 8
Phenytoin 79
Phoria 153
Phosphenes 59, 247
Photopsia 227, 264
Photoreceptor dysfunction 117
Photostress test 50b, 254
Pickwickian syndrome 226
Pineal region tumors 33
Pinhole visual acuity 2
Pink eye, chronic 265
Pituitary adenoma 98
    nonfunctional 98
Pituitary apoplexy 101, 133, 252
    syndrome of 101
Pituitary gland 93, 96, 97
    normal 96
Pituitary insufficiency 89
Pituitary macroadenoma 97f
Pituitary stalk 93
    section 99
Pituitary tumors 95, 99, 101, 103
Plasma regain, rapid 213
Plasmapheresis 211
Platelet-fibrin emboli 52
Poikilothermia 70

Poisons 109
Polioencephalopathies 47
Poliomyelitis 226
Polymyalgia rheumatica 81
Polyneuropathy, chronic
    inflammatory demyelinating 13
Pons 176
Pontine paramedian reticular
    formation 166
Ponto-mesencephalic damage 176
Post-lumbar
    peritoneal shunt 227
    puncture 227
Postovarian cancer surgery 265
Postrema syndrome 73
Potential acuity meter 42
Prednisolone 150
Presbyopia 141
Pretectal nucleus 44
Procerus muscles 205
Prolactin 99
Prolactinomas 99
Proptosis 208, 211-213, 247
Prosopagnosia 113, 114
Protein electrophoresis 50
Protractor myectomy 206
Provoked transient vision loss 49fc,
    50
Pseudobitemporal defect 258
Pseudodisc edema 14
Pseudo-Graefe lid sign 36
Pseudo-hemianopic defect 221
Pseudopapilledema 6, 14, 14t, 233
Pseudoptosis 201
Pseudo-sixth nerve palsy 142b
Pseudotumor 213
    cerebri 13, 225
        syndrome 225
    inflammatory 143
Psychogenic neuro-ophthalmologic
    disorders 218
Psychogenic seizures 218
Psychosis 117, 123
Psychosocial impact 237, 238
Ptosis 37, 178, 199, 206, 247
    aponeurotic 260
    causes of 200, 201, 201b
    congenital 201, 202
    evaluation of 200, 203, 204fc
    fatigable 259
    hysterical 201
    idiopathic 203
    on left-side, moderate 203f
    painful 260
    painless 260
    pupillary abnormality with 202
Pupil 188, 247
    bilateral

constricted 38
dilated 39
examination of 30, 32
normal 30
pharmacologic 36f
splitting prism test 219
status of 128
Pupillary abnormalities 33, 35, 35f,
    182, 247
Pupillary asymmetry, causes of 33
Pupillary defect 33
    relative afferent 32, 43, 45, 46
Pupillary disorders 32
Pupillary examination 30
Pupillary fibers 30
Pupillary inequality 32
Pupillary light reflex pathway 31f
Pupillary reactions 219
Pupil-sparing ophthalmoplegia,
    relative 131
Pursuit
    abduction lag phenomenon 178
    abnormalities 177
    dysfunction, testing for 167
    horizontal 167f
    paresis
        smooth 172
        unidirectional 172
    pathway, anatomy of 167
    subsystem 166

Q

Quadranopia, homonymous 25f

R

Radiation 233
    optic neuropathy 82
Rathke's cleft cyst 41
Raymond's syndrome 145
Rebound's nystagmus 194
Rectus muscle
    inferior 157
    lateral 157
    stimulation, superior 30
    superior 157
    weakness of right lateral 161f
Reflex 153
    distance, marginal 200
    eye movements 177
    near 30
Refraction 10
Refractive error 156, 246, 247
Refsum's syndrome 16
Reiter's syndrome 65
Renal cell carcinoma 18
Reproductive dysfunction 99
Residual neurological deficit 70

Retina 9, 21, 41, 43, 115
   photopigments of 50
Retinal abnormalities, congenital 17
Retinal artery
   obstructions 11
   occlusion 214
Retinal detachment 43
Retinal disease 221
Retinal disorders 45, 46
Retinal embolism 52, 55
Retinal fluorescein angiography 223
Retinal ganglion cells 30
Retinal hemangiomas 17
Retinal hemorrhages, location of 17f
Retinal metamorphopsia 118
Retinal migraine 119
   field loss 246
Retinal nerve fiber layer 4, 20f
Retinal phakomatoses 17
Retinal points 153
Retinal tear 119
Retinal toxicity 82
Retinal vein occlusion, partial 48
Retinitis pigmentosa 11, 17, 119
Retinochoroidal colobomas 18
Retinol 227
   binding protein 227
Retinoneural disturbances 156
Retinopathy 45
   central serous 62
   hemorrhagic 11
Retinoschisis 221
Retrobulbar hemorrhage 236
Retrobulbar optic
   neuritis 14
   neuropathy 45
Retrobulbar pain 227
Retrobulbar steroids 210
Retrochiasmal pathway 105
   damage, bilateral 105
Rheumatoid arthritis 71
Rheumatological disorders 142
Right eye, six extraocular muscles
   of 158f
Rituximab 74, 75, 211
Roth spot 17

S

Saccades 171, 175
   cortical control of 180b
   horizontal 164f
   hypermetric 184
   hypometric 171, 184
   memory-guided 163
   of distraction 195
   predictive 163
   reflexive 163

   spontaneous 163
   undershoot of contraversive 171
   velocity 184
   vertical 165f
   volitional 163
Saccadic
   abnormalities 177
   control 164
   deviation 195
   disorders 187
   dysfunction, testing for 166
   eye movement 178f
   paresis 171
   subsystem 163
   system 165
Sagittal sinus, stenosis of superior 233
Sarcoidosis 135, 137, 213, 226, 233
Scalp
   arteries, condition of 247
   tenderness 81, 247
Schwann cells 58
Sciatica 236
Sclera 213, 231, 250
Scleral ring 9
Scleritis 250
   posterior 213, 247, 248
Sclerosing panencecphelitis,
   subacute 110
Sclerosis, multiple 5, 47, 62, 63, 74
Scoliosis 236
Scotoma 264
   bilateral centrocecal 257
   cecocentral 22, 84
   central 21, 22, 45, 59, 87, 220
   centrocecal 45, 59, 70
   junctional 93
Seeking polycythemia 130
Seidel scotoma 28
Seizures 236
Sella turcica, normal 96f
Sellar mass 96
Sensorineural deafness 86
Sensory pain pathways 246
   convergence of 246
Serous meningitis 225
Serum prolactin level 99
Sickle cell disease 48
Sight loss 209
Simultagnosia 112
Simultaneous macular perception 154
Sinus
   disease 247
   stenosis 233
Sinusitis 211
   bacterial 65

Sixth cranial nerve 127
   palsy 142
      evaluation of 142
   unilateral 229
Sixth nerve palsy 131, 143, 229, 230
   acute isolated 262
   bilateral 262
   causes of 143b
   painful 262
Sjögren's syndrome 65, 71, 249
Skew deviation 141, 174
Skull fracture, depressed 233
Sleep
   apnea 226, 227
   deprivation 117
Slit lamp examination 60
Slow saccades, causes of 182b
Smith-Lemli-Opitz syndrome 202
Snellen's chart 1, 2, 41, 60, 155
   principles of 1
Soft tissue involvement 209
Somatostatin analogue 235
Spasmus nutans 191, 192
Spectacles 177
Speech 163
Sphenoid sinus, invasion of 97f
Sphenoidal
   air sinus 99
   ostium, natural 99
Spinal
   cord 71
   flexion 236
Spinocerebellar ataxias 184t
Squamous papillary subtype 97
Square wave jerks 180, 182, 184, 195
Squint 153, 155, 178
   causes of 156
   convergent 155f
   effects of 156
   latent divergent 155f
   nonparalytic 155, 156
Statokinetic dissociation 22
Stimulus deprivation amblyopia 157
Stomal stenosis 237
Strabismic amblyopia 157
Strabismus 102, 127, 147, 155, 162, 247
   infantile 162
Stroke 236
   cranial neuropathies 36
Sturge-Weber syndrome 18
Subtemporal decompression 235, 236
Sulcus, intraparietal 112
Supramarginal gyrus 112
Supranuclear
   eye movement
      abnormalities 182b

control 181b
gaze palsy 184
oculomotor disorders 163
palsy, progressive 171, 183
Susac's syndrome 16
Swinging-light pupil test 43, 44, 220
Swiss-cheese type 22
Sympathetic paresis 33
Syphilis 65, 213, 226
Systemic hypertension, malignant 233
Systemic lupus erythematosus 71, 226

T

Takayasu arteritis 82
Takayasu disease 251
Tay-Sachs disease 15, 172
Teichopsia 120
Temporal crescent, absence of 107
Temporal quadrantanopia, superior 93, 95
Temporomandibular joints 247
Temporo-occipito-parietal junction lesions 181
Tensilon 148
Tension glaucoma, low 28
Terson's hemorrhage 16
Tetracyclines 226
Thalamic lesions 181
Thiopurine methyltransferase deficiency 75
Third cranial nerve palsy 34, 133t, 134, 141
evaluation of 127
ischemic 129
isolated 128
nonisolated 127
Third nerve dysfunction, signs of 34
Third nerve palsy 260
causes of 128b
painful progressive 261
Third ventricular tumors 192
Thrombocythemia 48
Thrombolytic 79
intravenous 55
therapy 55
Thyroid
associated ophthalmopathy 208, 209
disease 149, 191
ophthalmopathy 149
Thyrotropin receptor antibody 211
Thyroxine 226
Tight-near dissociation 182

Tinnitus 228
Tocilizumab 75
Todd's motor paralysis 111
Tolosa-Hunt syndrome 129, 134, 136b, 213, 247, 250
diagnosis of 136
differential diagnosis 136
etiology 136
hematological tests 136
Tomato splat 16
Tonic pupil 236, 258
syndrome 23, 34
Tonsillar
ectopia 232
herniation, symptomatic 236
Tonsils 188
Topiramate 233, 234, 250
side effects of 234
Topographic agnosia 114, 124
Tourette's syndrome 204
Toxic optic neuropathy 62, 85
Toxins 233
Tram-track sign 212
Trance-like states 123
Transcranial doppler 53
Transcribriform plate 227
Transient vision loss, management of 54
Transthoracic echocardiography 54
Transverse
myelitis 68
sinus septum 233
Trauma 128
Traumatic direct carotid-cavernous fistula 266
Traumatic optic neuropathy 62, 88, 90fc
Treponema pallidum 137
Trigeminal
autonomic cephalgias 247, 248
nerve 230, 246
nuclear complex 246
Trochlea, enhancement of 250f
Trochlear
nerve 230
pain 249
tenderness 247
Trochleitis 247, 250
Tropia 155
Tropicamide 8
Tuber cinereum 93
Tuberculosis 213
Tuberous sclerosis 17
Tumors 47, 119, 128, 233
epithelial 97
intraorbital 248
Turner's syndrome 202, 226

U

Uhthoff's phenomenon 48, 60
Ulcer, marginal 237
Ulcerative colitis 65
Uncal herniation 33, 36
Upper gastrointestinal bleeding 237
Upper thoracic spinal cord 31
Usher's syndrome 16
Uveitis 247, 248, 250

V

Valsalva maneuver 212
Valve problem 227
Valvular heart disease 109
Vascular disease, recognize 16
Vascular system, proliferation of 11
Vasodilators 79
Vasopressors 79
Vasospastic amaurosis fugax 52
Vena cava syndrome, superior 226, 233
Venereal disease research laboratory 213
Venous collapse, self-sustained 226
Venous hypertension 233
Venous outflow, obstruction of 233
Venous pressure 237
Venous pulsation, spontaneous 10, 14
Venous sinus
pressure 226
thrombosis 233
Venous stasis retinopathy 52
Venous stenting 237
Ventriculoperitoneal shunt 235
Vergence dysfunction, testing for 168
Vergence eye
disturbances of 163
movements, disturbances of 182
Vergence subsystem 167
Vertebral artery dissection 250
Vertebrobasilar
arterial system 110
transient ischemic attacks 121
Vertical ophthalmoplegia, differential diagnosis of 141b
Vertical vestibulo-ocular pathways 168f
Vestibular disorders 175
Vestibular dysfunction 169
testing for 169
Vestibular nucleus, contralateral 190
Vestibular organ 187
Vestibular subsystem 168
anatomy 168

Vestibular system dysfunction 117
Vestibulo-ocular
   movement, horizontal 168f
   reflex 124, 168, 175, 177, 191, 263
Viral
   disease 62
   encephalitis 109, 226
   meningitis 226
Vision field defect, central 22
Vision loss
   transient 48, 50b, 51
   unprovoked transient 51, 51fc
Vision
   acuity of 1
   central blurring of 255
   central loss of 238
   continued loss of 236
   field of 107f
   impaired 117, 123
   multiple 119
Visual activity, endogenous 117
Visual acuity 2, 32, 41, 46, 229, 232, 246
   assessment of 1
   central 24
   distant 1
   dynamic 3
   interpretation of 2
   loss 83, 218, 229
      persistent 218
   near 2
   normal 1
   reduced 59
   subnormal 41, 219
   test 169
   types of 1
Visual agnosia 113
Visual allesthesia 119
Visual association areas, cortical pathology of 42
Visual aura 121
Visual conditions, types of 167
Visual cortex 167
   anterior 107
   primary 121
Visual disturbance 33, 204
Visual electrophysiology 222
Visual evoked potentials 61, 110, 218, 220
Visual experiences 117
Visual field 28, 46, 81, 84
   abnormalities 237
   constriction 220
   defects 27, 105, 117, 119, 238
      factitious 28
      inferior altitudinal 257
      progression of 101
      temporal 238
      types of 95
   examination 19
   generalized constriction of 238
   loss 218, 229, 230f
      bitemporal 24f
      persistent 220
      syndrome of monocular peripheral 107
   one-half of 107
   testing 19, 44, 232
Visual hallucination 121, 123
Visual hemineglect, severe 111
Visual illusions 123
Visual impairment 110
   retrochiasmal 105
Visual inattention 111
   recognize unilateral 111
Visual loss 41t, 80, 81, 85, 105, 111, 227, 235-237, 254
   acute onset 110
   bilateral 265
   causes of 46, 77
   central 10
   chronic 110
   despite medication 235
   progression of 255
   retrochiasmal 105, 109
   risk of 229
   sequential 256
   sudden monocular 254
   symptoms of 50
   syndromes 113
   transient 52
   unexplained 41, 254, 257
Visual obscuration, transient 13, 48, 227, 228
Visual pathway 3, 98, 112f
   disturbances of 117
   gliomas of 102
Visual phenomena
   negative 120
   positive 117, 118, 120
Visual prognosis 81
Visual release phenomena 117
Visual scintillation 51
Visual system 117
   disorder, nystagmus with 196
Vitamin
   A 226
      metabolism, abnormal 226, 227
   B12 86
      deficiency, role of 87
   B-complex
      absorption 87
      deficiency 87
   deficiency 87
   E deficiency 172
von Hippel-Lindau disease 18
von Wilbrand's knee 95
Vortex vein, posterior 10

W

Wallenberg's syndrome 123, 174
Wallerian degeneration 15
Weber's syndrome 145, 145f
Wedge-shaped scotoma, temporal 45
Wegener's granulomatosis 65, 137, 213
Weight loss 233
   surgically-induced 237
Wernicke's encephalopathy 144, 145, 172, 237, 263
Westphal-Piltz reaction 30, 36
Whipple's disease 171, 173, 174, 182, 193
White blood cell 69
Whitnall ligament 199
Wilson's disease 173, 182, 183
Word blindness 107
Wyburn-Mason syndrome 18

X

X cells 58
Xanthochromia 101
Xanthopsia 117, 123

Y

Y cells 58

Z

Zoopsia 122